FOCUSING-ORIENTED PSYCHOTHERAPY

THE PRACTICING PROFESSIONAL
A Guilford Series

Edited by
MICHAEL MAHONEY
*University of North Texas
and the Saybrook Institute*

SELF-NARRATIVES: THE CONSTRUCTION
OF MEANING IN PSYCHOTHERAPY
Hubert J. M. Hermans and Els Hermans-Jansen

FOCUSING-ORIENTED PYCHOTHERAPY:
A MANUAL OF THE EXPERIENTIAL METHOD
Eugene T. Gendlin

WORKING WITH DREAMS IN PSYCHOTHERAPY
Clara E. Hill

FOCUSING-ORIENTED PSYCHOTHERAPY

A MANUAL
OF THE EXPERIENTIAL METHOD

Eugene T. Gendlin

THE GUILFORD PRESS
New York   London

© 1996 The Guilford Press
A Division of Guilford Publications, Inc.
72 Spring Street, New York, NY 10012

Printed in the United States of America

This book is printed on acid-free paper.

Last digit is print number: 9 8 7 6 5 4 3 2

Library of Congress Cataloging-in-Publication Data

Gendlin, Eugene T., 1926–
    Focusing-oriented psychotherapy : a manual of the experiential
method / Eugene T. Gendlin.
        p.   cm. — (The practicing professional)
    Includes bibliographical references and index.
    ISBN 0-89862-479-7 (hard)—ISBN 1-57230-376-X (pbk.)
    1. Focused expressive psychotherapy.   2. Experiential
psychotherapy.   3. Mind and body therapies.   I. Title.   II. Series.
    [DNLM: 1. Cognitive Therapy methods.   2. Psychotherapy—
methods.   3. Professional-Patient Relations.   WM 425.5.C6 G325f
1996]
RC489.F62G46   1996
616.89'14—dc20
DNLM/DLC
for Library of Congress   96-4755
                                                                    CIP

Acknowledgments

I wish to thank Drs. Marion Hendricks, Kathleen McGuire, Mary McGuire, and Judith Malamud for their very helpful readings and comments on every part of the book, and Patricia Sella for many helpful discussions.

Contents

CHAPTER 1

Introduction

MANY METHODS AND STRANDS of psychotherapy are integrated in this book. Each is uniquely valuable in certain respects, provided the client–therapist relationship is given priority over anything else.

Focusing is a mode of inward *bodily* attention that is not yet known to most people. To learn it may require a few days of instruction, perhaps eight 3-hour sessions. Some people are able to do it immediately once they attend to their bodies in relation to a problem. During therapy a client can learn it over a period of months from occasional bits of instruction as shown in this book. What focusing is will gradually become clear in the first part of this book. General descriptions do not convey focusing. It differs from the usual attention we pay to feelings because it begins with the body and occurs in the zone between the conscious and the unconscious. Most people don't know that a bodily sense of any topic can be invited to come in that zone, and that one can enter into such a sense. At first it is only a vague discomfort, but soon it becomes a distinct sense with which one can work, and in which one can sort out many strands.

How long it takes to learn focusing seems to be unrelated to other variables. Some clients deepen their therapy immediately when they are invited to attend physically. Even therapists who do not know focusing can markedly improve therapy with some proportion of their clients, simply by asking how what is being discussed makes them feel *in the middle of the body* and then waiting quietly for the client to sense there. Therefore this is worth trying briefly with every client. But most people can discover focusing only with far subtler instructions over a period of time.

Focusing is a way to enter regularly and deliberately *there*, where therapeutic movement arises. In early research (Gendlin, 1968c, 1986) it was found that some clients begin therapy already knowing this way of bodily sensing, and

1

they were predictably more successful on the outcome measures. On the tape recordings their language often refers inwardly. For example, the client may say something like, "I sense it distinctly but I don't know what it is . . . yet." But most clients happen into this kind of sensing only very occasionally. So it is a great advantage if we know how to enable them to discover and employ it when they wish. It saves so much hapless work on the surface, or with emotions that may be very deep, but remain always the same.

Compared to what we can usually think and feel, what comes from the bodily sensed edge of awareness is characteristically more intricate and multifaceted, and yet also more open to new possibilities. We are not bound by the forms of the past, but contrary to what is often said today, we cannot "construct" just any narrative we like, either. Only certain further steps bring our concrete bodily life along with them. But all this cannot be said properly in an introduction. The words cannot yet mean what they need to mean, to say it. For example, the body referred to here is not the physiological machine of the usual reductive thinking. Here it is the body as sensed *from inside*, but the words "body" and "inside" will acquire a changed and more specific meaning as we proceed. Words alter their meanings in the context of situations, stories, and transcripts.

According to the experiential method, theories are neither true nor false (Gendlin, 1962). They are not true because the kind of entities they assert do not actually exist in concrete human experiencing. But they are not simply false, because they sometimes enable people to locate experiences they would otherwise have missed. The reality of what it brings out would remain even if we were to dismiss the theory.

In the experiential method theories, concepts, and words mean the actual experiences they have brought up, first in ourselves and then also in each next person. Of course everyone is different and can always be surprising, but we soon come to know and feel a range of experiences that each theory sometimes brings out. When we think of the theory, we think not just of concepts; we think of and feel the experiences. They are never simply what a theory asserts. Experiencing is always more intricate. And, it can lead to changes that seem impossible according to the concept.

One great advantage of using theories experientially is that we can think much further, and do much more by going on from experiences, than we could from the concept. For example, Freud's invaluable concepts seem to be about pathological entities from which no change seems to follow. But from the experiences they help us find, we can generate steps of change.

Another advantage is that we can employ all theories. They may contradict each other, but the concrete experiences they help us find do not. Experiences do not contradict each other. If we let theories, concepts, and words refer to concrete experiences, each can help at times. And when a theory leads to nothing that is experienced, we put it aside for the moment.

Experiencing is much more intricate and multifaceted than concepts and theories. Rather than remaining within the paucity and unreliability of a theory, we employ all of them to open whole reaches of human experience. One can then formulate more specific concepts that are also different in kind because they retain their link to an experiencing process that always exceeds them. But this will become clear only from the many examples I present in this book.

Chapter 2 is a consideration of clients who are not moving in therapy, a major concern of this book. Some only talk and do not enter into anything; others have intense but repetitive emotions, even large cosmic experiences but without a therapeutic process. Of course the process must arise from inside. No therapist or anyone else can make it happen. But we now know how to issue the small and unobtrusive but very specific instructions that engender focusing.

Chapter 3 gives eight recognizable characteristics of the small bits of therapeutic movement that typically arise from focusing.

In Chapters 4 and 5 each response in a transcript is examined to show where a small step of therapeutic movement happens, just what the client did to bring it about, and what the therapist did to help it to happen. I also discuss the aspect of the client's communication to which the therapist responded, and exactly how the response enabled the client to enter further into direct experience. This kind of direct experiencing can be clearly distinguished from repetition of the same feelings and emotions as before. It becomes clear just what sort of experiencing can bring something new and therapeutic. The examination of each response shows where the therapist's responses succeed and where they fail.

In Chapter 6 focusing is distinguished from other kinds of physical sensations, emotions, imagery, anxiety, hypnosis, meditation, Jung's four functions, and altered states. These distinctions will help. Otherwise, if one does not know focusing, one may assume that it is one of these other kinds of experience.

Chapter 7 at last takes up focusing as such.

Chapter 8 presents 10 excerpts in which focusing is being taught didactically (not to clients). Such teaching is not often useful in therapy, but it lets the reader observe focusing being more swiftly grasped.

Chapter 9 takes up certain difficulties in the teaching of focusing.

Chapter 10 consists of excerpts from a single case.

Part 2 of this book shows how other therapeutic approaches can and need to be adapted and modified so that they can be used in relation to the conscious–unconscious zone from which new steps arise. Each makes a unique contribution. But how can one determine what it is that is unique in each?

In Chapter 11 I present a new way to understand and organize the variety of therapeutic methods: by "avenues," that is to say by whether it is cognitions, emotions, or dreams that are employed as an avenue of therapy, or whether it is role play, actions as in behavior therapy, or bodily energy, imagery, values, super-ego messages, or client–therapist interactional events.

Chapters 12–22 each take up one avenue of therapy. I show how we can determine what is uniquely valuable in each, and exactly how the inclusion of focusing can enhance each method without changing it very much. More importantly, I describe how each can be modified as a part of focusing-oriented therapy, so that for example images, role play, and action steps *arise from* the edge of experience—and also *lead to* a renewed entry into the edge of experience. Therapy, I argue, does not consist mainly of the familiar, already defined kinds of experience, whether dreams or emotions, actions or images. Therapy is rather a process that centrally involves experience *before* it becomes one of these defined "packages" and again *afterward* when it dips back into the prepackaged zone at the edge of consciousness.

In Chapter 23 I discuss the aspects of the relationship and the presence of the therapist, which are crucial at all times throughout therapy. I then take up the occasional relational events and difficulties that provide valuable opportunities for therapeutic steps on the interactional "avenue."

The reader is advised to read all of Part 1 in order, as well as Chapters 11 and 12 of Part 2. After that one might go to the chapter on the avenue of greatest interest, although each of my chapters does retain and take along what was shown on previous avenues. Working on any one avenue involves the others because of their connection through the center point of focusing.

All types of therapist responses can be attempted without ever imposing anything on a client, and without obstructing the client's sense of ownership and active use of the hour. Whatever actually arises in the client is pursued, and anything else is quickly discarded, at least for the time being. That certainly includes focusing instructions, and any other therapist agenda. Remaining consistent with this principle permits the therapist to employ a great variety of kinds of responses, remaking each kind in a specific manner that enables it to contribute to the inwardly arising therapeutic process.

PART 1

FOCUSING AND LISTENING

CHAPTER 2

Dead Ends

Two kinds of dead ends can happen in psychotherapy: The first occurs when the therapy consists only of interpretation and inference without an experiential process. The second dead end happens when there are quite concrete emotions, but they are repeated over and over. In this chapter I discuss these dead ends further. I call the first a dead-end discussion.

DEAD-END DISCUSSION

At a party you may see an attractive stranger on the other side of the room. You want to approach this person but find it impossibly difficult. If you do approach the person anyway your actions will be awkward and you will feel the lack of your usual abilities. You might think, "My superego is too strong. It still identifies with my father who prohibited my sexuality when I was small. Now that I am not small, my superego should stop identifying with his prohibition, but it doesn't" (Freudian vocabulary). Or you might say, "I am afraid of being rejected. It's just an old fear. If I am rejected, I will be no worse off than if I go home without trying! I ought to try" (common sense vocabulary). But using this vocabulary and this logic does not change anything because you are engaged in a dead-end discussion. Your intellectual interpretation does not change your hesitation or awkwardness.

Therapists may draw people into dead-end discussions; we all do it at times. We may use Freudian theory to do it, or Jungian, cognitive, or any other theory, or just common sense. But a good therapist would not try to get a client merely to substitute a sophisticated psychological vocabulary for a commonsense one, if the words are the only difference. Seen in this way, no one would argue that the mere substitution of one ineffectual line of thought for another can constitute successful psychotherapy.

In our example a longer discussion might ensue in your mind, but it would still change nothing. For instance, is it your fault, your responsibility for your failure, or should you blame your parents? This is a very important question, but not one that would effect a change. Should you call it "cowardice" or a "dynamic" problem? Again, issues like these have great importance for how we view life, but in this case nothing would be changed by accepting either position. Should you adopt a sociological theory — the norm in your culture (or subcultural group) might be that one is not supposed to address strangers of the opposite sex, and that this is why it is hard for you? Perhaps this is a social norm that one is supposed to break, but it can be taught too well. Or should you say that your difficulty is a lack of "security," that your self-esteem would collapse if you got rejected? Any of these interpretations would probably leave you quite unchanged.

To bring this home I will ask you to imagine the dead end when one or another of these interpretations is accepted by a person. In our example, say that you became convinced of the truth of one of these interpretations. The interpretive machinery might be quite powerful, even fascinating. Then you say, "OK, if that's why it is this way, what can I do about it?" You now seem to know the "cause" but you still have no direct grasp of how to counteract it.

There was hope before: If only you could know the cause, you could do something to it, perhaps hack it apart, or break it, or fix it. But now you have found what the trouble is, and it is something you cannot directly get at. That is what I call a "dead end."

Much ineffective therapy is only an accumulation of many such dead ends without any direct contact or change. This lack of direct contact is often indicated by the word "must." One says, "I see; it must be that my father was too strong with me. I know he was. That must be what's doing this now." To say, "It must be" is an inference. People do not say "It must be" when they are directly in touch with the connection. They say, "It *is*," or "I feel." Of course this verbal difference only indicates the real difference. In the next chapters I will explain what direct touch is like and how it comes about.

There are still therapists who are satisfied with a plausible interpretation if the client accepts it. They do not wonder, nor do they teach their clients to try to sense inwardly, whether an interpretation is a dead end or not. To fail to wonder whether an interpretation brings direct inner contact makes everything a dead end and "therapy" becomes just "talk."

A good therapist should be very unsatisfied if the client agrees to an interpretation and then a dead end ensues. "Yes you are right; that is what it is," the client says. "But now what? How do I change it?"

Even worse than accepting a client's mere agreement, many therapists impose interpretations that seem plausible only to them, not to the client. Then they send the client home after an hour of arguing. Even if the client becomes convinced of the therapist's interpretation, change remains very slow and rare with this approach. There are many thousands of clients who experience no major change through years (9 years, 14 years . . .) of therapy, several sessions a week.

This critique applies not just to classical psychoanalysis. Some existential therapists also merely talk and argue. Instead of saying, "This is your oedipal prohibition," they say, "This is your failure to confront choices and encounter real others." With either kind of interpretation little or no change occurs.

Therapists who call their method "transactional" use psychoanalytic concepts, but in a more popularized form. Instead of the "superego" they talk about the "bad parent in your head." But many of them only argue that one ought to overcome that bad parent. If the client asks, "how?" the therapists have no answer. There again is the dead end.

More recent methods (such as "cognitive restructuring" or "reframing") show you how to think differently about a problem. They would help you (in our example) construe the situation in some new way, for example as a challenge, or as an occasion to practice overcoming your obstacle. This sometimes works, and sometimes not. To determine whether the reframing is effective, you must sense whether it has brought a *bodily* change or not. You must sense what actually comes in your body in response to a reframing. A real change is a shift in the concrete bodily way you have the problem, and not *only* a new way of thinking.

The field of psychotherapy today is very diverse. In recent years it has been increasingly recognized that interpretations are not sufficient to bring change because they usually lead to a dead-end discussion. The newer therapies all have ways to engender actual experience, which can bypass dead-end discussions. (These therapies often fall prey to the second dead end; I discuss it in the next section.) Some therapists of the older orientations are also adopting the newer techniques. Some contemporary psychoanalytic authors are quite aware of the pitfall of dead-end discussions and add ways to cope with it in their methods. Kohut's addition of Carl Rogers' "reflection of feeling" enables patients to sense their concrete present experiencing and enter further into it. Many Jungian therapists have added Gestalt therapy's "two chair" method (see Chapter 13). In every method there are some therapists who are concerned with "the process" of therapy, that is to say, with just how anything concrete actually happens.

In each method there are some therapists who know the bodily dimension I speak about and some who do not. We are going to discuss exactly what client and therapist can do when there is a dead end discussion in order to bring about the concrete steps of experiential processing.

First Conclusion

Moment by moment, after anything either person says or does, one must attend to the effect it has on what is directly experienced. Does a given statement, interpretation, cognitive restructuring, or *any* symbolic expression bring a step of change in how the problem is concretely, somatically experienced? If it does, the directly sensed effect must be pursued further. If there is no effect, we can discard what was said or done. We can thereby avoid a dead end discussion or try to curtail it if one ensues. This bodily checking should apply not just to verbal interpretations but to most anything therapists or clients might do. All therapeutic interventions require the client to check for the intervention's concrete effects. Some interventions have a genuine effect and some do not. Similarly, what clients themselves do or say needs this bodily checking. It is often difficult to show clients how to check inwardly, in a bodily way, whether what they have just said has had a bodily effect or not. We will discuss how to help them to do this.

The first conclusion is not new in itself; only how to bring about the inward checking is new. Freud emphasized that the aim of interpretation is to bring up the missing experience. Interpretation is mere "scaffolding" like that which is put up around where a building will rise and taken down when the actual building is here.

The psychoanalytic author Otto Fenichel (1945) has also described this process:

> In giving an interpretation, the analyst seeks to intervene in the dynamic interplay of forces, to change the balance in favor of the repressed in its striving for discharge. The degree to which this change actually occurs is *the criterion for the validity of an interpretation.* (p. 32, emphasis added)

Effective psychotherapists from Freud on agree unanimously that a concrete experience must occur in response to an interpretation; otherwise nothing has been achieved by the interpretation and it should be at least temporarily discarded.

But despite the fact that Freud so long ago said that a therapist had to attend to the effect of an interpretation, this requirement has not been well understood. One implication of it that is often missed is that a therapist can use many interpretations and many methods, not just one! Because there is an inner touchstone that will show the success of any intervention, namely whether a bit of movement comes, a therapist has the option to try interpretations or procedures derived from many methods and theories. If one of these fails to move something in the patient, the therapist can try a technique from another method or theory. With the multitude of theories and methods that exist today it is arbitrary to choose one theory and then impose it on one's patients. Checking for a physical effect happens to be a nonarbitrary touchstone. With it the therapist can make use of what the various approaches have to offer — and *swiftly discard* anything that does not have a physical experiential effect.

At times the therapist may want to continue with an interpretion, even when it has no immediate effect. But most of the time, if there has been no experiential effect, the therapist can discard whatever was said and bring the person back to the spot just preceding. ("Oh I see, it doesn't do anything to say that. Well, as you were saying . . .") In that way a whole hour (or even 5 minutes) need not be lost in arguing or confusion.

To keep the clients' process on its own natural track is the easiest way to avoid dead-end discussions. A therapist must know that it does a great deal just to keep a client company with the exact sense of what the client is expressing. When that is achieved the bodily-sensed effect in the client is one of "resonating." A safe and steady human presence willing to be with whatever comes up is a most powerful factor. If we do not try to improve or change anything, if we add nothing, if however bad something is, we only say what we understand exactly, such a response adds our presence and helps clients to stay with and go further into whatever they sense and feel just then. This is perhaps the most important thing that any person helping others needs to know. It is also the easiest way to avoid dead-end discussions.

But such responses (called "reflections of feeling") need the physical checking I just discussed. The client must inwardly check: "Are we together now, with this? Does what the therapist says back to me encompass what I was just now struggling to convey?" When it does, the client will feel a bit of physical relief. Hearing back what was said, the client feels that that much has indeed now been said. What has been understood exactly need no longer struggle to be heard. *Now it can just be here.* It can breathe. When that happens, there is also a little bit more room inside — room for the next thing to come up from there.

Without the client's inward checking, the method of reflecting the client's messages can become mere words. Then it is a dead-end discussion, although brought about by the client rather than by the therapist's intervention.

After anything the therapist has done or said, the moments immediately following reveal whether there has been an experiential effect. By this I do not mean that the person has agreed with the therapist's assertion. The question is rather whether what therapist or client has said connects with what the client senses concretely. If not, then what has been said is not on the mark.

If there is an inwardly sensed connection or any physically sensed response to what was said, it is vital to attend to it and stay with it, because further steps will come from *there* — from the inward response, even if it is only a slight stirring without words. (Many theapists do not know to look for such an effect, let alone train and ask the person to look for it. They talk right on through such an effect even when there has been one!) If there *is* an effect therapist and client must instantly stop talking. The client needs to attend silently to it, stay with it, and pursue it.

For example, suppose client and therapist have been stuck at the same spot for some time (minutes or months). Both people have said numerous things that made no difference; nothing budged. The therapist has said this and tried that, but what the client sensed has remained unmoved. Let us suppose that the therapist has many more things to say. Suppose one of these (at last) brings a slight loosening in the client's sense of the problem. Something stirs in there, in that heretofore dead place. Shall the therapist now go right on talking so that the little bit of movement is lost again? No, we want to stay with what stirred in that place. We want to attend to it, sense it, let it open, and allow it to move in a new way.

I will show exactly how a therapist can aid the client to enter that place where concrete experiential change can come. The need for this has not been understood by many therapists. They might agree that whatever is said needs to have an experiential effect. They might agree that such an effect is the purpose of the work being done. And yet they do not seem to know how one finds it directly. And if it does come, they will fail to notice and pursue it.

The failure to pursue such a directly sensed opening leads us to the second kind of dead end I mentioned.

DEAD END: UNCHANGING FEELINGS

People in therapy often have strong emotions and "gut feelings" that are quite concrete and experiential. They are not just talking or intellectualizing. Yet despite the fullness of their emotional content, it does not change; they feel the same feelings over and over again.

The central theme of this book concerns what can be done about the dead end of unchanging feelings: how to obtain the little steps of experiential change that characterize psychotherapy when it works.

There are now many psychotherapeutic methods for engendering deep physical feelings, both from the past and in the present. These methods often result in intense emotions being felt and expressed, yet these feelings often do not change for many months and years. Others of the newer methods tend to flood the person with emotions but leave what would be called the "ego" as small and brittle as it was before. Sometimes these flooding methods are combined with "integration sessions" — mostly old-fashioned discussion. But the steps of actual change are to be found neither in mere verbal discussion nor in flooding experiences, nor in mere emotional intensity.

Dead-end feelings arise and remain unchanged most commonly because they seem quite clear and final; there is no murky edge to them that asks to be explored. The client does not say, "I'm scared but I don't know why; there's a lot more to it but I don't know all of it." Instead, the client says, "I'm scared of it," and the therapist responds, "Tell me more about it. Please go into it further. Just what is it like to be scared in this way?" The client says, "I'm scared, that's all. Can't you understand that? Haven't you ever been scared? Well? That's what I feel."

Now what? Of course the client can talk about why the fear seems to happen, when it happens, early memories, other times of being scared, and so on.

But the fear may remain just as it is, as if it were a completely packaged, finished experience, without internal complexity.

Although every therapeutic method has some way of moving past dead end feelings, and these methods sometimes work, sometimes they also fail. And despite their differences they share the same goal: therapeutic movement. The therapeutic movement is described in terms of the various contents of which personality is supposed to consist according to the different theories. But people do not really consist of the contents the various theories posit. Nor does therapeutic movement come in the gross forms in which it has been so variously described. Rather, it comes in tiny steps. I will show how we can employ all the extant methods, despite their contradictions, once I have shown how the little experiential change steps work. We will then also see exactly how they are sometimes brought about in each method.

The change steps will also let us think about human experience in a new way: Every bit of human experience has a possible further movement implicit in it. Human experience is never complete. It is never just as it appears. It never consists only of already-packaged things.

One of my favorite psychoanalysts once asked me, "After one has been in analysis one knows where all the things are, and one can get in touch with them and reopen them again. Just what are you saying that's more than this?"

He asked me this question because he heard me speak of a process whereby the client does more than become familiar with emotions and experiences and learns to touch them again and again at will. My assertion that there could be more than this puzzled him. In his own analysis his inner contents did not change; they only became known, touched, and capable of being touched again. Of course, as Freud said, this is in itself a great development. To have touched something experientially many times does liberate energy, and it does engender enlarged perspective and new behavior. Nevertheless Freud missed the little steps of change that can occur inwardly in what one "touches." Either this process had not occurred in his analysis, or perhaps he did not describe his analysis well.

The change Freud looked for was limited to a coming to awareness. No change in the content itself was expected. The content was thought to be perhaps an infantile wish, or something that had occurred in the past. Freud held that the content does not change, but in coming to awareness it "loses energy." The "ego" gains this energy. This description does sometimes fit, and with some things it may describe all that is likely to happen. But all of psychotherapy, change, and growth cannot be understood merely in terms of energy loss by otherwise *unchanged* "contents."

In Freud's theory pathology consists of packed pieces. If our problems were packed pieces, then indeed they might not be *able* to change; they might only be able to lose energy. But this theory leaves some vital theoretical and also some very practical issues unaddressed.

As I will show, when therapy is effective we soon also observe something else: steps of change in *what* the content seems to be. We want to know how to engender such steps of content change.

Theoretically, we want to understand how experience and events are not fixed packages, that is, how change-steps are even possible.

Present experiencing is not just an assemblage of past pieces of experience. This is a widespread error inherent in the current mode of "explanation." One explains an event at a later time by going back to some earlier time and finding there the same units. The event of the later time is "explained" as a certain rearrangement of the units from the earlier time. We are accustomed to this kind of explanation from physics and mathematics. If we are to get an answer of 96, we require that the answer come from 96 units, whether it be 6×16 or 3×32 or 8×12 or 1×96 or $192 \times \frac{1}{2}$. Also, in physics, the sum total of energy and matter in a reaction is "conserved," so that any change can be traced back to some energy or matter or forces that were there before and are still here now, only rearranged. When something changes we break it down into smaller pieces that did not change — that were only rearranged. When we can locate these unchanged elements, then we feel we understand; we have an explanation.

But there are other kinds of explanation that do not require this assumption of packaged pieces or units that remain the same. For example, we can explain an event by showing how it fits into a larger picture. Say someone does something puzzling. When we know the broader situation, we may see how the behavior makes sense. Then we say we understand; we have an explanation. But these are not the only kinds of explanation and understanding. From the change-steps I will describe, we will see a different kind.

Mathematics and logic work only with fixed units. In multiplying or in logical deduction one must not throw in extra units, or lose any that one had at the start. But experience and situations do not come in neatly divided and fixed units. Any situation can be cut up in a great many different ways to get very different logical inferences. One can always notice one or two additional elements, so that what seemed a logical proof falls apart. That is the reason why logic does not give necessarily correct conclusions about human experience. If you slice the facts a little differently, logic is overthrown.

For therapy and change it is of course very fortunate that nothing past or present is ever packaged so as to have only one shape with fixed results. Therefore nothing is ever quite finished. All events and experiences can be carried further, and when this happens there is also a change in what they had been. Such changes could not follow logically from what they seemed to have been at an earlier point, and yet these changes are truthful and not in the least arbitrary. But they usually have many more facets than their earlier form.

The past is not a single set of formed and fixed happenings. Every present does indeed include past experiences, but the present is not simply a rearrangement of past experiences. The present is a new whole, a new event. It gives the past a new function, a new role to play. In its new role the past is "sliced" differently. Not only is it interpreted differently, rather, it functions differently in a new present, even if the individual is unaware that there has been a change. To say it pungently, present experiencing changes the past. It discovers a new way in which it can be the past for a present.

The present is always a new whole, even if the individual is explicitly reliving a past. Emotions and memories from the past come as part of the *present* person. The past changes in a new present. Even if the past is wholly implicit and unnoticed, it can be carried forward into a new whole as part of the new, the process of present experiencing. Events of the past are not thereby falsified retroactively as was done in the Soviet Encyclopedia, but their role in the body can acquire a new function.

Second Conclusion

Every experience and event contains implicit further movement. To find it one must sense its unclear edge. Every experience can be carried forward. Given a little help one can sense an "edge" in the experience more intricate than one's words or concepts can convey. One must attend to such sensed edges because steps of change come at those edges.

We will discuss what to do when there seem to be no edges and therefore no steps. In a seemingly complete experience, how does one find where it can be carried further? How does one help a person find this edge, this sense of intricacy more than one can as yet say? We will discuss exactly how to find the edge, and how to engender the steps of change that can come at such an edge. Change hardly ever comes in one step; rather it consists of many small steps and now and then some large ones.

I have tried to describe two typical dead ends: the dead end discussion without experiential concreteness, and the dead end of emotions and feelings, directly contacted, but repetitious. In contrast to these, we want to be able to recognize and bring about a series of experiential change-steps. What do such steps look like? What exactly can one work with, when such steps are not happening, to bring them about?

15

CHAPTER 3

Eight Characteristics of an Experiential Process Step

To understand the change-steps of the therapy process we must consider them from inside. We examine the patient's process and we postpone discussion of therapist interventions.

The view from inside may be unfamiliar to some readers. It is the standpoint of the person sensing, coping, and struggling with an outer and an inner field of experiencing. There we find thoughts and perceptions, and along with them there is also some directly sensed bodily experience. The bodily experience becomes more distinct if attention is paid to it.

THE DIRECTLY SENSED "SOURCE"

Something can emerge from the unconscious without one's being able to sense its source. For example, one may recall a dream, a thought may come, an image may "pop in," strong emotions may suddenly well up. Actions and role play may arise spontaneously. It is commonly assumed that these come from "unconscious levels" so deep that one cannot sense their source. But it is also possible (at various depths) to sense the source directly. There can be a direct awareness of the "border zone" between the conscious and the unconscious. For example, if one cries, one can turn one's attention inward and sense "the crying place" from which the tears are welling up. Or if a strong emotion comes, one can focus on the inward sense of which that emotion is a part. An image that "pops in" need not remain only visual but can be accompanied by a physical sense, a quality perhaps, an aura. Such an image is not purely puzzling and incomprehensible or explainable only by interpretation. There will also be an inward understanding that is not conceptual and cannot be spoken. The image can lead to its own direct sense of significance.

Even in simple conversation an individual can attend inwardly so that something directly sensed can come in. One can stop and sense the place that one is trying to "get at," the place that one is speaking from. This sense is always much richer than what one says in words, and one cannot know all that it is or could be in it. This is what I mean by "the implicit."

Without such direct sensing of the source the client can experience only what has emerged. Then one can only add interpretations to it. The client has no direct experience of the source and no direct impetus to further steps. There is only the material and the therapist's interpretations.

Instead we will see here that the source of what emerges can be directly sensed. It will turn out that this can make very important differences in therapy and in the development of a person. In what follows I will try to describe the characteristics of this direct sensing.

THE INITIAL LACK OF CLARITY

The direct sense of the implicit source is always *unclear* at first: vague, fuzzy, not recognizable as a distinct emotion or a familiar feeling. Nevertheless it is sensed distinctly.

To experience something that is as yet unclear differs from experiencing an emotion; we know clearly that we are angry, or sad, or joyful. It also differs from familiar "feelings" even when these do not fall into universal categories. "How I feel when . . ." may be quite familiar. What one senses at the "border zone" is unclear, in that one does not know what to say or how to characterize it. Yet it is definite in that one senses unmistakably that it has its own unique quality. One cannot be talked out of this unique, unnamed quality, and one cannot be talked into feeling it as something else. In that respect it is very definite.

Consider a person who tells you about a problem. After 20 minutes perhaps the person stops. Everything that can be said about it seems to have been said — and yet . . . . . the problem is felt as more than that. The edge is felt but it is unclear. At the moment the person may not have been able to enter further into that edge, but it is there. The discomfort of the problem is the edge; it is more than could be said. The person may now fill the time with talk because remaining quiet is uncomfortable. During such talking the person may lose the bodily sense of that edge.

We can see the unclarity of the edge with the fear in our example about approaching the attractive person at the party. For some people it would have this unclear edge: "I think I know what goes into that fear; it's that I've always been scared just to make a decision on my own. I'm scared it will be wrong. But . . . uhm . . . " This person has a sense of the edge. "Uhm" is the felt sense. Or, if nothing seems to be there a distinct but unclear sense can soon come in.

Sometimes a person's experience does not seem to have any edges for a long time. More often the edges seem missing because the pace of the person's talk is too rapid. To stay with something directly felt requires a few seconds of silence. It can be anxiety producing. People are likely to go on talking, and to move to something else, and soon again to a still further point. In that way people mostly stay outside of themselves. Another way clients stay on the outside of themselves is to berate themselves as if they were an external critical voice. They are angry at the trouble and although they sense it directly, they do not invite the direct sense of the trouble to speak to them further. They ignore the edges and repeat the main packaging (Hendricks, 1986).

But I will show how we can help them to stop, to enter inside, and how to help the coming of a directly sensed, unclear edge.

IT OCCURS IN A BODILY WAY

A direct sense of the border zone occurs *bodily*, as a physical, somatic sensation. It is sensed in the viscera or the chest or throat, some specific place usually in the middle of the body. It is a special kind of bodily sensation, and I will describe it more exactly later. It is sensed inwardly, not as an external physical sense such as tight muscles or a tickle on the nose (these do play a role, but a different one).

Oddly enough, many people cannot sense their bodies from inside. For example, some people can sense their toes only if they first move them. Some say they must press their toe against their shoe. Certainly these people also have intense emotions, but they locate them "all around," or in and around their head. Without some special procedure in these cases, the body may remain uninvolved in the therapeutic process. But such a person can soon learn to sense the body from inside ("How is it in your chest or stomach now?") and will then discover that every concern can form a unique bodily sense. It is characteristic of this sense that it is at first unclear, but soon it proves to be the source from which the experiential complexity of any given concern will emerge.

Freud's term "preconscious" referred to something different from this: what we *can* be aware of if we choose, such as available memories and feelings. In contrast, he thought that "unconscious" material *cannot* be sensed anytime we

18

like. Freud thought in terms of the content, the "material." For him the pre-conscious was the realm of available material.

What I am referring to is the layer of the unconscious that is likely to come up next. This is at first sensed somatically, not yet known or opened, not yet in the "preconscious." Freud had no term for this layer. Nor has there been a term for it in the common language. We now call it a "felt sense." Sometimes I have called it a "direct referent." Freud's free association and Jung's active daydream techniques sometimes lacked this somatic character. Other times it was included but not specifically noted. For example, in free association a "block" would occur; Freud would then interpret the block. Implicitly the patient focused on the block — perhaps a directly sensed discomfort that seemed at first impenetrable. But this direct sensing was not emphasized. A correct interpretation might then shift and open the block.

To some of my readers the inward attention examined here will be familiar. They will know how it is to turn away from one's words and thoughts to attend in the body, or at least attend to feelings. Other readers may need a little help following it. As an example, sometimes you decide you are hungry because you have not eaten for a while. But usually you sense directly in your body whether or not you are hungry. Similarly, you can check directly to see if you are comfortable inside.

A direct, at first unclear bodily sense at the border zone is not quite the usual bodily sensation; it is not an emotion, not a thought, not a definable content.

Our usual way of thinking divides experience into discrete entities: thoughts, feelings, memories, desires, body sensations, and so on. In our example at the beginning of the chapter, you *think* there is nothing to lose by approaching the person. You *feel* tense and scared, and also angry at yourself. You may *remember* other times this has happened and perhaps some childhood memories as well. You *desire* the person or you want to make an approach. You have an *image* of doing so. You have the physical sensation of your heart pounding.

These experiences are cut apart from each other. If you were now to say to yourself, "How do I *physically* sense this situation *as a whole*?", even the question is confusing. It involves an unusual way of sensing. We are used to letting "physical" and "body" refer to just sensations. Can we *physically feel* a situation? We usually think of "situation" as outside, and we split that off from our inside.

Suppose your belt feels too tight. You loosen it and feel better. The tightness was the physical sensation. But suppose you loosen your belt and the tightness remains? Then that is your physical sense of a situation.

By "feel" we usually mean well-known emotions such as being "scared" or "angry." But one can also have a very distinct feeling that has not yet opened to reveal what it contains. That is a bodily felt sense.

Sometimes we have experiences that cross the lines between thought, feeling, desire, image, and sheer body sensation, but not often. Nor is a felt sense a combination of these many together. Although it can come along with any of them, and also lead to any of them, a felt sense differs from them all. It is a bodily sense of some situation, problem, or aspect of one's life.

Usually a felt sense must first be allowed to come; it is not already there. A felt sense is new. It is not already there as a bodily-sensed object. It *comes* freshly, in something like the way tearfulness or yawning *come* in us.

The felt sense in our example is not the scared feeling — though the scared feeling is part of it, as is every other aspect of the whole problem. It is not the heart pounding, not the memories, not the desire to approach, not the anger about your inability. If attention is put in the middle of the body, the felt sense can be allowed to come. It comes, so to speak, "around" or "under" the anger or "along with" the heart pounding or as the physical quality that the memory brings with it.

With some amount of practice one can let this odd kind of experience come, which we now call a "felt sense." Many people in psychotherapy and outside of psychotherapy have learned this or found it (see Gendlin, 1981). With some commitment of time it seems that any type of person can learn to isolate the felt sense, from hospitalized persons labeled "psychotic," to college students, children, and creative artists — seemingly anyone.

THE FELT SENSE IS A WHOLE

A characteristic of this felt sense is that it is experienced as an intricate whole. One can sense that it includes many intricacies and strands. It is not uniform like a piece of iron or butter. Rather it is a whole complexity, a multiplicity implicit in a single sense.

With the emergence of such a single bodily sense comes relief, as if the body is grateful for being allowed to form its way of being as a whole. The bodily sense becomes something in and of itself, a fact, a datum, something that is there. The person *has* that "something that is there." It is something you *have*, but not something you are. Before you *were* that way of being. Now you are the new living that is ongoing, as you sense how you were. How you were is now something you *have* in front of you. It has become the object to which you attend.

CHANGE-STEPS ARISE FROM THE FELT SENSE

When a step comes from a felt sense, it transforms the whole constellation. It might be a big dramatic step or a very small one, but it is a change in the nature of the whole. Such a change or "shift" is experienced unmistakably in the body. One has a sense of continuity, the sensed whole is altering, and one senses this altering directly and physically.

A STEP WILL BRING ONE CLOSER TO BEING ONESELF

In such a step or shift one senses oneself differently. There is more to be shown about what "self" means in this kind of experiential step. Such a step is a (perhaps small) development of the centered whole of the person.

As one comes to have a sense of this whole as an object there comes to be a difference between oneself and that sense. "It is there. I am here." There is a concrete disidentification (that is one way of putting it). "Oh . . . I am *not* that!" A felt sense lets one discover that one is not the felt sense. When one has a felt sense, one becomes more deeply oneself.

STEPS ARE IN THE DIRECTION OF GROWTH

A step has its own *growth direction*. One cannot legislate the direction. Yet it helps greatly to know what a direction of growth is.

For the moment I am content if the reader wishes to interpet my claim that there is a direction to the process as a value that I (and therapists like me) read into the process. Let us postpone the argument as to whether I put it in, or whether it emerges. Either way it is a necessary characteristic. It is the development of the person.

A contrast with catharsis will help convey what I mean. Suppose a person is awash with intense anger and fury, more anger than the person can possibly control or manage. In therapy this may involve screaming, kicking, or beating a pillow. Later the person may feel better. People also find that anger does not destroy them. But during the expression of the anger the person may feel swept away like a nutshell on an ocean.

In contrast, when a person's central core or inward self expands (i.e., in a direction) it strengthens and develops, the "I" becomes stronger. The person — I mean that which looks out from behind the eyes — comes more into its own. The increasing strength and development of the person is essential to a successful therapy.

With catharsis the person can also develop, but frequently it leaves the person feeling as small and tenuous as before. Then the person may be "in touch with feelings," even very "bodily" ones, and yet growth has not happened.

One develops when the desire to live and do things stirs deep down, when one's own hopes and desires stir, when one's own perceptions and evaluations carry a new sureness, when the capacity to stand one's ground increases, and when one can consider others and their needs. The last item here is not contradictory to the others. One comes to feel one's separate existence solidly enough to want to be close to others as they really are. It is development when one is drawn to something that is directly interesting, and when one wants to play. It is development when something stirs inside that has long been immobile and silent, cramped and almost dumb, and when life's energy flows in a new way.

But how does this growth first come about? Of course, if the growth continues for a long time, we can easily notice the result. But how can the beginnings of that growth be recognized, so that we can aid it, or at least not get in its way? What are its first green shoots? What is the person doing that might not look too dramatic but leads to this result?

Before such development is obvious, there are many small stirrings, many tricklings of energy that strive to live and develop. They can come with most any little step. We can see it in the following example from a first interview:

Client: She said I was insensitive. She said it for years before we were divorced. And it's true, she'd see all kinds of things in other people, and I wouldn't see anything.

Therapist: It seemed true, what she said.

C: Yes, it was true. I would like to change my insensitivity. It's one reason I'm coming into therapy. I don't want to be an insensitive person. *I've come a long way, though. When I was young I didn't know anything about feelings.*

T: When you look back you feel pretty good about how far you've come.

C: I've also made it to my present job, which is near the top, and I'm not known to be a hard person.

T: You've done it without being a bad person.

C: (*Cries*) I'll be damned. I don't know why I'm crying. That's dumb.

T: Something wells up in you that says, "I'm not a bad person!"

C: Is that what it is?

Some therapists would not have known to pick up on how he feels he has already come a long way (see the italicized statement above). Then he would not have said the other positive things. Some therapists are accustomed to work only with what is wrong; they often ignore the positive stirrings of the person.

In this example it is easy to see what I mean by growth direction because he said more positive things, and because the result was dramatic. His inner being comes alive as his good motives and efforts are recognized by the therapist and by himself. As he is inwardly moved, he cries.

One need not take sides; the therapist did not say that he is not a bad person, or that his ex-wife was wrong. It was enough to respond to the client's perceptions as distinct from those of others. One finds that those perceptions have internally coherent meanings. Here this much criticized person is given some recognition of his own perceptions. It leads him also to give his own perceptions some recognition. As a result, his inner being, long put down and silenced, wells up. He is surprised and does not know how it happened.

But something like this effect can occur less visibly. It is generally good to take in and say back positive things clients manage to say of themselves. This also applies to anything clients are especially interested in, anything they love, or anything that is unique about them. We may or may not see their inner being stir, but we can sense that responding to those things makes a moment of contact with the person inside.

Nothing is more important than the person inside. Therapy exits for the person inside; it has no other purpose. When that inner being comes alive, or even stirs just a little, it is more real and important than any diagnosis or evaluation.

In the transcript I present in the next chapter, you will note that the therapist actively suggests certain values. I think you can probably judge that this is not what causes the result. Later we will discuss this question carefully. Here I am concerned only about showing how a growth direction is a characteristic of the process.

We do not need a metaphysical assumption that human process always moves toward health. We do not want sloppy optimism. With so much suffering and destructiveness all around us, optimism is an insult to those who suffer. But pessimism is an insult to life. Life always has its own forward direction, whatever else may also be occurring.

To follow or encourage a growth direction is very different from promoting a set of values, an idea of "good" or "bad." Contents do not stay static. What seems bad soon opens and alters what we think is bad. Therefore good and bad must be rethought just as all notions of content must be rethought.

Theory cannot direct the process we are discussing because it has its own direction. But theory (a new kind of theory) can find this "direction" even though it is not definable in terms of its content.

I am aware that it is unconvincing to say that the bad will open into something good. I would remain unconvinced myself if all I had to go on was what I have said here. The transcript I present in the next chapter will enable us to study such a step in detail.

STEPS CAN BE EXPLAINED ONLY RETROACTIVELY

What a process step will be cannot be deduced or inferred in advance. It is almost always much more specific and finely textured than any theory would infer, even in the rare cases when one guesses correctly. In retrospect once a step has occurred, it is possible to interpolate logical steps retroactively, to relate to how the problem appeared before the step was taken. After the change one can understand the progression. But in advance one cannot prefigure it. One has to wait for the step to come concretely.

Here is a summary of the eight characteristics of a felt sense:

1. A felt sense forms at the border zone between conscious and unconscious.
2. The felt sense has at first only an unclear quality (although unique and unmistakable).
3. The felt sense is experienced bodily.
4. The felt sense is experienced as a whole, a single datum that is internally complex.
5. The felt sense moves through steps; it shifts and opens step by step.
6. A step brings one closer to being that self which is not any content.
7. The process step has its own growth direction.
8. Theoretical explanations of a step can be devised only retrospectively.

CHAPTER 4

What the Client Does to Enable an Experiential Step to Come

LET US EXAMINE an instance in which a processing step occurs to see the role of the directly experienced, unclear felt sense. In the next chapter we will examine the same segment, to see how the therapist helped the coming of the felt sense and exactly what helped the individual to stay with the felt sense so that the step could come.

The segment occurred at the start of the hour. I have ended it after the moment when the step occurs. Of course the therapist and the client went on from there, and this led to further steps. I only briefly summarize the earlier sessions, but I will microscopically examine the section in which the step occurred.

On the right hand side there is enough information to help you follow the transcript. It may be necessary for you to read over the transcript first to understand it, and then examine it more carefully for our purpose here.

Let me say in a general way what the excerpt is meant to illustrate. I would ask the reader to notice that the excerpt begins with a dead end discussion. The client has been thinking in a certain way about the issue; it is a line of thought she has often pursued. The therapist is therefore familiar with it. Despite the client's conclusions, the problem is not moving toward a resolution. The reader can easily imagine an hour spent in such a discussion without any effect.

Also notice the eight characteristics of a step, which were outlined in the last chapter:

1. At various moments the client will turn her attention to something implicit that she directly senses. At those moments she senses the border zone between conscious and unconscious.

2. What is sensed in this way is at first unclear, murky, puzzling, not fully recognizable. She can address this only by temporarily shelving what she had been saying or thinking. When the therapist first asks her to do this she is unwilling to let go of what she was thinking and still wanted to say. In the excerpt I point out that moment.

It is not necessary to decide if her perspective is wrong or right in this process, nor is there any denigration of thinking here. The process moves between thinking and bodily sensing; both are required. But to find the bodily sense she does have to turn her attention away from the old information, away from what is clear. Instead, she turns to what is felt unclearly around the clear feelings, and beneath them.

You will notice that there is a time during which nothing specific emerges from the unclear felt sense. The client does not instantly discover an answer or move ahead. This uncomfortable period of time endures for a minute or two before something happens.

3. You will also see that the sense exists bodily for the client; she is attentive to her inward physical state.

4. What she discovers is a whole, a single entity. And yet, when it opens we can see that there was complexity implicit in it.

5. The actual step involves a shift, an opening in the felt sense. Until then the felt sense had remained closed, silent, and unmoved. Now it shifts and opens. This shift also includes a feeling of physical relief, a bodily indication that what was said, or recognized, is directly meaningful as it emerges from the murky sense. This does not mean that what was said is ultimately true or right. Neither the therapist nor an experienced client would assume that it is. Later steps are likely to further change what now seems to be true. What is apparent is that the murky sense of the issue is directly affected by what has been said. These statements "speak for it" or "from it" whereas much else that was said and thought had left the unclear felt sense untouched.

Such a step feels good; it releases energy. What one finds may feel good or bad, but its emergence — the step of finding — always brings relief, like fresh air. This kind of effect does not make something painful more painful. I call it a "felt shift."

The felt shift changes the constellation of the whole problem and the person's attitude toward it.

6. Notice that although the client discovers a deep part of herself, it is not herself that she discovers. That is, she is interested in it and sympathizes with it,

but she remains separate from it and greater than the part that is there. In this deeper sense of oneself, the person is not the content.

7. What has emerged was not the result of the client's values or purposes (that is, her desire for competence or her desire to reach out rather than pull back). The values she had condemned the fact that she sometimes pulls back; nevertheless, what emerges does not arise from these values. Nor does it arise from the therapist's values, although he actively puts them into the process. I believe that neither the client's nor the therapist's values made any difference here. But what emerges is not arbitrary; it has its own direction and its own values.

8. In retrospect one can make sense of what emerges, and one can form a theory and invent logical steps that could have led to it. Once we see the step, we can understand the statements that led to it in a new way, so that the step can make sense coming from them.

What happens in a step cannot be predicted from what is said or thought before it occurs. And although it remains logically related to the same topic, problem, or issue that brought it forward, the problem has changed from how it seemed. We call that "content mutation."

THE DEAD-END DISCUSSION AT THE START

In earlier sessions there had been a good deal of dead end discussion, occasionally a bit of focusing, which the client had learned to an extent. The dead end discussion concerned her negative evaluations of herself and her great concern with how she appears to others. With regard to men, she had said much about being unsure of whether she is attractive and described her preoccupation with this question. She had also expressed annoyance at being so concerned with this and lectured herself for not upholding her values, according to which appearances should be unimportant. She criticized herself and used words like "insecurity" to describe her feelings about herself. She described what happens with men and people in general: She said she becomes "withdrawn."

She had talked about her grades in school (having gone back after some years), her various academic interests, and her boredom with and rebellion against what goes on in the classroom.

She was angry at the block she felt in herself, and it made her angry at herself. The block got in the way of living her life. Sometimes it was an extreme withdrawal, an inability to be with people at all. She had been sent home from college the first time because she had "freaked out" in a crisis that was much like a breakdown.

She had failed to hand in a paper, which remained unfinished because she felt it was not good enough the way it stood. This would set her to wondering why she was so concerned with being brilliant, good, and attractive, and the discussion would come full circle. Being tested or evaluated were too important to her and she felt forced to avoid those situations.

If you happen to be unfamiliar with the client-centered way of responding, called "active listening" (Rogers–Kohut), you may think that this therapist is very passive. You might see it as inconceivable that a therapist would spend most of the time intent on receiving and reflecting back so exactly only what the client conveys. It is actually an extremely active and powerful way to make deep and unobstructed contact every few moments. It is a way to keep the client in the driver's seat most of the time. If you teach someone to drive a car, you cannot do the driving yourself. Occasionally you may need to take the wheel and show the person something, but if you spend most of the time doing that, the person will not learn to drive.

In the next chapter and later in the book I will discuss other kinds of therapist intervention. But those interventions should not take up a lot of the free space of the hour. Most of a therapy hour should be spent with the client confronted with the spaciousness of the hour, uncharted and waiting to be filled by something coming from inside. If what is received and reflected, the client can return to this inner waiting.

What can be done, however, if the client fails to turn inward and await the next step from inside? Then what comes will only be something verbal, a next thing to say, and a dead end conversation is likely.

As you read the beginning of this excerpt, please imagine how easily the client could have spent the hour in her own dead-end discussions, talking about how badly she performs in school, and how she avoids men. Imagine that you are about to be presented with a long transcript of such a discussion. She is concerned with how she seems to others, and she would argue with herself over whether that should be important to her. She would pursue how she came by such poor values, how everyone in her community is concerned with appearances, how society encourages that, her rebellion about it, and some vignettes to bring her point home. She would also discuss the evidence that shows that she does have some distinct intellectual abilities, and that she is attractive, against the evidence to the contrary.

This excerpt should be understood as an example of an alternative to this type of dead-end discussion. Look for exactly what was done instead.

C1: I was thinking about . . . on my way over . . . I don't seem to think a hell of a lot of myself.

C1: It is the beginning of the hour, and this is what she thought about on the way here.

T1: So . . . you're asking . . . why do you have such a low estimate of yourself.

C2: Well, uh —

C2: What he said does not fit.

T2: Or, maybe not asking, exactly.

28

C3: I had a dream . . . I was alone with this guy, ah (*silence*) . . . and the dream was real nice, it was a real nice relationship. When I thought about it next day I thought, why don't I have a real one! I don't think he could really see anything wrong with me. I was also thinking why I was absent in school so much. When it comes to the end of the line I don't have a paper, I hold back, I get jittery and then I pull away from it.

C3: By "end of the line" she means when the time comes to hand in the paper or actually get involved with a man.

T3: You're saying there is something similar about those two things.

C4: Yeah. I have all these excuses about why I never do my best, uh . . .

C4: "Never do my best" — that is, it will not be a real test.

T4: You come right up to the line and then something holds back.

C5: Yeah.

T5: And "jittery" is the best word for it.

C6: Yeah, yeah. Uh . . . I pull back.

C6: She means that "jittery" is not the best word for it. "I pull back" is.

T6: "Pull back" is it.

C7: The jittery is more a surface than the pull back. The jittery comes when part of me says, "Well, you know, you really have to do it now."

C7: She gets jittery when she thinks she will force herself to do it. But feeling jittery is not what prevents her from doing it.

T7: So we don't know what pulls back, it's not the jittery that pulls.

C8: No, the jittery is a result.

T8: So we don't really know what the pull back feels like, what it is that wants to pull back.

C9: Well I think it's . . . ah . . . that I don't want to test myself. And I'm afraid, ah, the bad things will be confirmed.

C9: She is not willing to let go of what she is thinking and to sense what the pulling back feels like, as he invites her to do. Rather she repeats what she said in C3 and C4, which he does not want to hear, and did not respond to. She thinks she avoids a real test for fear that she will find out that she is not that brilliant, or that she is not attractive to men.

T9: Can you feel the pull back if you imagine yourself going ahead?

C10: Yeah, I can feel the pull back now. . . . The pull back is into weed, that's what it does.

C10: She can feel her desire, right now, to pull back into marijuana. She might mean she wishes she could smoke some right now. Or, she might mean that her pulling back often pulls her into using dope.

T10: Into weed.

C11: Marijuana, that's the perfect place to pull back.

T11: That's a perfect place to pull back to.

C12: Yeah. But if I don't go to the line, then I don't have to pull back.

T12: As long as you don't really go across the line, there if no testing of it, there is no proof, good, bad, and you're suspecting that you're afraid of actually finding out.

C13: Right!

C13: This was a strong "right!" Finally the therapist attended to her view of the problem. Until now he had ignored what she had been saying (because it was similar to what she had said before, which led nowhere). But he should have responded as he did in T12 sooner.

T13: I was interested also in just the feel quality of it, for a minute you could feel the pull back.

C14: Yeah, I could feel it.

C14: As she says this, more quietly, she seems to be sensing the pulling back right now.

T14: Let's just tap it lightly, and see what it turns up.

(*There is a short silence.*)

C15: Scared . . . it's like the world is going to bite me or something (*laughs*).

C15: This describes *the quality* of the unclear sense of the whole of it. It's "scared," and more exactly, this kind of scared.

T15: Um hmm. Yeah, yeah.

(*More silence*)

C16: It's very strange. Feeling this feeling underneath it, and trying to talk, right now.

C16: She describes having a felt sense. She finds it odd. There is the presence of "this feeling," which is "underneath," so

30

T16: Sensing the feeling directly and trying to say what it is. And it's scared.

C17: It's very interesting, the fear is right underneath it. Now I'm content to just sit there with the withdrawn, and feel apathy until I . . . end up with the feeling, then I withdraw into the nice apathy again. (*Laughs*)

T17: Mmm, the apathy is more comfortable and the fear is right under it, so you just push down and ah . . . there it is.

(*Silence*)

T18: Well, let's be friendly with the fear, and sort of say, that's all right, right now we're not doing anything. We'd just like to hear from it. What it's so scared about.

(*Silence — 3 minutes*)

C19: This is an all good part of me but it would rather be dead, than come out to . . . um . . . being tromped on.

T19: It's all good, but if it's going to get tromped on, it would rather be dead, or stay pulled back.

(*Silence*)

T20: Now, can you really be glad that part came out and that it's speaking to us? Can you welcome it?

C21: It's like . . . when you're just being nice to a person, and someone watching later tells you that you were just trying to buy that person.

that she cannot very well talk without losing hold of it. She also makes it clear that there are no words to express it. It is an unclear, single "this."

C17: She describes going back and forth, sensing the "scared" feeling, pulling back into apathy. She calls it "the nice apathy" and laughs because, of course, she does not really want the apathy, but she can sense directly how it is more comfortable.

C19: Now the shift has taken place. Something new has opened, and it turns out that this is an "all good" part of her that pulls back. She senses the reason for the pulling back from *the inside of* the pulling back, or more exactly, from inside this newly sensed "all good" part of her. It would rather be dead than be received like that, but she senses this part of her that seems much more significant than simply being the reason for the pulling back.

C21: She describes why it pulls back. The good of this part is received by others as bad. She gives the flavor of that in an example. She was nice to someone. Another person watching accused her later of "trying to buy that person."

T21: Inside you it's good and then they make something bad out of it?

C22: Yes.

(*Silence*)

C23: Well, that sure is different.

C23: She means that her pulling back has turned out to be something very different from what she had expected, and said earlier. Rather than being negative, "what pulls back" has turned out to be a good and loving part of her.

Let us cut the excerpt off right here so that we can examine exactly how this step (this felt shift) occurred. The hour of course continued and the client remembered other instances of this kind of experience, and various aspects of her present life were illuminated. She got to know this "all good" part of herself better.

I do not want to speculate about the client, and I would ask you also not to do so just now. Some of my readers may find it difficult to do what I am asking, so I must emphasize it. Move your attention away from the content and examine instead the process. This may be difficult, but it is what I would like to ask you to do.

Let us look at exactly *how* a step like this developed here. Put aside for the moment *what* you might have pursued that this therapist did not. Instead, go along with me in thinking *how* this step came about.

In the next chapter we examine just what the therapist did to bring the step about, but first we will discuss the client's step.

In the first part of the excerpt the client has what I call a "dead end" analysis of her problem. She thinks the trouble must be that she is afraid of a test — she asks herself, "Why should I be afraid?" She thinks that she must fear finding out that she is not as smart or attractive as she wishes. That is what she means at C3–C4 and C9. She gets "jittery" when she thinks of forcing herself to hand in a paper, or to get with a man.

With this as her analysis the problem itself has not changed. She is in the position of my earlier example in which I asked you to imagine yourself too shy to approach a person of the opposite sex whom you do not know but wish to know. In that example the dead end analysis was that you are afraid of rejection, or of looking foolish, but that analysis does not change the concrete feeling; the way your body *is* and acts. Therefore, if you forced yourself to approach the person, you would be clumsy and tense, and would not do it well.

Analyses of this kind are dead ends not only because they do not change the problem as it exists concretely in one's body but, more importantly, because the sort of answers they provide offer no *direct* leads. The leads are in what gets *actually, physically* in the way when one tries to do what one wishes to do.

The client in the excerpt has not only the analysis but a "feeling" that gets in her way. She calls it "my fear of a test." As long as she treats this as plainly defined by the terms of her dead-end analysis, a known thing, her fear of tests, it will seem to keep that shape.

What occurs here to help her move beyond the terms of this dead end analysis? It happens when she says, "I pull back." She refers to the actual bodily version of the problem. Such freshly coined phrases often indicate that something concrete is being described. She would not say "I pull back" if she did not actually sense it in herself. The therapist therefore instantly responds to the new feeling, and refers to it as an "it," a "something." He calls it "the pulling back."

Of course it is not certain early on that she senses "the pulling back" directly as being "something there." The therapist need not be certain that it is. He simply invites it to be there, as a felt sense. If that is not happening and does not happen, he will try to do the same thing with a different feeling later. Suppose she treats the pulling back also as having no leads, nothing implicit: she might say, "I pull back, that's all. Haven't you ever pulled back from something?" The therapist might return to listening, and try to help a felt sense come at a later point.

But the pulling back became a felt sense. Let us examine it according to the eight characteristics of an experiential process step (see Chapter 3).

1. At C14 the client begins to *sense directly* what it is in her that pulls back. Instead of inferring, she senses the pulling back itself. Or, we can say, she senses the wanting to pull back. Her sense of it is direct: The "pulling back" becomes a felt sense, a separate thing, an "it."

Such an "it" was not simply there all along, just waiting to be attended to. Rather, when she first said she pulls back she meant it only in the specific behavior she was observing. She said that *she* pulls back. She pulls back from handing in anything to the teacher and she runs away from men. But as we have seen, the pulling back can be directly sensed as an "it." The pulling back has become an "it." It has come only just now as a felt sense.

2. Although she has a well-worked-out set of *ideas* as to why she pulls back, she does not yet *know* what meaning might be in the pulling back. It feels like something meaningful, as if *it* knows why it pulls back, but she does not yet know.

By C14–C17 she "has a handle on the felt sense" (as I put it). She has the word "scared," the quality of which she described: "The world is going to bite me." (Again the freshness of her description indicates that she probably senses this quality quite directly.) She now calls the pulling back by that tag, "the fear."

Have we seen the second characteristic of a felt sense, that it is at first *unclear*? It might seem that we have not. It is crucial to notice that "fear" is much more than just fear. There is an unclear "it" here, and this "it" is afraid. The whole of the problem is implicit in it. If it were just the sensation of fear, and not an unclear whole, nothing further would come of it. We all know what it is like to be afraid. But this "it," however, pulls back from something. She senses herself pulling back from the fear (into the nice apathy) and then again contacting the whole thing. Back and forth.

This is time when nothing seems to be happening. She spends time with this directly sensed, but unclear "it" that pulls back. We call the spending of such time "focusing." By "focusing" we mean spending time with something bodily sensed but unclear (until it comes "into focus.")

3. Is the pulling back a bodily sense? In this example there is no obvious indication of it. But how else, and where else would one sense the pulling back? Later examples will show its bodily character more clearly.

4. Was the felt sense an internally intricate whole? Yes, the pulling back is *one* thing, and contains implicitly a great many strands. It contains the reason for pulling back and what it pulls back from. It contains many instances when the same thing happened, and it also pulls back from them. It can provide an answer as to what it has to do with men and sex, and with situations in which there may be a lack of competence. All this and much more is implicit in one whole, and can emerge from the feeling of pulling back. Some of it emerges here in this step.

It is all sensed in one "feeling," which she touches, from which she then withdraws into apathy, and then touches again. It is an implicit complexity, sensed as a whole.

5. Have we seen *a step*? Yes, suddenly "it" opens. From being unclear and closed, it has shifted and opened. Now the whole complexity is understandable to her but it is characteristically different from the usual kind of "understanding." It is a direct kind. She can feel that *this*, which now makes sense, is continuous with the previously closed felt sense. Now she retroactively understands the felt sense that was closed before. Such understanding usually leads to a fresh phrasing, since no common phrase exists to say it. She calls it "an all good part of me."

In such an understanding an intricate mesh with many strands makes sense as a whole. All that intricacy "was" already implicit in the previous felt sense, but it could not be entered. She could not feel her way into it. It was closed. Now it is all open. She can feel into it and it all makes sense. What, why, and with whom, and many remembered instances are all now available together.

So it is not just that this part of her is "all good." Why it pulls back is now also available. It pulls back from a specific way that she might be responded to, namely as if she had been bad. It pulls back from being "tromped on."

As is so often the case when a felt sense opens, the general words do not convey the exact quality. One must express it with a specific example. ("When

34

you're just being nice to a person, and someone watching later tells you that you were just trying to buy that person.") One tells a little story to convey it exactly.

Like most puzzling feelings and behaviors, the pulling back was not just irrational or negative. Rather, the pulling back always did make sense. The pulling back knew why it pulled back. Now she experiences this: Of course it would pull back if it were accused of being ill-willed, selfish, or bad.

The incident in the story had happened recently to the client. That incident was obviously not the cause of why this part of her expects a negative response to a positive intent. The incident only lets her express the quality of what the pulling back pulls back from. No doubt many memories of such incidents are now also available, all recoverable from the pulling back, which has now opened and now makes sense.

Subsequently memories of similar incidents came one by one, and she talked of them. But the step we are examining here is not a memory. It is a shift in a whole complex texture. The pulling back implicitly includes many memories and other experiences. The step consists of the pulling back itself opening and letting her sense — from inside "it" — what part of her it is that pulls back, and why.

This part of her is very different from what she had thought must be the pulling back in her. It is not an avoidance of the outcome of a test. Rather, it is the feeling of expecting a wounding reaction, of being tromped on.

Along with this shift, the client's whole attitude and manner of experiencing has changed. She has compassion for this part of her which feels that it gets "tromped on." Of course she still wants to come out, not to pull back all the time, but only now does she feel the "all good" character of the feeling which pulls back. Is it obvious how this seemingly small step is a change in the whole constellation of how she is?

6. As she senses this "all good" part of her, *she* is moved by it, and has sympathy and understanding for it. This little step has put her "more deeply in touch with herself," as the saying goes.

And yet, let us observe carefully: Her "self" *is not* this "part" nor any other part of content. Rather, *she is the one who senses it*, can speak for it, understands it, and senses its all goodness. The self is not any specific content.

7. This excerpt is a good example of what I mean when I say that *the process has its own direction.* The therapist is inclined to welcome anything, and the client happens to be very critical of this "pulling back." But neither set of values account in advance for the fact that what came surprised her by feeling "all good." Why does she sense this bad thing as all good? It is not because of new values she imposes or that the therapist decided that it is good.

The experience itself brings its own evaluations. What came out has its own implication. Being "nice" to someone and then being seen as selfish generates its own evaluation. My point is that being nice to someone has its own inherently rightful demand to be received lovingly in its own terms, and it carries its own refusal to accept being received as bad or selfish.

I am pointing out that the process has its own direction and valuation. This is a characteristic of the steps of experiential process I am examining. If someone wants to call this internal direction good or bad (self-actualization, narcissistic), that is a different issue.

Of course I think that one aids the process by knowing about its positive direction, by going with it, and even by preparing for it in advance — looking for it, expecting it to come.

8. In *retrospect* we can see that the shift was not just arbitrary. It was not an abrupt shift to something else. The step was not just a reframing, or a new interpretation. Rather, we see the *continuity* of the process before and after a shift. Although what the problem was seems utterly different than what it seemed before, we can understand it as still "the same problem." But the phrase "the same" now refers not to a self-same definition, but to something experientially continuous: in terms of its definition the problem is now not the same. This kind of continuity has "*carried* the problem *forward.*"

From the new step we can freshly understand what went before. Now we see that this new step could have been incipient in the events that preceded it. But such a step could not have been deduced in advance. It must first happen in a bodily way. Then, in retrospect, it is not hard to insert logical steps to account for how the problem of pulling back from men and school "was really" the problem of a loving part of her that did not want to come out unprotected for fear of being tromped on.

But notice how different the problem is now! The issues are not about her competence, not that she might find out she is not as good as she hoped. The problem can no longer be discussed in terms of getting a good grade or being attractive, nor is she any longer annoyed at caring about these things. These things are not what "it" cared about all along when "it" pulled back. Instead, she comes to know and appreciate this vulnerable and all-good part of herself, which she had not known or sensed as such before.

Am I saying that direct contact brings absolute truth? No, because further steps will also be changes in the whole texture, and what comes of those may lead to an alteration in what was said at an earlier step. This process of steps has truth at every step, but it is not the kind of truth that can be stated in verbal propositions at each step. It is a truth of change and development in the whole mesh of experience.

HOW MUCH OF A CHANGE IS A SMALL STEP OF THIS KIND?

Is it clear that this process step has concretely altered the client? Without having more examples to look at, it would be easy to miss the concrete change. It might seem that she only got a new perspective here, perhaps a more correct interpretation. Is it not likely that this "part of her" will still pull back and block her?

The answer is: yes, it might still block her. A large problem is not solved in one step. But the step is a small bit of concrete change. Let us see exactly how what was doing the blocking has changed.

If we speak in terms of parts, we can say that her relationship to the part that had been pulling back has changed. Now it is open to her; she senses its meanings; she sympathizes with it; she grasps its good sense and its goodness. But this vocabulary of "parts" must not trap us into thinking they are *static* parts. They are parts of temporary constellations.

She is not this or any part, nor is she all the parts. She experiences a sense of warmth, of flowing, of goodness, softness, and a desire for a positive response to her own inner being. In directly sensing what she thought of as an avoidance of people, *she* moves forward, toward coming out.

The process step involves a change in the content, and a development of the self as well, a little movement of the whole person toward life.

In this step we see the very moment of an actual change. The change has not yet gone very far. Before the step, "it" was an avoidance of life. But even now "it" still says that it would rather not live than come out and be tromped on. So it has not changed into something else, nor has the change gone so far that we can no longer understand how it could have been the way it was before. We can still easily see that what came out had been hidden in a refusal to come out, and that was all that had been visible.

This example includes a reliving of something from the past, yet it clearly shows that there is change and *new* formation. I want to show that such steps are not just emergences of what was already there; rather it is the whole texture that changes and develops.

Could one argue that there was no new formation here, only an emergence of what was already there? Before this step, "it" would have been called a pathological block representing an angry withdrawal from life. Was it that she has merely construed as positive something that had seemed pathological before? After all, people often try to recast things positively, without much effect. A step that is concrete is needed, and it must actually come. The step must be a change and a new development.

Before the step this part of her was stuck, silent, hurt, resentful, refusing to live, and that was all that could be felt. Now as this part of her comes to be sensed more, the wanting in it stirs, moves, and speaks. Now its wanting *flows forward* into being felt and lived. Is this not a great change?

As a small child and growing up, had she felt the things that are now clearly sensed without knowing it? So many people who experience a step wonder: "All this feeling which now emerges, was it all there while I felt so little of it?" The answer is yes and no. This question about hidden feelings is answered if we understand the implicit texture of experience. It does not consist mainly of formed contents. Feeling responds to present living; it is not a hidden package underneath. To feel is to carry something further into present living. What was quite stuck was *not* felt, but as it flows forward into further experiencing it can change and can come to be felt. This further experiencing was *not* there before.

Let us not reduce the implicit texture of experience either to the old or the new form. It did not already contain everything it now seems to have contained, nor did it contain only what we now think it contained. Rather, all packagings are temporary organizations. The seemingly simple contents arise from the whole texture and tend to contain its intricacy in them. That intricacy is always ready to be carried forward as a whole, and new contents can form.

According to my theory a "pathological content" *is* nothing but the lack of a certain *further* experiencing. In our example it would be the client's experience of having her "scared" feeling come out and *not* be tromped on, not stopped and turned into withdrawal. Rather, her reaching out would *continue* as a reaching out, and reach someone. Without that further experience, the whole texture is halted; it is "stuck" and does not flow further. One can misread this being stuck as a pathological package: the negative tendency to refuse, withdraw, and avoid. But the idea of a negative package does not lead to the implied further experiencing because the concepts of pathological packages are negatively wrapped, so that they are only what they now are — they cannot develop into what they could be. What is missing cannot be deduced from a negative, pathological conception.

When the missing further experiencing happens, I call it "carrying forward." But carrying forward is not just something we express verbally. It is the actual experiencing that would allow the whole to be as it inherently needs to become. We see this carrying forward here in this change:

What has functioned as an avoidance of life continues, becoming what it would have become if it were not stopped. It has now actually become a desire for life. In the minutes during which the client felt it directly from inside, she allowed it to continue into itself. She spent those minutes living with this pulling back in a very different type of *process* than she had lived with it before. In these moments she appreciates (allows, gives room to, lives, has, is . . .) the pulling back so that it can continue into what it really is, the loving in her.

For a moment, assume with me that all *content* really results from the process of living, or more exactly from the *manner* of the process of living. When the manner of living is different, the content also becomes different. Because her manner is to let the pulling back be and not respond to it as bad, therefore the erstwhile content — the good that is responded to as being bad — is no more. In this manner of living the content becomes the good that needs to be responded to as good. This is a new constellation.

Had the client's manner of experiencing been an angry rejection of this part of her (if her attitude had been "it is no good and blocks everything I want"), she would have remade the content of her experiencing in the same way. It was first made by the rejecting response from others and then maintained by her own rejecting response to it. (That is why the therapist, worried that she might reject "it," urged her to "welcome it," but he need not have done that. In this example she welcomed the formerly rejected part of herself of her own accord.)

Had the client taken a cold and distant approach to "it," then it would have remained as it was (my "vulnerable" part that gives me so much trouble). One *could* merely come to have contact with something within, which then remains the same — but not if one's manner of living it becomes exactly the positive opposite of the old negative manner which had made that seeming package in the first place.

I do not mean to argue only for a theory. Rather, I would like you to see exactly what is happening. If you see it, then you can think about it in your own way and formulate your own theory. If you do not like or agree with anything I have said here, please look again at that part of the transcript and formulate from it a theory for yourself.

Perhaps I have gone on too long here with a theoretical explanation. What matters to the project of this book is that you see what happens at such a process step. In fact, my project fails if you agree with the theory but see only the theory. The project is to note the observable details of the change step as it is happening.

We want to know exactly what to do to enable such a step to come. First let us notice again just what move of her own brought the client's step about. Then in the next chapter we will examine what the therapist did to help bring it about.

The client let herself directly sense *that* in her which was doing the blocking. Her crucial move was to give it room, to let it speak and move. My approach is to say, "let us hear from the opposition." Perhaps it seems odd to attribute speaking and moving to an "it." You might find a better description. What matters is that you notice exactly what I am referring to: She is up against something inside that stops her. She has made inferences about it according to various hypotheses. The thing inside makes trouble for her. It is the opposition, the enemy, that which defeats her. All of this leads nowhere.

Now she turns and does something else. She gives the supposedly bad thing itself a hearing. First she lets it be sensed. As she does, there is that period of time when it is definitely there but has not yet opened. She describes what it feels like to be just touching it, backing away (into "apathy") and then moving forward to touch it again.

This "it" has stopped her from doing what she very much wants to do, so it has been a bad part. It had avoided life's confrontations; it feared failure; it shied away from a test. It had been the opposition. Now instead, she has asked "it"; she has let the actual pulling back come forward, be here, be sensed more, and she has then let it open so as to show her its internal meanings.

What I call "the opposition" is that which does the opposite of what she tells herself to do. She tells herself to hand the paper in, to "get with" a man. The opposition is against those things and prevents them. It seems irrational.

In therapy clients spend hours berating themselves, describing themselves from the outside, criticizing themselves, always speaking only from their own side to deplore an inner obstacle without ever stopping to sense it and see if it is indeed as they surmise, and let it speak to them. That is the crucial move which brings the step.

When the opposition is allowed to come in so that it can be sensed and can open and speak people are usually surprised at what was implicit inside it. Once in a while one finds just what one expected — but even then it will be full of fresh detail which could not have been found through inference. Sensing from inside is totally different from surmising something from the outside.

Here is another example. Note the difference between surmising and direct asking, and the resulting surprise:

C: I'm mad at Tom [her new husband] for doing that. I want to push him away.

T: What does that pushing away feel like?

C: Hmm . . . Like I want to shove him into that big black case my cello is in. *I think I must* want to shape and cut him to some mold of mine. I do that to people.

T: Well, sense it a little longer.

C: Hmm . . . Oh! (*surprise*) It's like putting him away just now, but knowing that I will want him back later — keeping him in a safe place like a precious object.

Exactly how do inference, interpretation, or surmising differ from directly sensing the trouble, asking *it*? In a surmising one says, "It *must* be . . . [that I fear what the test will show]." Something surmised lacks *direct* contact. Mere interpretation is helplessly up in the air. There is no corroboration of it, no way to choose between many different interpretations. Many different interpretations are always possible.

To get an inference we must leave the troubled feeling and go to our minds for ideas about it. In contrast, in order to ask our questions of the concretely experienced trouble itself we must go to it. We must pause and let it come in more. We must sense it more clearly. We must touch it, tap at it, and wait for *it* to open and answer our questions.

CHAPTER 5

What a Therapist Can Do to Engender an Experiential Step

HERE IS THE SAME TRANSCRIPT as in the preceding chapter. This time my notes on the right explain the reasons behind what the therapist is doing.

C1: I was thinking about . . . on my way over . . . I don't seem to think a hell of a lot of myself.

T1: So . . . you're asking . . . why do you have such a low estimate of yourself.

T1: He *wishes* she were asking this.

C2: Well, uh —

T2: Or, maybe not asking, exactly.

T2: He sees from C2 that what he said in T1 was not the case.

C3: I had a dream . . . I was alone with this guy, ah (*silence*) . . . and the dream was real nice, it was a real nice relationship. When I thought about it next day I thought, why don't I have a real one! I don't think he could really see anything wrong with me. I was also thinking why I was absent in school so much. When it comes to

41

the end of the line I don't have a paper, I hold back, I get jittery and then I pull away from it.

T3: You're saying there is something similar about those two things.

T3: Notice the word "something." (We will discuss it later.)

C4: Yeah. I have all these excuses about why I never do my best, uh —

T4: You come right up to the line and then something holds back.

C5: Yeah.

T5: And "jittery" is the best word for it.

T5: He thinks "jittery" is the quality word that would let her sense the whole of this.

C6: Yeah, Yeah. Uh . . . I pull back.

T6: "Pull back" is it.

T6: Although she says, "yeah," the "uh . . . I pull back" lets him know that "pull back" gets a hold of the whole of this feeling more deeply.

C7: The jittery is more a surface than the pull back. The jittery comes when part of me says, "Well, you know, you really have to do it now."

T7: So we don't know what pulls back, it's not the jittery that pulls.

T7: He would like her to sense that, right there, which wants to pull back.

C8: No, the jittery is a result.

C8: She does not do what he hoped she would do.

T8: So we don't really know what the pull back feels like, what it is that wants to pull back.

T8: He tries again to ask her to let the "what wants to pull back" form right here, so she can sense it. If she sensed it, that would provide a fresh opening.

C9: Well I think it's . . . ah . . . that I don't want to test myself. And I'm afraid, ah, the bad things will be confirmed.

C9: Instead, she tells how she thinks about the problem.

T9: Can you feel the pull back, if you imagine yourself going ahead?

T9: He ignores what she says. He invites her to imagine going ahead, so that the pulling back will come to her right now, concretely.

C10: Yeah, I can feel the pull back now. . . . The pull back is into weed, that's what it does.

T10: Into weed.

T10: He does not understand what she means.

C11: Marijuana, that's the perfect place to pull back.

C11: She explains that she can now feel how smoking marijuana is, for her, a perfect way of pulling back from living and from situations. The role of marijuana in her withdrawing becomes clear to her, if she had not known it before. She finds it here: the pulling back is into a drug.

T11: That's a perfect place to pull back to.

C12: Yeah. But if I don't go to the line, then I don't have to pull back.

C12: She reiterates what she has been trying to say.

T12: As long as you don't really go across the line, there is no testing of it, there is no proof, good, bad, and you're suspecting that you're afraid of actually finding out.

T12: At last he responds exactly to her own analysis of the problem.

C13: Right!

C13: She gives him a strong "right!" She feels that this time (at last) he took in what she thinks about it.

T13: I was interested also in just the feel quality of it, for a minute you could feel the pull back.

T13: He tries again to turn her attention to the feel of the pulling back itself, right now. He says "I was interested also . . ." because he is aware now of having ignored what she had wanted to say. So he owns up to this being his own interest here — his way, not hers.

C14: Yeah, I could feel it.

C14: Now that she is no longer trying to say something that has not been heard, she is willing to try what he is asking for.

T14: Let's just tap it lightly, and see what it turns up.

(There is a short silence.)

T14: This is an instruction to sense "it," not to impose anything on it, but to wait and see what comes from "it." (She has learned to do this previously, so he does not need to explain it to her.)

C15: Scared . . . it's like the world is going to bite me or something (*laughs*).

C15: She is sensing the feel quality of the pull back, as he asked her to do at T13. The quality is "scared, like the world is going to bite me."

T15: Um hmm. Yeah, yeah.

(More silence)

C16: It's very strange. Feeling this feeling underneath it, and trying to talk, right now.

C16: She finds that she cannot talk at the same time. In order to talk she has to let go of the direct sense of the quality. This

43

T16: Sensing the feeling directly and trying to say what it is. And It's scared.

C17: It's very interesting, the fear is right underneath it. Now I'm content to just sit there with the withdrawn, and feel apathy until I . . . end up with the feeling, then I withdraw into the nice apathy again (*laughs*).

T17: Mmm, the apathy is more comfortable and the fear is right under it, so you just push down and ah . . . there it is.

(*Silence*)

T18: Well, let's be friendly with the fear, and sort of say, that's all right, right now we're not doing anything. We'd just like to hear from it. What it's so scared about.

(*Silence — 3 minutes*)

C19: This is an all good part of me but it would rather be dead, than come out to . . . um . . . being tromped on.

T19: It's all good, but if it's going to get tromped on, it would rather be dead, or stay pulled back.

(*Silence*)

T20: Now, can you really be glad that part came out and that it's speaking to us? Can you welcome it?

C21: It's like . . . when you're just being nice to a person, and someone watching

direct sensing is still new and strange to her.

C17: She moves back and forth, withdrawing into apathy, then forward to sense the fear, then back to apathy again. Or, perhaps we should say the fear comes, goes, and comes again.

T17: He responds to her laugh (the realization that the apathy is "nice"). He understands her to say that the fear is right where she can touch it whenever she wants to.

T18: The silence being long, he worries that she might not be welcoming whatever has come, or that she might be angry and rejecting of the fear. He shows her how to form a friendly space, a little distance, so the "scared" can open. This long silence of 3 minutes after T18 is not interrupted by the therapist. The client is looking down. Apparently she is sensing inwardly, being with what is there, waiting for it to open. This could not happen without some periods of silence.

C19: This shows that she probably did not need T18, although we cannot be sure.

T20: He structures a welcome reception for what has come. At last this part that pulls back has opened and the therapist is worried that she might react rejectingly toward it. But her calling it "all good" makes this therapist response seem unnecessary.

later tells you that you were just trying to buy that person.

T21: Inside you it's good and then they make something bad out of it?

C21: Yes. (*Silence*)

C23: Well, that sure is different.

THERAPIST TECHNIQUES FOR ENGENDERING PROCESS STEPS

Listening for and Checking Each Nuance

At first glance it might seem that this therapist responds *only* by reflecting back what the client says. But that is not all he does. First let us briefly discuss the procedure of reflecting or mirroring. Then we will note at least five other quite different kinds of responses this therapist also makes.

Reflecting, or "listening" (as we call it) includes saying back exactly what the person is trying to convey. The therapist attempts to grasp *exactly* how each moment of her experiencing feels to her. He wants to be in contact with every turn she takes and with every one of the meanings she finds. Of course every therapist will misunderstand at times and inadvertently ignore some messages. As soon as the therapist realizes that this has happened, a fresh effort to understand has the first priority. Whatever else the therapist may do is not done without recognition of exactly what the individual intends to convey.

But a person cannot usually grasp exactly what another person means the first time something is said. The therapist needs to be open to corrections. A kind of rhythm develops. The client says something; the therapist reflects it; the client corrects it; the therapist restates the reflection now corrected. Then the client senses inwardly: "Does that reflection say just what I meant?" There will generally be a nuance that the therapist has not grasped. The client repeats the missed nuance. Now the therapist reflects only the missed nuance. The client senses and asks inwardly: "Does that now state it as I feel it? . . . Ah, yes, that says it." What the client was trying to say need not be said anymore, because it has been said and heard. Now there is room inside the client for something further to come. But nothing more is ready to be said. There is a little silence. The client sits in that silence at the edge of what could be said. When the next thing to say does come, it often comes from a deeper level.

The therapist is a separate, different person and may say and do many things, but what should always come first is for the therapist to receive the client's communication just as it was intended.

The therapist keeps the client company with each nuance. She does not

45

need to argue with him about what her experience is at any given moment. How it seems to her is what he wants to understand.

Recall now how it feels to *you* to try to sense further into your direct experience while you are with someone who does *not* understand you and does not want to sense your experience as you sense it. You have to fend off the other person's desire to deny or ignore what you feel. The person has some other way of viewing it. That other way of viewing it might even be correct, but you have to swim upstream, trying to sense your own experience while having to hear and consider efforts to make something else of it. You may also be a little hurt because what you said very carefully has not been taken seriously. Indeed, it was not taken in at all by the other person. Everyone is familiar with this kind of interaction.

Under such circumstances you might do one of two things. You might take some time to consider the other person's ideas about you. If you try to understand these ideas inwardly, you might find some way in which they fit. Yet the person (who is not really listening) may not want to hear exactly how you made the ideas fit, or what you found freshly in yourself as a result. The person may not understand the place in yourself to which you applied the ideas. A second way to deal with a person's ideas about you is simply to ignore what the person has said. You can sense how it actually is for you inwardly, in spite of the other person's outlook. You can do this only if the person will keep quiet for a while. This type of miscommunication occurs often in therapy when the therapist does not reflect the client's feelings.

To reflect is thus a rare and powerful way to let clients enter further into their own experience. It is a way of being as close as possible to someone without imposing something on them.

Responding So as to Create a "Something There"

Therapists usually wish that clients would do what I describe in this book. They are pleased when the patient senses inwardly and senses especially the exact spot where an opening might occur. But most therapists do not know very clearly where such a spot would be, or that it comes first as an *unclear* sense. So they do not know very well how to invite or aid clients to focus their attention where such a sense might come.

Another difficulty is that many clients do not go to the border zone and do not know about it. Instead of sitting in silence at the edge where they cannot say more, they avoid silences of that sort. They try to find something else to say, and something else again, to fill the time with conversation.

Clients might make roughly correct inferences about their troubles, and they might say and repeat these, but not know how to profit from them. Similarly, the therapist might offer interpretations that could have experiential effects, but if the client does not know to take in the interpretation and check it inwardly there is little or no effect.

As Freud wrote in *Beyond the Pleasure Principle* (1928/1959), patients often accept a therapist's interpretation in a way that has no effect. There is no "dynamic shift" and nothing emerges. Freud gives a theoretical explanation for this (the repetition compulsion) but does not tell us how to respond so as to deal with this problem in practice.

How may we help a person to find and attend to that unclear edge in the border zone between conscious and unconscious? One way to do so is to respond in a pointing way toward an unclear "something." For example, in T3 the therapist does this. He says, "You're saying *there is something* similar about these two things."

The therapist could have reflected the same message without pointing at a "something." For example, he would not have been pointing in this way if he had said "not handing papers in is like not getting with a man" or "in both instances you avoid." Neither would he have been pointing if he had interpreted this way, for example, "You are unable to give up even a little bit of control," or "Isn't this an angry withdrawal from living?" The client might have agreed to these or other possible interpretations, or she might have argued with them. But these responses would not have pointed to an unclear "something" that she might directly sense.

At times the client might already sense a "something." The similarity between school papers and men would then no longer be just an idea. She would feel the similarity as a "something" that is concretely present in both situations although as yet unclear. But usually no such "something" comes to the client concretely. Because no "something" is there, the therapist may seem to respond to something that is not there.

But the therapist's response (T3) points the client's attention to where such a "something" might come. This makes it more likely that the client will find a concrete something there when she checks his response.

But his pointing fails; at T3 she does not look. As so often happens, she ignores the pointing and goes right on talking about herself in the usual externally observant way: "I have all these excuses. . . ."

There is no great let down when a pointing response fails to work. In this case the therapist simply follows the client and tries again a little later. A therapist practicing focusing can point very frequently in this way. Eventually one response will succeed in helping a something to come.

Notice at T4 that he does it again: "*Something* holds back." It is an invitation to her to sense such a "something" if it can come.

Almost anything can be phrased in such a way as to point to something. Let me use a trivial example: "I liked that movie." "You can sense a liking there; something in you likes that movie." Of course, if someone liked a movie we would not ordinarily respond in this way. We would probably do so only if it was puzzling how anyone could possibly like it. The effect is to point the person's attention inward to something that is directly sensed. The response also turns something that was clearly defined into something that is still unclear and could therefore lead further.

Not only can we point in this way, we can also think about the client's experiences in terms of an unclear felt sense. To be able to think in this way during the hour with the client is a great advantage. When the client in our example compares drawing back from men and her difficulty handing in her papers, the therapist does not conceptualize the similarity in words. He could formulate it variously in terms of many psychological theories and vocabularies. Since so many are possible, he would lose most of them by choosing one. Instead, he lets them all remain open and implicit for him. Thereby he has a verbally unexpressed sense for something similar to the client's sense. He knows that it would also exist for the client as an unclear sense at first. In this way the therapist's sense of the client's experience is not lost, however many hypotheses and would-be interpretations the therapist may find coming to mind as well. The actual experience is responded to concretely.

This kind of response can occur every few minutes in therapy and will eventually have its desired effect. It does not need to lead to focusing every time. (No one can spend a whole hour focusing anyway. It would be far too intense.) And the therapist willingly goes with the client wherever she may lead, until his pointing invitations begin to work.

Many other examples of pointing responses will be presented in the transcripts to follow. In technical language we call a felt sense a "direct referent."

Finding a "Handle" Word or Image

Once a felt sense has arrived, therapist and client can both try to find a word, phrase or image to describe it. When this succeeds we say that the client has a "handle" on the felt sense. As with the handle of a suitcase, which brings with it the whole weight of the suitcase, the whole weight of the felt sense is brought forward by that one word or phrase when one repeats it to oneself.

Notice that in T5, having spoken of the "something" that "holds back" in T4, the therapist goes on to try to get its best handle. He thinks it is the word "jittery." He imagines that the unclear sense of holding back has a jittery quality.

He is wrong, but the attempt to get a handle has the desired result: it invites the client to sense the quality of the something. She does that at C6, and states it as, "I pull back." The therapist at T6 immediately drops "jittery" and adopts "pull back." He has no investment in which of the words best helps to hold on to the unclear sense. If "pull back" does it, he wants that phrase, and drops the earlier one.

However, as often happens when the therapist is wrong, the client feels compelled to explain more exactly why he was wrong. Clients tend to be polite and so they do not easily discard what a therapist has said, even if it was wrong. Can you see here why we would wish her not to have to stop and explain at length why "jittery" was not right? To explain that to him, she must leave her direct inward sensing and may not easily find it again. Therapy becomes easier when clients know that a therapist wants them to disregard therapist statements that are not right.

Sensing Whether the Handle Word or Image Resonates

The therapist cannot decide which of the person's words brings the felt sense along with it. Clients must sense for the physical effect of what they say. They check to see if the handle word (proposed by either person) speaks for the "something there" and helps to hold it.

At T7 the therapist shows her that he has fully taken in the fact that the word "jittery" is not the handle word. But he also tries for a "something"; he phrases it, "*what* pulls back." This does not work because she is still attending to the fact that jittery was *not* it. So at T8 he tries again, inviting her to sense "what the pull back feels like." He goes even further in establishing this "something": he gives it a wanting of its own. He says they do not yet know "what it is that *wants* to pull back." He is doing more than just finding a "handle" word. She must check to see if the word or image that might be the handle word *resonates* with the unclear sense of what is blocking her way. "Pulling back" does that.

Explicitly Inviting the Client to Let a Felt Sense Come, and to Focus on It

The therapist can sometimes do more. The client can be asked, "This, which you just talked about, can you feel it *now*?" Or, the therapist can ask, "If you put your attention in your body, there in the middle of your body, can you feel this?" These are explicit instructions to let a felt sense come, and to sense it.

At T8 the therapist explicitly invites the client to attend to the unclear felt sense. He says, "We don't really know what the pull back feels like, what it is that wants to pull back."

Again this fails to work. Instead of sensing inwardly to answer his question, she tells him her hypothesis.

Another method to help the coming of a felt sense is to ask the client to imagine the situation vividly, and to imagine trying to do what they have trouble doing. Then the concrete felt sense of what is in the way is likely to come.

For example at T9 ("if you imagine yourself going ahead") the therapist asks the client to imagine herself going ahead with a man. He hopes that if she imagines going ahead with the man the felt sense of the pulling back might come in strongly and distinctly.

A therapist can engender a felt sense more elaborately than this. For example, suppose the client complains about procrastinating: "I have this task to do and I really think I want to do it, but somehow I can't get started." The therapist can say: "Imagine that you are just now going to start. Make it very vivid to yourself. Imagine where you are going to do it, and that you are just now going to begin. . . . Now put your attention in the middle of your body, and notice: What sort of sense comes in your body as you try to start?"

Once in a while such instructions help the client discover where a felt sense comes. But elaborate instructions should only be given rarely. They turn the therapist into a sort of master of ceremonies and this can shrink the spaciousness of the therapy hour. Also, if the instructions fail to produce anything, the client can get discouraged. A simple pointing response creates no such difficulties. For example, the therapist may say: "When you try to start, *there is something* that doesn't want to start" or "As you imagine starting, *something* won't let you."

What the therapist ought to have done at T9 is respond to what the client said! But he was too involved in his own project (to get her to focus on the pulling back).

She does as he asks at C10 and finds in the pulling back her desire for marijuana. This lets her sense directly that marijuana is a place she pulls back into. She feels her desire for a joint *right now*. The pulling back is here now. It is now not only the pulling back from men and handing in her papers, but also her wanting to pull back from the immediate therapy situation. Perhaps she wanted to pull back from the therapy situation because he pushed her to sense the pulling back directly (while she was still trying to say her thing and he would not hear it). She wants to withdraw right here and now, but not in a way that lets her focus further on this wanting. Rather, the desire to pull back seems to be only the desire for weed.

All therapists come to this kind of juncture: It is very good that the problem is now concretely in the room as an issue between client and therapist. But now, how can it be handled so that something new happens. One quick way is simply to spend a little time receiving the client's side of the communication. That lets the interaction be one in which the client succeeds at being active. Such interaction will usually move past the blockage, because most pathology consists of failed and stuck interactions.

This illustration shows very well how interaction is the wider context within which the clients *inward* change process happens. The manner of interaction needs to be different before the client's inward process can become different.

In this respect it is important that the therapist in our example had always warmly received anything the client said or did, regardless of its goodness or badness. It now turns out that this kind of reception is a positive opposite to the emotional package that seemed negative. Here is an interactive situation in which she feels welcome as she is, with whatever she finds inwardly. Hence the contents of what she finds can change from being the stuck results of not feeling welcomed into what they always should have been: some sort of continuation of the desire to live.

Because content depends on the manner of experiencing, the interpersonal relationship is vital. To understand the steps of the change in content we must examine not only the client's inner process but also its interactional context. After all, the inner process occurs not only inside the client but also inside the interaction with the therapist. The client experiences herself in the interaction. If the interaction is troubled, negative, or blocked, the internal contents will be formed from that manner of her experiencing.

We cannot usually get people to shift their attention if we ignore what their attention is focused on. Usually we must first respond to that. Having been heard, people are free to let go of whatever it was and take in what we say. But as long as their own message is not taken in and acknowledged, they will keep sending that message and cannot easily take anything else in.

Or, if people do comply, their manner of interaction is passive; it consists of a compliant response to being pushed. That kind of interaction frequently occurs between people, and such pushing is often how people interact with themselves. Because pushing is the usual manner of interaction it brings forth contents in their usual form. To find the contents changing inside, one must experience onself in a different manner of interaction, and one must also approach oneself inwardly in a different manner.

At C12 the client tries once again to say what the therapist ignored before. This is typical also. What is not heard is usually repeated over and over. Some people in close relationships, such as a marriage, say the same things over and over for 30 years. It is because the other person never takes it in for what it is intended to mean. It is not that they agree or disagree; they just fail to hear it and take it in. If it were ever fully heard as it was meant something different would be able to arise in the person.

At T12 the therapist recognizes that the client is reiterating something that he has previously run over and ignored. He takes it in and reflects it fully ("as long as you don't really go across the line . . . "), saying it just as she means it. For this he gets a solid, heartfelt "right!" (C13).

Now, her attempt to be active and tell him something has succeeded, and she is no longer passive nor does she feel imposed upon. She need no longer struggle to tell him her side; now she is free to hear his suggestion and decide to try it.

It also helps that he phrases his suggestion (T13) in a way that indicates that it is *his* thing that he is interested in. When things get tangled, it helps for therapists to be very honest and take responsibility for whatever they are doing. At T13 the therapist can feel clearly that *he* wants her to focus, and that this has been a slight disjunction between them. By "disjunction" I mean the familiar feeling that one person is trying to get the other to do something that the other person does not want to do, but both people pretend not to notice this and continue in a friendly fashion. A therapist should always try to notice this sort of "slight" disjunction and should not let it continue for more than a few responses. *The manner of the ongoing interaction is always more important than any other consideration such as whether focusing is occurring or not.*

One easy way to restore the connection is to reflect the other person's side (T12) and to allow time for the person to experience that their side has been fully taken in. In the transcript we see the connection restored only when he got her strong "right!" (T13). Only then does he return to his own side and explicitly marks it as his own by saying, "*I* was interested also in. . . ."

Now they are together again. Her active effort has succeeded, and what is hers and his have been clearly marked. She can decide to try his thing, now that hers is not being ignored. She does so just after he says, "*I* was interested also in just the feel quality of it, for a minute . . . feel the pull back."

In this example the client becomes both willing and able to focus very quickly. So it is easy to see the progression. With some people many sessions might be required before they are able to focus. Some people need to be given quite formal and didactic focusing instructions. A therapist can mark off a period of time in the hour for focusing instruction. ("I want to show you something for a few minutes. Tell me when I can do it. It might help or it might not. Can we try something?") In Belgium and Germany some therapists arrange to teach focusing to each other's clients. But most people can learn it quite naturally as it is described here, with very small short bits of instruction that do not require the client to be passive and do not preempt the client's sitting freely before the wide open spaciousness of the hour.

"Resistance" is often a reaction to the therapist's behavior. Resistance is aroused or increased when a therapist wants to push into an area in which a more intricate process is required. To disentangle from a client's resistance it is best for a therapist just to listen and reflect the client's communications exactly.

Of course resistance can be a reaction to past experiences with others. It can also be an inward phenomenon, arising from the client's own efforts to enter a place in which a more intricate process is needed. The way out of this situation is for the client to hear from the opposition. Let the resistance speak. For example, the client says, "I ought to get into this but somehow I don't want to." Then the therapist may ask the client to sense the bodily *quality* of this unwillingness. "Is it heavy, or jumpy, or like walking in glue, or how?" By focusing on the bodily quality, the client can come directly to the concrete feeling of not wanting, and can then hear from it further. "Let *it* tell us why it doesn't want to."

Sometimes dissociation will occur at a certain juncture. ("If I try to go on, I feel strange and everything gets foggy. There's no road there.") This probably means only that it is not yet time to go further in that direction. Some other steps may need to come first. I have often observed that a few months after such issues were initially raised they are ready to be processed. If this is also thought of as resistance, it should be honored for the time being.

But in our example there is absolutely no question of resistance. In this excerpt genuine focusing happens very swiftly and easily. The client only wished the therapist to understand and take in what she said. This is not resistance. Nor would it be resistance if she happened to have much more difficulty getting the wholistic felt sense of the "pulling back." For many people it takes quite some time to learn how to *let* something as odd as a felt sense come in. It is hard to know how to dispose one's attention so that a felt sense may come. It is rather like attending to something that is not even there yet. It is not an obvious mode of attention at all.

Providing Instructions to "Tap It Lightly," Sense It, Be with It, Stay Next to It

In subsequent transcripts you will see many versions of instructions to stay with an unclear felt sense. It is difficult to keep one's attention on something unclear. It may come and be concretely present, but then vanish again.

Once again I want to say that therapy can proceed even without focusing. Even if there is only talking, some new edges and new feelings and memories do come at times. Focusing is a systematic, knowing way to let something implicit open.

In the example we have been working with the client had done focusing before, but it was still early in her therapy. Notice that the therapist was not sure she would understand his instructions as phrased. He was therefore ready to rephrase it in several versions. Her understanding is shown both by the silence that followed his rephrasing and by the fact that she did not look puzzled or appear stuck. One could see that she was silently doing something of importance to her. Of course the therapist could not be certain until she spoke again that what she did in the silence was indeed what he had asked for. Whatever she did and said, he was ready to receive it and respond to it in his usual way. He was also ready for the typical pitfalls: she might not have understood the instruction; she might have become impatient with the fact that the unclear felt sense had not opened up right away; she might have become angry at the unclear felt sense ("that's so dumb, it makes me miss what I really want in life . . . "); she might have identified with it ("there's no 'it' here; I want to pull back, that's all.") None of those pitfalls happened here.

To stay with a felt sense requires feeling both distinct from it and near it, next to it, able to return to it again and again during a long minute or so. That is exactly what the client does in this example.

Look again at C16 and C17. What the client does here is exactly the aim of the therapist procedures we have been discussing.

C16: It's very strange. Feeling this feeling underneath it, and trying to talk, right now.

C17: It's very interesting, the fear is right underneath it. Now I'm content to just sit there with the withdrawn, and feel apathy until I . . . end up with the feeling, then I withdraw into the nice apathy again (*laughs*).

One might object on theoretical grounds to my ways of describing what is happening here, and it could be restated in any number of ways, but what the client is doing here is what matters, however one chooses to describe it.

I have chosen this therapeutic interaction as the first excerpt because the client describes the process in her own words. C16 and C17 put into words exactly what it is like to stay next to a felt sense. The felt sense is right there, she can feel it "underneath," she can sense it, and she can move back from it and then let herself sense it again.

The client is inwardly tapping and feeling into the felt sense at the edge of what she knows. This is just what the therapist has been trying to bring about. Without any pressure his responses tend to bring it about. Reflecting back each message invites her to check his restatement. Such inward checking tends to let the client encounter the felt sense. Since he senses what she says in this way, he easily responds to the "something" — an implicitly meaningful datum, a referent that might be there. The same thing happens when the client tries to sense which "handle" fits best ("pull back" or "jittery"). To decide this she will probably sense what she has there as a whole, to see to which word "it" responds. And the therapist also explicitly invites her to attend to what is sensed unclearly, to tap it, touch it, and wait and see what it will show if it opens. All these therapist responses aim at just this process, which happens during the silence, and which she then describes in words in C16 and C17.

Let me point out one more major consideration. The therapist's aim is not the client's direct sensing of just any kind of feeling, especially not a familiar feeling. The aim is rather to invite the client to attend to what is directly sensed but is more global and unclear than the usual — something at the zone between conscious and unconscious.

We can see the difference between the usual recognizable feeling and a felt sense. The client has a familiar feeling she calls her "apathy." She pulls back into that, away from the unclear feeling, the "it." She calls the apathy "nice" with a laugh. She means that it is more comfortable. But soon, again, she senses "this feeling underneath" which she calls "the fear."

But the feeling is not just fear. We are (wrongly) accustomed to dividing human experience into discrete entities, as if experience consisted of separable things. Once we think of it that way, everything seems known and static. Then the client's apathy seems fully known: It is simply the avoidance of the fear. The fear seems to be a complete entity, something that can be known apart from what it is the fear *of*. Then the fear is just fear, and there are no leads from the fear. The fear seems clear enough, and familiar, but its "object" is unknown. Dead end.

But these are not two separate things: the fear and what it fears. Rather, "fear" names *the whole thing*, and she touches this intermittently. The implicit complexity has a fear quality.

In the next chapter I discuss the difference between an emotion as such and the broader fabric of the felt sense, of which emotions are only a part. If what is there were simply just fear, the client would not sense something unclear and implicit in it. It is a puzzling, unclear, wider whole that surrounds and accompanies the fear.

Many people do not at first sense an emotion in this way. The fear for them would have nothing more in it, and they could only speculate about its cause. Therefore more therapist instructions and more time would be needed to point a client toward the discovery of the broader unclear bodily quality that comes with the emotion.

Of course all therapists would like their patients to sense the more global whole that accompanies such a fear. But to bring that about, most therapists know only to ask their patients to "say more about" whatever they bring up. But it can be much better if the theapist knows from where the right kind of "more" is likely to come.

Our goal is to become more exact and specific about how to engender this inward coming of an unclear whole. Later I will present the more exact instructions we can use when focusing has not happened as easily as it has in this excerpt.

Being Friendly toward a Felt Sense, and the Friendly Reception of Whatever Comes from It

Just as the therapist does from the outside, it is important for clients to take a friendly attitude toward their felt sense.

Some people find it odd and difficult to be friendly toward something troubling. They might say, "How can I be friendly toward this fear which has caused me so much trouble? I hate it!" But being friendly does not mean denying that one feels angry or impatient with it. The point is not to try to feel "accepting" when one feels unaccepting. Rather, being friendly toward the felt sense means that one makes a separate space for the anger and impatience, appreciates them, and lets them flow through, but also makes a protected space for the felt sense. One does not deny the anger but one does not let it prey on the felt sense and cause it to shrink back and disappear. We might not like what we hear from the felt sense but we want to be friendly to the messenger, or else we are not likely to hear more. So instead of criticizing or attacking "it," the client learns to be friendly toward it and glad about its arrival.

At T18 and T20 in our example the therapist tries to insure this, as the client had previously been quite critical and annoyed at her tendency to pull back.

He hopes that she can put that aside and be friendly toward the as yet unclear felt sense of being "scared."

With more experience of process steps this friendly inward attitude becomes easier. With repeated experience one comes to know that what appeared negative contains positive life energy that is only twisted or blocked. One comes to expect it to change its form as it is carried forward in further steps. So one can prepare to feel friendly toward the feeling before it opens.

At T20 the therapist appreciates the shift from how that part seemed (a pulling back from life) to what it now seems to be (a loving, coming forward). But he is not sure that the client will appreciate or welcome that step. A client may need help, especially when something loving, forward moving, or freeing is trying to come. A frequent therapist error is to be interested only in negatives and things that are troublesome. Explicitly welcoming every new positive life energy is more important. Therapy *is* the coming forward of the person. We work on the negatives only because they block it.

But can all negative things be carried forward in steps that let them become inherently positive? What if there had been an angry, destructive part of the client that she had happened upon, instead of what she found? Well, what she found was a "destructive" part until it opened and shifted.

It may not be reasonable to *assume* that nothing in humans is ever inherently destructive, but we do not require such an assumption to be able to go forward. It is enough that we have frequent observations of such change steps as the one that happened in this transcript. The process we want, the process we are working to engender and carry forward, is a process toward more life. If other processes are equally basic in human nature, we still want to engender this one.

Let us assume only that in seemingly destructive contents there *may well be* positive life energy. For example, there may be self-assertion; self-defense; an affirmation of one's being; wish to be protected, or to laugh, or play, or be close to others; and so on. It is important to carry these aspects forward, whatever one assumes about the fundamental nature of human beings. Whether it is human nature or just our own choice, responding to life-affirming moves helps to carry forward the kind of process we want. When a "felt sense" forms, the "self" becomes, in a new way, free and different from that whole. The *formation* of a felt sense is itself a new bodily step, a bit of a new kind of living.

CHAPTER 6

The Crucial
Bodily Attention

IN THIS CHAPTER I WILL discuss how a felt sense differs from
more ordinary kinds of experiences. By contrasting it with more familiar experiences, I hope to describe the felt sense more exactly.

FELT SENSE VERSUS EMOTION

Autonomous Coming

A felt sense is not the same thing as an emotion, but they do resemble each other
in certain ways. Both have a life of their own — we cannot fully control what
emotion we shall have, nor whether it will come or not. An emotion may come
unbidden. All we can do is to dispose ourselves to its coming. For example if we
vividly recall certain events, we *may* experience the fresh coming of the actual
emotion. Even if the events happened long ago, recalling them can recreate the
emotion. Or not. Emotions have their own autonomous *coming*. To find out if
the emotion came we have to see if we feel it there. If not, it did not come. This
is similar to a felt sense.

The Differences

The first and main difference between an emotion and a felt sense is that an
emotion is recognizable. We usually know just what emotion we have. When we
are angry, sad, or joyful we not only feel it but we know what it is. But with a felt
sense we say, "I can feel it, right there, but I don't know what it is."

A felt sense has its own meaning, but it is usually more intricate than we can express with the usual phrases and categories. Yet is is very definite in that we sense immediately when something does not fit. The felt sense seems to object, to shrink, or to respond by being utterly unmoved or unaffected. The wrong words cause the felt sense to have a stuck quality. The felt sense does not stir in response to those words.

In contrast when the right words are found, the felt sense opens; it flows forward. Where before it was stuck, now it flows into the meaning of the words. These words become continuous with the felt sense. With them the felt sense moves and opens.

A felt sense is the wholistic, implicit bodily sense of a complex situation. It includes many factors, some of which have never been separated before. Some of those factors are different emotions.

A felt sense contains a maze of meanings, a whole texture of facets, a persian rug of patterning — more than could be said or thought. Despite its intricacy, the whole felt sense also has a focus, a single specific demand, direction, or point. It can "add up to" or "come to" a single further step. Then we know and can say "what it really is," and saying this seems to carry the whole intricacy. Or, with a problem, sometimes we can say "what the worst of it is." One single thing, one statement, or one next step can arise from the whole of it all, if we allowed it to form.

Actually all human situations are much more intricate than our concepts and phrases can capture. A simple statement can say what the situation is, but only because the statement brings the intricacy along with it. I say that such a statement *carries forward* the intricacy of the situation.

When there is a felt sense, only certain phrases or actions will resonate with the felt sense and carry it forward. Until such phrases or action-steps come, we do not know what they will be. Even when we know a lot about what went into it, a felt sense includes much that is not known. It is the unique sense of a whole intricacy, and so it does not fall into a familiar category.

Another difference between an emotion and a felt sense is that an emotion is less reliable than reason, whereas a felt sense is more reliable than reason. When we act in anger, we often feel sorry later because we reacted only to a part of the situation. When we are calmer, we recall the whole of the situation. That is why an emotion is usually less reliable than reason.

In contrast, a felt sense is more reliable than reason because more factors can be sensed in it than reason can manage. This does not mean one can discard reason and responsible choice in regard to the felt sense. On the contrary, we always need both the felt sense and rationality. What forms as a next step is often only a first bit of a process that requires more steps. One cannot just go out and do or say any option that one step brings. Some quite wild things to do or say may come as next steps. Therefore, to let a next step come freely, one needs to assure oneself that the responsible power of choice and action is retained. Then whatever comes can be welcomed. One need not immediately act on something that emerges. There will be time to make choices at a later moment. For now, suspending rational judgment, we can let "it" speak and welcome what it says. It is only *one* step; there will be more, and we can be assured that further steps will change everything again and again. Therefore one need not reject what may seem to be an irrational step, but allowing such a step to come and to spend some time letting it be here does not mean that one discards reason.

For example, I suppose I think I know what I ought to do, but I cannot seem to make myself do it. I let my inability to act generate a felt sense. From it I might get a first step: "No, it isn't right to do this." Rationally I still think I should and that I will. But I let this sense of its being "not right" be present. From the fresh felt sense of it my next step might be: "It would be right to do it if . . . I had a plastic bubble all around me." Of course this seems unrealistic; I cannot protect myself with a plastic bubble nor would I want to. But the step has utterly changed the whole way in which I have the problem. Now I need no longer argue with myself about whether the action is right or not. It *does* seem right, but not in my present state of vulnerability. This little step points to where the trouble is: Somewhere I am left unprotected. Where, or in what respect am I so vulnerable? My next few steps will show me the answer to this question, and when that emerges clearly I will know better what to do and how to do it. Or I may find that "vulnerable" means something else. Perhaps it leads to a step of seeing that I am angry and would blow up at the wrong time if I were simply to go ahead.

With a felt sense one does not know in advance just what will emerge. Over a series of steps the whole situation will change, and we cannot know how. But we do know in advance that the felt sense includes *more* factors of the situation than we already know. In contrast, an emotion is a reaction to less of the situation than we already know.

There are other differences between an emotion and a felt sense. See Table 6.1 for easy comparison.

A felt sense will have a certain bodily quality, such as, jumpy, heavy, sticky, jittery, or tight. At times the bodily quality might best be described in words that are also the names of emotions, for example scared, shameful, or guilty. Even so it contains a whole intricacy of elements, not only what the emotion of the same name would contain.

When a felt sense shifts and opens, emotions may emerge along with thoughts, perceptions, memories, or a more holistically sensed aspect of the problem. A felt sense often contains emotions. Thus one does not find a felt sense by avoiding or trying not to feel emotions. Rather, if there is already an emotion, one lets the wider felt sense form as something that can come with, under, or all around the emotion.

In a felt sense emotions are not split from other facets of experience such as thought, observation, memories, desires, and so on. As these contents form and emerge from a felt sense, they become separated. Then they become rec-

TABLE 6.1. Emotion versus Felt Sense

Emotion	Felt Sense
Clearly recognizable. An emotion is easily named.	*Not clearly recognizable.* A felt sense is not clearly categorized at first.
Narrower. When an emotion occupies my body it shuts out much of what I already know about the situation.	*Wider.* When a felt sense forms I am in direct contact with more than I know about the situation.
Internally uniform. If I enter into the emotion of anger I get angrier and angrier. That is what is *in* anger — more anger.	*An internal multiplicity.* If I enter into a felt sense I will see that it contains many different facets of the many situations implicit in it.
Single cue. The emotion arises in response to a specific event.	*Many strands.* The felt sense can be brought forward by any of the elements that compose it, including what led up to it, what is expected, sought for, or avoided.
Past. Although we feel it now, many emotions come from the past, recreated now as they were then.	*Present.* A felt sense is always a new total of what composes it, and since it is always changing, it is uniquely in the present.
Example. Something makes me angry. The emotion is anger, indicated by the increased heart rate and perhaps a muscular readiness to hit someone.	*Example.* Something makes me angry. The felt sense includes the anger but also all the many facets that went into making me angry, all that has happened, what people did, what I am like, why I cannot easily change that, and all that goes with the incident — all as one uniquely sensed quality.
Always the same. Anger always has the same felt quality; it always makes me want to hit, kick, and stomp.	*Always different.* Each felt sense is a unique quality. It is the sense of this unique situation or concern.
Kinds. There is a known catalogue (sometimes called the "keyboard") of emotions. In a given culture everyone knows a certain set of possible emotions.	*Kinds.* Unknown — each felt sense is just the whole it is. No catalogue of them is conceivable.
Universal character. The basic situations that cause the basic emotions are always the same. For instance, I expect something and it does not happen, I am disappointed. I love someone and someone else attracts the loved one away from me, I am jealous. I am laughed at, I feel ashamed. It is all universal in any given culture.	*Individual differentiation.* "Beyond the human patterns that are the same for everyone, I find my own meanings. I do not invent them. They emerge. They may seem to have been there all along — but actually they change and form as they "emerge." They are new, different, and exclusively mine."
Can be easily named and explained. We can explain our emotions in terms of common phrases and patterns of situations.	*Hard to find a fitting word or phrase.* New phrases (sometimes poetic sometimes clumsy) must be devised. Aspects of situa-

The person says, "Wouldn't you feel the same way if this happened to you?"

Stays the same. For example, if I become angrier and angrier, the anger stays itself; it only increases in intensity.

Intensity. Emotions are very intense. They pull our attention toward themselves. They are hard to get rid of.

tions that are not usually differentiated arise.

Changes. If I stay with a felt sense (or an emotion as part of a felt sense), it shifts. Change steps come from it. Bodily changes comes along with such steps.

Not intense. A felt sense is not usually intense. One has to concentrate one's attention or one loses hold of it (Quite intense emotions may arise from it.)

Both

Both come in a bodily way. We can say, and wish, that we felt an emotion or a felt sense, but we cannot control its actual coming.

Both form in something like the same bodily "place." A felt sense seems "deeper" because it is more clearly located down in the chest and stomach, and (in another meaning of "deeper") because it is found "under" emotions. But the felt sense may also be said to be "all around" an emotion. It is a wider, a more wholistic sense of more than I can say — all that is involved and goes with an emotion, or with any other content.

---

ognizable as either emotions, memories, desires, thoughts, observations, dreams, or feelings.

A felt sense is not the combination of these other psychological elements, although it implicitly contains them. "Implicitly contains" means that, with further steps, these other elements may arise from the felt sense. But they are not there as such, as things are in a box. Rather, the term "implicit" says that they emerge as such only if *further* living, speaking, and interaction *carry forward* the felt sense. What the steps reveal was not there, as if under a blanket. Rather, it is further made in further steps. What is still "implicit" is never the same as further steps render it.

An important difference between felt sense and emotion can be seen in the way you feel an emotion more and more intensely. No matter how strongly you feel the emotion, it does not change or reveal new aspects. If you are angry and dwell on it, if you become angrier, your body wants all the more to hit, kick, or pound, or something of that sort — and that is always so, regardless of how different each anger generating situation may be.

In contrast, the felt sense implicitly contains all that has made you angry, the sense of the whole situation, all that led up to it, and how it involves you.

The anger is not the felt sense. To let the felt sense come, you have to become quieter. The felt sense is not as intense as the anger. From the felt sense, when it comes, you can find more than you knew about what made you angry, and what you are involved in now that this (whatever it is) has happened. The felt sense is a multiplicity, sensed as one. It also has its own focal point — the worst, best, or most important, salient "upshot" — the next needed step in thought or action.

When acting according to an emotion you act on fewer factors of a situation than you would normally consider. The felt sense includes more than you have yet thought of or noticed as such, and more than you *can* think of or notice explicitly. (Of course it is not omnipotent and may still fail to include quite a lot: e.g., some of what other people sense and know.)

Currently the expression of emotional intensity is much in fashion. People have freed themselves from the older emphasis in psychology on intellectual analysis because it was not effective enough. Now many people are convinced that reaching an emotional catharsis is the best method of psychological healing. (We will discuss this below, and in Chapter 15.) A pitfall of catharsis is that one tends to regenerate the same emotions over and over. There is an erroneous theory that emotions can be "emptied out." Actually emotions are generated each time catharsis occurs. They do not just lie waiting as if they were finished things that could be gotten rid of, thrown out, or pushed out. The organism has the capacity to generate the same emotions again.

To be sure, it is valuable to feel and express long-blocked emotions. Many people repress some of their emotions and cannot feel them — they live without knowing how they feel. Turning toward emotions and letting them be felt is a great relief. That this has been recognized is a great personal and social development. But once an emotion has been completely felt and expressed, no change in the person will come from repeating that emotion.

When asked to find the felt sense that may underlie an emotion some people might object: "I don't find anything unique here. What intricacy do you want me to explore? When I am angry I know why. What makes me mad would make any sensible person mad." The answer to this is, yes, we usually do know the event that made us angry, and some of the reasons why. That is true. And perhaps it seems that this sort of event would evoke the same emotion in any person. And that is as far as an emotion goes. A felt sense goes further. For instance, "I feel sad. Why? Because my cat died. Wouldn't anyone feel sad if their cat died?" With this truth, it may seem pointless to ask, "Exactly what is it about my cat dying, that makes me feel so sad?" And yet, in going deeper you may find that guilt (about not taking enough care of the cat) is one component of the sadness. And this "not enough care" is part of a much larger mass of regrets, of things done wrong and things that might have been — a heavy weight. "Yes, if I had done something sooner, I wouldn't feel so sad about it now." This does not mean there would be no sadness, just that one part of the sadness is also this heavy weight of guilt, which was just found. Another person might feel lonely, and then also the lack of "something that held me together," and a fear of emptyness and falling apart.

Or there might be a helpless feeling left from reaching to another being, hoping to do something so that the being is not left alone, unaware of what is happening, and baffled as its body refuses to function anymore.

If we attend to the physical quality of the whole situation, we will always find intricacy. And we also find what it is that makes the situation especially hard for us, in exactly what respect it "gets us" is unique to us, and is embedded in an intricate texture. As we find and articulate what gets us, the felt sense is carried forward and the intricacy opens, sorts itself out into strands, and changes.

FELT SENSE VERSUS IMAGERY

In the rest of this chapter I contrast and compare the felt sense to a number of other kinds of experiences. I do not pretend to treat them adequately. My purpose is only to show by contrast what a felt sense is.

An image is a visual experience, a picture before you. Or, it could be an auditory image, the sound of a bell or the sound of words you hear. It is that perception of the external sight or sound.

A felt sense is a sensation in your body, like the queasy sense that lets you know that some problem, to which you seem to have an answer, is not solved.

An image can lead you to a felt sense, if you stop to sense the impact that the image has for you. But such a bodily sense is not usually immediately available. You have to remain quiet for a few seconds, and attend in your body for what comes in response to this image. That is the felt sense, not the visual experience or sound.

Chapter 14 goes into detail about working with imagery.

FELT SENSE VERSUS MORE USUAL PHYSICAL SENSATIONS

A felt sense is a bodily sensation, but it is not merely a physical sensation like a tickle or a pain. Rather, it is a physical sense *of* something, of meaning, of implicit intricacy. It is a sense of a whole situation or problem or concern, or perhaps a point one wants to convey. It is not *just* a bodily sense, but rather a bodily sense *of* . . .

Some physical sensations are similiar to a felt sense, so that one cannot always tell the difference. For example, indigestion can seem like a felt sense in the pit of your stomach. Then you might not know whether the feeling has to do with the situation or is just indigestion. You can find out if you imagine that the situation need not be coped with right now. You pretend that you will not have to deal with it till next year. Your stomach eases. Then you do the reverse; you imagine that you will deal with the situation right now. If your stomach tension returns you know it is the situation that is making you feel this way; you have a felt sense.

There are physical sensations that can be caused by a situation that gives rise to a felt sense. Tense shoulders or a crawling on the skin can certainly be due to that type of situation, *yet they are not felt senses*. The difference can be seen in that these sensations are not implicitly intricate. I mean that pain is only just what it is, for instance, a stab of pain. The intricacy of the situation is not found in the stab of pain. The small of one's back may hurt without containing in it the whole emotional situation it indicates.

Physical sensations occur around the periphery of the body, whereas the felt sense is usually (with some exceptions) in the center, the abdomen, the solar plexus, the chest, or the throat: Nevertheless the peripheral physical sensation can be quite useful. If one might ask, "What would my painful shoulders say?", something can come forward even without experiencing a felt sense. The shoulder pain exists as part of a whole mass of experience. Attending to a pain in the shoulders can also help one find that mass of experience directly. One can get a felt sense if one senses for the quality that comes *in the middle of the body*, in relation to the shoulder pain.

Also, once the felt sense has been carried forward through enough steps, there is a release. The pain in the shoulders should have also eased. Peripheral indicators provide an extra barometer to show when one has made an advance.

It is good to let a felt sense come, especially if one suspects that a psychological problem causes a physical trouble (psychosomatic symptoms). Some might say all physical illness is like that. We do not know.

FELT SENSE VERSUS ANXIETY

A felt sense is not anxiety, but it may include, or form quite close to, the anxiety. It can be the sense from which the anxiety arises and what is involved in it. Anxiety itself is very uninformative. It gets in the way of sensing even what one already knows, feels, thinks, and observes. With anxiety it is hard to let a felt sense form, but if it does it is instantly rewarding because the anxiety decreases. One may not like what one finds in a felt sense that accompanies anxiety, but each step further releases some of the anxiety. From the felt sense one may be led to find and touch the worst spot, and oddly enough that lets one breathe again.

Anxiety compares to the felt sense much as emotions do. It could be classified as an emotion. Anxiety is often said to be the royal road to self-knowledge. That view comes close to saying that the royal road goes through what we sense but fail to recognize. However, the anxiety as such does not contain the intricacy necessary to explain itself. Concentrating just on the anxiety will only make us more anxious. After a while we might become adapted or desensitized to it, but nothing new develops. Getting more and more anxious means becoming less and less able to sense what one does not yet know. Anxiety is not a felt sense.

But as with every other kind of experience, a felt sense can form from it or near it, as the holistic sense of the situation.

FELT SENSE VERSUS HYPNOSIS

Quite apart from the benefits of specific hypnotic suggestions, being in the state of hypnosis can be very helpful to a person. One is deeply rested. I am not opposed to hypnosis. I am only distinguishing it from focusing on a felt sense.

The coming of a felt sense has little resemblance to hypnosis. Only in the first moments of becoming quiet are they similar. Instead of further relaxation, with a felt sense one remains near the normal level of relaxation. Staying at that level is quite the opposite of hypnosis. At the felt sense level hypnotic suggestions are not effective. The body does not obey them; instead it talks back — and for focusing on the felt sense that is just what we want!

For example, suppose you say, "I feel fine about this problem." Under hypnosis such a statement works as a suggestion, and it will be obeyed. You will feel fine. In contrast, during focusing if you say, "I feel fine about this problem," saying it may actually help a felt sense to come. The body talks back by producing the felt sense — something does not feel fine about the situation.

In hypnosis a felt sense will not usually come because the body is silenced. That is why hypnosis works: The bodily knowing which forms a felt sense is knocked out. The body seems melted, gone, and ready to produce whatever bodily sensations are suggested.

What is called "spacing out" differs from a felt sense for the same reason. Rather than letting the bodily sense of one's concrete living come in one's body, so that it can talk back and correct what we think, in spacing out one floats away from the body.

Of course someone might use the term "self-hypnosis" to describe doing something like focusing on a felt sense. I am not concerned with fighting about words. The concrete differences are what matter. Even a little bit more relaxation than the right amount makes the coming of a felt sense impossible. If everything slows, becomes still, and thickens inwardly, so that it becomes difficult to pursue one concern rather than another, one has relaxed too much to be able to focus on the felt sense. Once one relaxes that deeply, deliberate moves with one's attention are hard, even painful, and focusing is not possible. (See my article on this, Gendlin, 1996b.)

FELT SENSE VERSUS MEDITATION

If the word "meditation" is used very broadly, then the process steps I am examining can be said to be a kind of meditation. There are of course many kinds of meditation; why might this not just be called one more kind?

In one widespread type of meditation, meditators relax too deeply for a felt sense to come. After a lot of practice their attention moves down to that deeply relaxed level as soon as they turn inward. They have a descending elevator that bypasses the level where a felt sense can form. I want to tell people who practice this kind of meditation that a felt sense forms halfway down. The elevator can stop halfway down.

One needs the felt sense and its steps for one's personal development. At times one needs it even for meditation itself. In meditation when the atmosphere is gray or in some way unfree, it is better to come up, let the sparkles subside, move the shoulders a little, and come to a normal level. Then go halfway down and get the felt sense of whatever is off kilter. After a few steps, when that felt sense releases, one can return to meditation and find it much better than before.

I want to communicate this precisely; focusing involves deliberately attending down where activity arises and staying with something. One should keep one's attention on the unclear discomfort, on the felt sense that comes in response to one's deliberate seeking. One seeks the whole sense of what is wrong at the moment (or, in a given concern). This is clearly different from one of the common meditative states in which one's inward activity is altogether quiet, and one senses a deep, thick "no-thing." (See McGuire, 1984, "Making a Space"; Gendlin, 1984b.)

FELT SENSE VERSUS JUNG'S FOUR FUNCTIONS

Jung distinguished four kinds of "functions" (as he called them): sensation, feeling, intuition, and thought. A felt sense is none of these. But Jung also thought there was a fifth, the "transcendent function" in the center of the four. To a point his description of this fifth function corresponds to my definition of a felt sense. Whether or not Jung's transcendent function is a felt sense we can see that a felt sense is not one of the four functions. Or, we could say that a felt sense is a special kind of each of the four. It is sensed bodily like sensations. It is also felt as we feel feelings and has an evaluative character. Like intuition a felt sense brings us information beyond what we currently possess. And certainly a felt sense implicitly contains something like cognition and it also includes all that we have thought. But it would be a special case of each of the four.

What Jung says about the transcendent function is instructive: He tells us to give our word-making power over to "the affect," to let it speak. He also instructs us to let it make images. He says that the sort of "affect" that can do this is not the feeling function.

But Jung seems to miss the directional character of a felt sense — its way of leading to a next step and more steps after that. He thinks you must "accumulate" the "material" that arises from letting the effect speak, and then interpret it (using his concepts). The felt sense, on the other hand, provides its own interpretation by pointing you in the direction it wants to go — toward the next step.

FELT SENSE VERSUS CATHARSIS

With cathartic methods (such as primal scream therapy and other "discharge" therapies) people reexperience past events and the emotions they invoke. As I said before, if these emotions were blocked and never fully expressed, then their reappearance is new and helpful. But clients in cathartic therapy aquire the habit of instantly shifting to the past from any present feeling. Cathartic therapists do also emphasize experiencing "in the present," but they mean present bodily feelings about the past. They wish their patients to repeat the past concretely in the present. As soon as they feel something in the present they let the memory of a past experience come and take its place. Usually the past event is one they have already screamed about and discharged many times before. This method can make clients miss the sense of their present life, as if nothing in their present experience needs attention.

The cathartic method is not meant to have this result. Those who advocate its use are often misled into assuming that the past must be "worked through" whenever it is still found in present experience. But it is the nature of experience to include the past implicitly in the very makeup of every present. Other therapists make the opposite error. They wish their clients to concern themselves not with the past, but only with the present.

In contrast, a felt sense has a different kind of present. The current talk about the "here and now" neglects how time relates to experience. Experience is not divided into pieces that are *either* past *or* present *or* future in a linear sequence. Each moment is a new constellation in which the past functions implicitly — and hopes for the future, along with hopes for the future from the past, are recontextualized. That is also true of every kind of past experience. The past is newly remade in every ordinary present experience, and also in every felt sense. The past is implicit, but not as itself, in unchanged pieces such as memories. When memories are explicitly experienced the present is not. For example, we cannot attend to the present while we remember the past or relive past events. But usually, when the past is not itself present, it is implicit in a present experience. The present is as it is partly because of the past — and it would be different if the past had been different. In that way the past is always implicit, and cannot be separated from the present.

An imagined future is also an essential constituent of any present experience. I do not mean events that will happen later; I mean events that we hope will happen or we expect to happen. This is a future that is here now. The implied future we imagine now is always part of the meaning of the present. (See Gendlin, 1996a.)

FELT SENSE VERSUS ALTERED STATE

Other therapeutic techniques bypass the person's present life by encouraging the person to enter "altered states," unconnected to how one is living one's life. Such experiences are gigantic, yet they may bring little change beyond some initial widening of perspective. The experiences can be large, yet the person can remain small, easily disorganized and often swamped. However valuable the experiences may be, they do not absolve or relieve us of the need to develop ourselves as persons. And that happens in small steps.

A felt sense comes at the border zone between ordinary and altered states. Some relaxation is involved in letting it come and sensing it again and again, letting something come from it. But once the sense has come one is instantly back in the ordinary, reacting to what came, asking further what it is, or what is in it. On the old map of conscious, unconscious, and border zone, a felt sense is on the border. One might say it is the border zone itself. Through it one can sense how the whole of the organism is, just now. In comparison to the awareness in altered states it is very close to an ordinary kind of awareness, although at the edge of an altered state.

In the next chapter I describe how one finds the border zone.

CHAPTER 7

Focusing

How is the border zone concretely found? Where does one enter it? What if no edge, nothing like a border zone seems to be there?

Sometimes unconscious material emerges spontaneously, for example, when odd images or long repressed memories come. They must have crossed the border zone, but now that they are here they may seem to be like anything else, so they do not reveal this zone nor what more lies behind it. Contents like this may be of little help because their coming may bring no change in the person's present experiencing. With these or any other contents we would want to ask, "Where are the 'edges'? Where is that unclear, implicitly intricate mass of experience from which the steps of a process of experiential change can come?" If it is not already evident, how can an individual find this direct bodily sense, the edge, this "entry point" into the experiential process we have been describing?

Because every method of psychotherapy intends to work at the edge, every method will be more effective if we know how to engender its presence.

In a long series of research studies it was found that some clients in therapy do work at such an edge, and they are the ones who have successful outcomes (Gendlin, 1968c, 1986c; Hendricks, 1986). The findings have been widely taken to mean that psychotherapy is exclusively suited to those people and will always succeed if they are the only clients we select. But the findings raise a much more interesting question: How can we enable others (who are much more numerous) to do what they do not know how to do of their own accord, namely, to focus their attention in this odd way, on what is at first not even there, and then is unclear when it does come?

We can now teach people what we call "focusing": how to let a felt sense come, and how to work from it. Focusing has been taught to large numbers of people in and outside of therapy. Its applications far exceed psychotherapy.[1]

As we saw, a bit of focusing might take just a minute or two. The whole process of focusing can take 5 or 10 minutes. Sometimes it is necessary to stop focusing when one is quite stuck and try again a few hours later. Walk about, make some tea, and wait for the next bit. Perhaps, in midst of doing something else, a next bit will suddenly come.

Focusing can be engendered in therapy without teaching it explicitly. The therapist can provide small bits of instruction periodically that spread the teaching of focusing out over some months. But to understand focusing, you will have to learn it. It is a special, teachable skill and it is best to see how the focusing process can be taught as a whole.

Focusing seems simple. Unfortunately learning it is not. Certain pitfalls are frequently encountered. Because the "territory" of concrete experience is so finely patterned and organized, nothing said in general is sufficient. We have developed in recent years a whole panoply of helpful specific techniques, but because there is no end to the specificity of experience, there will always be room for more. Despite all the instructions and notices of possible pitfalls, learning to focus will usually require some 3 to 8 hours of teaching in person. Most people will encouter some difficulty and confusion that need individual attention. We now have teachers of focusing in most cities in the United States and in many other countries.

Our teaching consists of six steps, with many details grouped under each. The divisions are of course artificial. No living human process breaks down into six steps. The six steps are useful only for teaching. In a way, because focusing enables one to discover one's own inward source, there is a considerable contradiction in "teaching" it at all. Because of this, teaching focusing requires a dual perception from everyone. I call it "split-level instructions." We say to people: "Try the steps exactly as outlined — but the moment they do not feel right, stop, back up a little, and see what does not feel right. Either you discover focusing because our instructions work, or you discover it by sensing why our instructions do not work. Do not do any violence inwardly even if our instructions seem to tell you to do so."

Why are split-level instructions not more widely known? The teaching of many processes requires use of them. What we teach may be invaluable — but *only* if each individual will use it to come into more contact with what actual experience shows itself to be, directly. Ultimately this must be the case with everything that is taught.

With focusing, at least, people rapidly find that following instructions can differ from pursuing one's own inward experience. Beginners often report: "Oh . . . I was trying to do it 'right.' That got in the way." This is accompanied by a laugh which indicates that the person has already found that focusing originates inwardly and is essentially different from something imposed on us from the outside.

But since focusing is new to most people, it does require instructions. And it requires putting aside one's preconceptions of what focusing is, and also what one is accustomed to doing inwardly to help oneself.

So please hold in abeyance how you usually deal with feelings and problems and keep them in reserve in case you absolutely need them. I ask you to go beyond reading the descriptions and let actual experiences come in accord with them, as I shift to illustrating how to engender focusing.

If something I seem to ask you to do *feels* hurtful or denies what is *directly* there for you, or if it becomes scary or if you have to force something — then please stop. Back up just a little, and try to sense exactly what feels wrong.

CAN YOU SENSE FROM INSIDE YOUR BODY?

Today people are evenly divided as to whether it is easy or very hard to attend within their bodies. Some can do it in an instant; others require some practice. Both groups can learn focusing, but the latter group must first learn to sense the body from inside. In case you happen to be in the latter group I ask you to follow these preliminary instructions.

- Can you sense the inside of your stomach and chest? What do you sense there? Take a minute or two . . .
- Is it something like a sense of wooly comfort, is it fluttery, tense, or how? It need not have a verbal description, so long as you can say, yes, that quality is there. Take a minute or two . . .
- Did your attention succeed in getting in there?

Many people are helped by beginning at the bottom. Try this:

- Put your attention into your right toe inside your shoe. Can you do it? If not, move the toe, then it is easy to sense inside it. Then hold it still. Now you are sensing inside your toe. Do the same with the knee and then the chair pressing on you from below. Then come into your stomach and chest. What quality of body feeling do you find in your stomach?

If sensing inside the body has become easy, we can begin focusing:

Clearing a Space

Begin by taking a minute to just rest and be friendly with yourself inside. See what stands between you and feeling fine. Each one of us carries several problems at a time and it is usually a mix of these. It helps to sort them out in the following way:

- Put your attention in your stomach or chest, and (knowing it probably is not so) say something like, "My life is going just fine these days. I feel totally fine about it." Then attend to the middle of your body and see what comes there.
- Your mind may quickly answer this question before you manage to put your attention in your body. If that just happened, begin again.
- Did a not-so-good overall body feeling come, as if to say, "No, I'm not totally fine, rather, something like *this* . . . "?
- Whatever actually comes, say, "Hello, yes, that's there," and get ready to sort it out. Usually the not-so-good feeling has to do with more than one thing. Ask, "What is one thing, one part of my life, that is in this mix?" If you can find one part of your life that the overall sense is about, promise it that we will come back and work on it later. Right now, for a little while you want it to wait — a little distance away — so you can take an inventory of the rest of what is here.
- You may want to decide just how far away it should wait; right in front of you on the floor, perhaps quite far away in another state, or just below the horizon. What is the right distance so that you do not lose hold of it, so that it will not go underground, so that you can stay related to the problem, and yet not sunk in it?
- Now attend again in your body. Except for that one problem, do you feel okay about how life is going?
- You should find that the overall sense that comes now is somewhat relieved compared to the way it was before. If it is not different, then ask more forcefully, "What would come in my body, if that problem (somehow, magically) came to be all OK?" Then wait and see what actually comes in your body.
- Then see again, except for this thing, can you say you feel all fine about how life is going? Wait. A lighter sense should come, leading to more things to place at the right distance.
- Now pick *one* of these concerns you found. It can be any one of them. If you are new to the focusing process, pick a relatively small one.

A Felt Sense

Whatever you may know about the concern you have chosen, since it is a problem it also has an unresolved edge, a *felt sense* of unease, unresolvedness, or implicit richness that is more than you can fully comprehend. To find this unclear edge do the following:

- Attend in your stomach and chest and see how the whole thing makes you feel, *there*, what bodily quality it has there.
- Just say, "I feel *all* comfortable about this," putting your attention in your body, and wait. See what comes if you say that.

- The fuzzy, murky, unsatisfyingly vague sense that comes might seem like nothing at all. Can such a fuss be made here in this book about this mere nothing? Yes, if it is there, that is the felt sense. It does not seem very promising — I agree.
- Perhaps now you have lost hold of that felt edge. Let your attention return to the middle of your body. Once the feeling comes again, be willing to be with that unclear sense for a minute (a minute is a long time). Touch it again and again.

This step is the hardest part. You need to sense something quite concrete and more meaningful than you can as yet say or define. If nothing has come as yet, try the following.

- Imagine standing in front of a big mural. You have to step back to see it all. This mural will be an image of the whole thing. Wait for that picture. What picture comes? Now sense how that image makes your body feel.
- If the image has not given you a concrete felt sense try to say one true thing about the problem. Then say that over and over, and see what comes in your body, in response.

Getting a Handle on It

Try to find one word, a phrase, or an image to capture exactly *the quality* of that felt sense.

Some quality words are "sticky," "stuck," "heavy," "antsy," "helpless," "burdened," "worried," or "jumpy." Or you might find a phrase that exactly fits, such as "stuck in glue," "lost on the prairie," or, as in the example, "it is not jittery . . . 'pulls back' is what it is." Find the word, a phrase, or image that fits exactly.

Resonating the Handle

If the word, phrase, or image really fits, there should be a little relief to be had, just from how well it fits. That little relief can come several times. Ask your body "Does _____ really fit? Is it _____? Is it like that?" There should be a little relief, a bodily signal, that says, "yes (*breathes*) that's it all right."

Asking

Now, just as if you did not know anything about it, ask in your body, ask the felt sense itself, what it is. Try these ways of asking one at a time:

- If one has some effect on the felt sense, stay with that effect. Leave the other questions for another time. (Before you try this question let us make sure first that the felt sense is there again. Remembering it is not enough.

If it is not there you cannot possibly ask it directly. Can you still sense it? Use the handle word or image to get it back. Is it there again?)

- Ask it this question, "What about this whole thing is so _____?" (Put the handle word, phrase, or image in the blank.)
- Or, "What's really *in* this _____?"
- Or, "What's the worst, the most _____ about this whole thing?"
- Or, "What would it need to feel OK?"

As long as nothing moves, give each of these questions a minute and then go on to try the next. Make sure each time that you first have found the felt sense again.

Most people find quick answers coming in from what is already known or can be surmised. Let all thoughts just go by if the felt sense does not stir in response to it. Asking the felt sense takes more time. Before there is any effect, there might need to be a whole minute of tapping the unclear felt sense, touching it, perhaps backing off, and then touching it again.

Asking the felt sense is somewhat similar to trying to recall something you have forgotten, when there remains only a felt residue of what it is. Something is still there, but it does not open easily. This is not a question of remembering, but rather of letting the felt sense itself *respond* to your question. It will respond by first stirring a little inside. Is there *any* effect when you ask the question?

This takes practice.

If you can spend a little bit of time with this directly felt sense while not yet knowing what it is, you are focusing. At a certain point it will open and give you a step. It does that when it will; you do not control that.

Receiving

Whatever comes with a little stirring in the felt sense, please welcome it. It is not the final answer, only a first step. You do not need to believe it, just take it as a first thing your body wants to say. Be pleased that it speaks. Let it be a step — knowing that it is not an ultimate answer.

Try not to let your critical capacity knock out that first little step. To be sure, you will not know for a while if it is real, if it is right, if it is realistic — a crowd of questions often springs to mind just after a little step comes. Push these questions aside; they have to wait. You cannot answer them now. Only after more steps will you be sure that this was really a step. You are not assuming that the step is right; you are only listening to it.

If the step indicates a direction that feels life enhancing, permit the step to remain in your mind even though it is unrealistic at the moment. It may be only a direction, a first hint of something that will become much different and realistic later. Letting your body live in that direction can be very helpful even if this first statement or image is not realistic.

Look back and see if you have "edited" what first came, if you have added, changed, or cut it in any way that spoiled its bodily effect. Sometimes, if you restore it to be as it first came, you can get the good new bodily energy again.

To "receive" in our sense means to let the step be, give it a space to be in, not to reject it, however odd or wrong it may seem in itself. It comes with a little bit of bodily felt release, a breath, a bodily sense that something is right about it, and that is what you want.

CONCLUSION

These steps constitute one round of focusing. Any serious problem requires many such rounds. A small problem might have been completely released by one round.

If focusing is new to a person it is unlikely that all the steps would have happened just on these first instructions. Nearly everyone runs into certain difficulties.

These focusing instructions can be printed in two short pages. But all the variants, additional instructions, and details could fill several books. *Focusing* (Gendlin, 1981) has a special chapter for each of the most typical difficulties.

In the next chapter I offer a number of transcripts of people being taught focusing. These are examples for us to examine.

NOTE

1. Focusing has been described in a learnable way in a separate book (Gendlin, 1981). It is there presented in extremely simple language for every type of reader, and I say more there than I can here. In this book I want to present its use in psychotherapy. I also want to present fine points of how to teach it, and some theoretical reflections.

CHAPTER 8

Excerpts from Teaching Focusing

THE EXCERPTS IN this chapter show focusing being taught specifically, not in the context of standard therapy. In the next chapter all excerpts are from standard therapy. Those involve much more than focusing (because therapy is more than just focusing). But here it is focusing that is being taught.

The first group of examples come from therapists twice removed from myself. They were trained in focusing and listening by Dr. Mary Hendricks at the Illinois School of Professional Psychology. A few are experienced therapists who returned for additional training; most have little experience. These therapists are all new to focusing, so these excerpts do not show the more sophisticated ways of teaching it. Paradoxically, this makes some of what happens in focusing all the more visible.

These therapists are new also to reflective listening. The people whom they worked with had not been instructed in focusing before these sessions.

EXCERPT 1

Transcript

T1: OK. If you could go inside your body for a moment again. Stay there for a moment and ask your body, "Is it rage, is that it? Is that the right word for it? Is that, is that really it?" And again ask your body to see if that really captures for you what this is, this thing that you call "rage." Is that really it? And let your body tell you.

My Comments

T1: The therapist is asking for bodily attention. This is not just to check the word "rage," but also to let the next step come from the body.

C2: It's interesting. I can still see, I can see kind of a division, where when I ask my body, or it's kind of like I ask this other part of my body, "Is this it?" All I get is visualizations. [T: Um hmm] You know I get pictures.

T2: Pictures of rage.

C3: Yeah.

T3: So it is rage, does that feel like that's it?

C4: Yeah. It's rage but it's not just the word, it's the visualization and the word. [T: Um hmm] And the visualization is stronger than the word, if you know what I mean. It's not just simply the word.

T4: You get a picture —

C5: Yeah. And the word is just kind of a word to me and the picture is really what's real.

T5: The picture is more real than the actual word "rage." [C: Um hmm] Um hmm, uh huh. And what kind of picture do you get here?

C6: Just uh, uh, kind of a whirling, kicking, you know, wild, wild man. [T: Um hmm] That, uh, just kind of mindless wild man. Just going berserk. Just going nuts.

T6: Totally out of control.

C7: Oh God, yes. [T: Um hmm] There is nothing, no real frame of reference around me, it's just that thing — just out of control, just gone, you know. [T: Yeah] Moving as fast as possible, just kicking and hitting and —

T7: Very, very erratic. Very powerful.

C8: Yeah. Moving so fast it's hard to see. You just see kind of a blur of motion.

C2: The client says all he gets is visual imagery.

T3: The therapist seems stuck on the word "rage" and pays too little attention to the image. Like words, images can lead to the bodily sense *they* produce.

C4: The client points again to the image as being more than the word, and more important here.

T5: The therapist grasps that the image needs to be responded to and worked with.

T6: The therapist tries to respond to the quality of the image.

T7: This misses the quality of anger in the image. A phrase like "hitting and lashing out in all directions" might have been better.

[T: OK] Tremendous noise. [T: Um hmm, um hmm]

T8: Can you go inside now and just sense for a minute and just feel that feeling, for a moment. *(pause — 30 seconds)* And what is the worst of this thing, that you call rage. What is the worst of this image, this uncontrollable lashing-out monster. What is the worst of all of that for you? Then wait for your body to stir to give you the answer.

(pause — 15 seconds)

T8: To ask what "the worst of this" is, is a question of the whole. To answer it one attends to the whole of *this*. One senses it as a whole, so as to sense what about it is so bad. One waits for the body "to stir" as its answer, rather than trying to decide anything.

The 15-second silence was enough to let the client sense what he describes at C9 and at C11.

C9: Really the worst is control. Um, I could only let myself experience parts of it. It was just like it seemed, kind of let it bounce out, and it would have to bounce back. Because if I really allowed myself to experience it, I would really start doing it. [T: Um hmm, um hmm]

T9: There is a fear if you really got into it —

C10: To me, it's not a fear. It's a fact.

T10: Um hmm. It's very real.

C11: If I, if I let myself really do it, I would just get up and like throw the chair through the window and just start turning shit over and throwing things around and breaking things and just, I would just kind of go berserk. The rage would just, you know, it would just be there.

T11: Just, pull all the stops.

C12: Yeah.

T12: Um hmm. Yeah. And that's pretty frightening.

T12: This response is an invitation for the client to return to the inward body sensing, to check, as indeed he is doing, throughout this example.

C13: Yeah. Well, *when I get in touch with it, it's not frightening*, it's a very powerful feeling. You know *when I'm in touch for now, it's like very powerful and very strong.*

C13: It feels "powerful," not frightening.

T13: So frightening is not the word for it.

C14: Not at this moment. It's uh . . . I . . . I, *in fact, I really like that feeling. I like that feeling of power.*

T14: There's some aspect to it that is attractive for you.

C15: Oh God, that's a real omnipotent thing. You know, it's like *hey, nobody can fuck and hurt me.* [T: Um hmm] You know if I let that happen, there wouldn't be anything that could hurt me. [T: Um hmm]

T13: The therapist understands only here that "frightening" is wrong.

Discussion of Excerpt 1

This brief excerpt contains just one small step, of course, not a complete working through of the anger. But it is important for us to see exactly the kind of step it is. There is a mutation of content, *from* an out of control berserkness *to* a sense of an owned power ("hey, nobody can fuck and hurt me").

Before we discuss how that change happened, let me make sure that we realize its importance. This step of change is a growth or development of the person. He is living in a new way as the owner of power — powerful, rather than swept up in uncontrolled affect, or with suppressed energy as before.

What we have said earlier in general is demonstrated here in this short example: We cannot be satisfied with the simple emergence of unchanged experience. We want more than just the anger to come out — as it was and had long been. We want to understand how, along with the emergence of an experience, the person can develop and grow, and how what emerges can change as it emerges.

In this excerpt there is some emergence of anger. At first the client says, "All I get is visualizations," but in the 15 seconds of bodily attending that comes later he clearly senses his anger directly and senses what it would make him do.

From the viewpoint of mere emergence there is not very much here. Only a minor direct emergence happens. But from the viewpoint of therapy, an important step has happened. The client has become stronger; he has had a new experience of sensing himself as powerful, and the anger that would have made him berserk, the actual content, has changed into owned power.

From our point of view it is very desirable that the individual find a step like this coming.

The client is unlikely to find himself being repeatedly swept up by anger considering that this one little process step has already changed it into owned power. In steps such as this, each bit that emerges changes, and not only does the content change, the client develops right along with it.

Now how was this attained?

It is not up to the therapist to decide that the anger should or should not emerge. Whatever comes is welcomed, nothing pushed away, but the anger is not elicited further as mere anger. Instead, what the therapist asks for is the whole body response. The therapist asks the client to pay direct attention to the bodily sensed whole, in the spirit of "checking" the step with this bodily whole.

At first the client has only words and images, no bodily felt sense. One way the therapist helps the coming of a whole felt sense is to seize upon the main word or phrase, attempting to find a single handle for the implicit whole. Determining that the expression (it could be verbal or an image) does or does not capture the whole requires the client to check inwardly. If indeed the word describes the whole, it is likely that such checking will let a felt sense come.

Another way to invite a felt sense forward is for the therapist to instruct the client, saying, "If you ask your body . . ." or "Then wait for your body to stir to give you an answer. . . ."

For the client in this excerpt the coming of a bodily sense "of the whole thing" is something quite new. It is not a long repressed feeling only now emerging. It is created, in the present, by the adult's body. The coming of a bodily sense of the whole *is* therefore a forward movement, a new way of living, freshly formed content; it is not from the past.

A felt sense also lets one be a stronger "self." Because the felt sense is a self-enclosed whole, I who have it am freed in a certain way. To have this whole makes the person bigger than usual. In contrast, an emotion overtakes and sweeps the person along. When swept along by an emotion, there is a temporary diminution of self. So closely identified with the affect the person is temporarily less than usual. Of course emotions are also vital, especially if they are new. But it is also vital that the sweeping emotion, be accompanied by inward checking which is something the person does actively. In response to checking, a fresh new whole comes. The development of the "self" in relation to this new whole requires more than merely, for example, saying, "How do *I* feel about this anger that I just acted out?" The whole organism needs to live further, in a holistic way that includes the emergent content. Otherwise there will only be the old "I" and the old anger, with its out-of-control quality.

We do not want to know (in this example) how the client feels about being out of control. We can imagine that. What we want is a concrete bodily bit of holistic living, a felt sense in which the content of the anger will mutate, and the self will grow and develop.

This kind of change, of which we have seen a small step here, was brought about by letting the bodily sense of the whole come, by doing so again and again via "checking" with it at each juncture, and by waiting for it to stir and respond.

C1: I'm not sure. What do you mean, "How does that feel for me now." It feels frustrating!

C1: The therapist had asked "How does that feel for you" and the client does not know what to do with that question. The client has a "dead-end" feeling. It is frustrating; that is all.

T1: OK . . . *does that really feel like what it is now,* is that pretty much all?

C2: Um hmm, . . . I think, also angry.

C2: By "checking" the word, the client senses something more.

T2: OK, check with that feeling and see if that's the crux of it for you now. Really try and let your body sense the whole, all about that, frustration, that anger, does that seem to cover it?

T2: Notice: "let your body sense the whole . . ."

C3: Yeah, I, I, the image, I get an image (*pause*). [T: um hmm] . . . And the image is like a cartoon, like an animation, um, of a woman . . . with ah, I don't know how to describe it, like almost pulling her hair out and tears kinda squirting out all over the place (*laughs*).

C3: An image has come. The quality of the image is sensed in a bodily way. There are no words for it. This is quite characteristic; the individual has to invent metaphoric language: notice the word "like" in "I don't know how to describe it, like almost. . . ." This indicates a direct sensing that is not verbal and can only be a sensed quality. Notice the laugh when she succeeds in finding an expression that fits. The laugh is a bit of bodily release which comes when what one says fits.

T3: You have an image, then, of a woman who's pulling her hair out, and tears are just coming out all over the place.

C4: Um hmm, do you know what I mean, like, you can just see the anguish in her face?

C4: She continues to try to describe the quality, which means that she is sensing that quality the image gives her.

T4: Um hmm, . . . now can you take that image . . . of the woman who has anguish in her face, *and check that with that body feeling you have,* and see if that image really can match that feeling?

T4: The therapist returns her to the body sense.

C5: Yeah, it does (*laughs*), really well (*laughter*).

C5: This causes more laughter, as the image indeed does "check out." It resonates, touches, moves that whole body sense of the "frustration." There is a bodily release.

T5: OK, good . . . that matches what feels right for you. . . . And how's that make you feel?

C6: Well I'm laughing; that's how it makes me feel good (*laughter*). It's funny to look at it, you know cause it's looking at it differently . . .

C6: She says it feels "good" even though at C4 she had said, " . . . you can just see the anguish." She comments on how different this is from how she had been seeing the problem previously.

(*Silence — 10 seconds*)

Discussion of Excerpt 2

This excerpt begins with a dead end feeling. "Frustrated" means just that, frustrated. The client does not even grasp the therapist's question. She says, "I'm not sure. What do you mean, 'How does that feel for me now?'" After all she just told him how it feels, namely frustrating. It is as if she had said, "Don't you know what 'frustrated' means?" She has no access to any edges, to anything that is experienced as unclear, as something that could lead to more. There is no entry into something further. So she is puzzled by the therapist's question. She could say more about why, but as to what she feels, "frustrated" is just frustrated. How, from that, does she get to a process step in six responses?

The therapist gets her to "check" that word, and so makes a distinction between the word and something she can check it against. In this way the direct datum she has named becomes independent of the word.

By using pointers, the therapist also helps her to find the direct bodily access. He talks about "what *it* is now" and also uses the word "all," which leads her to sense it as a whole. The therapist works for the bodily whole ("Really try and let your body sense the whole, all about that . . .").

The image comes from *that* with a new sense. The image taken as such is of sorrow, anguish, and agitation. But her sense of the image brings a physical change in her. She laughs, and struggles to make up examples to express the sense that the image gives her.

The change came with the image, but the change is not the image itself. It is in her body. The image and the body change is a new step in how she is. It is and includes the past, but in a new and changed way, as a new and different bit of holistic living.

This image came from bodily sensing the implicit whole, in the checking of "frustrated." The image is not merely a picture from unchanged content. Rather, along with the coming of the image there is a physically felt change. It is not as if something first comes unchanged, to which the individual then reacts. Rather, the image comes as part of a new bit of bodily being. It is not only emergence but already a step of change.

In many cases (though not here) when an image comes, it is necessary to ask the person to attend directly to the body sense that image brings. So often people attend only to the image, without attending to its bodily effect, thereby preventing a changed way of somatic being from coming. One needs to let the implicit sense come, which the image can facilitate.

EXCERPT 3

C1: The problem is seeing _____ tonight, and the fact that I have some guilt feelings about not writing, but I realize part of that is . . . um, that my friendship with her is not really what I thought it was. That I have some ambivalence toward her and that I don't trust her.

T1: OK. That's a whole lot. *Just let that be there, the whole thing.* OK. That problem about seeing her, that you're going to encounter her, that your relationship isn't what you thought it was, and it is some other things, right? And just leave it there, and you stay where you are, and try to get what that is. Don't go through a list of all the things it is, but just, *let it be there and let it come to you, what it feels like. Get a sense of the whole thing.*

C2: (*Smacks lips*) I feel anxious about it.

T2: OK. Is that the whole feeling? Is that what comes from the feeling when you feel that problem?

C3: Also anger. 'Cause I don't know how truthful I can be with her.

T3: So there's some question about your honesty in this, your truthfulness in this.

C4: Um hmm.

T4: Can you get, without going through a list of stuff, or forcing any words on it, just let yourself sit with that whole feeling, the whole thing — your part in it, her part in it, the situation, and from the outside,

T4: The emphasis on getting the sense of the whole is phrased here as "from the outside." I do not like that phrasing very much but they seem to understand each other, as the last response (C38) shows.

83

just look at the whole thing and see what you see there. You may get, you may get something. Let what you get come straight from the feeling.

C5: You're wanting me to describe a feeling, or an image, tell you what I see.

T5: Yeah, if you see something, or if you get a phrase that's close to it.

C6: Strain.

C6: From anxious (C2) and anger (C3) it has mutated to "strain" here. Strain always has a holistic quality, and indicates that the individual has attended in the bodily way one feels such qualities.

T6: Strain.

C7: Yeah.

T7: OK, you're nodding.

T7: There is often an involuntary nodding to oneself, when one senses more deeply and recognizes what one senses. The therapist is drawing the client's attention to her own *body* responsiveness, to getting the handle-word: strain.

C8: Uh huh.

T8: Does that seem like that's it?

C9: That's it.

T9: Can you check the word "strained" against that original feeling you had?

C10: The original feeling of being anxious with her?

T10: Yeah, yeah. Does it exactly fit?

C11: Hmm, the "strain" feels more real, Carla.

T11: Uh huh.

C12: A strain, a guardedness.

T12: Is the image of you being guarded?

T12: This seems confused here. The therapist seems to think the strain is an image, instead of a body sense.

C13: Uh huh. Me being guarded and her being probing. Mmm.

T13: Can you go even deeper into that — what the feeling is of you being guarded and her being probing? Is there something underneath that?

C14: The trust issue. And that bothers me. There's things I'd like to tell her, and I don't think I can 'cause I don't trust her.

T14: So, is that another piece of the image?

C15: Sure. That I'll be drinking a glass of wine, and I'll be wanting to tell her things and I feel guarded about what I can say. (*Silence*) It's hard for me to be assertive with her. That's it. It's hard for me to tell her, "I just can't talk about that person with you, or I don't want to give you the goods on so and so."

T15: So all this is hard for you, the whole, the whole scene.

T15: This therapist response is too round and general. It misses the step she got. It should have been something like: "It's hard to be assertive and stand your ground with her."

C16: Uh huh.

T16: OK. Without going through, you know, too much stuff from your head about what it means, can you just sit there with that image, that picture, and see if anything else comes out of it, get a sense of the whole thing, everything that's in it.

C17: It's change. Hmm.

T17: It's change in it.

C18: Yeah, I can describe that. You want me to do that?

T18: Well, maybe just, what's the change? Yeah. What is all that change?

C19: Our relationship. That I'm not, the one that she helped promote to her old position. Hmm.

T19: That's what the change is.

C20: Uh huh. And I don't owe her anything more because of that. It's a feeling of obligation, or something.

C20: Here is another mutation in content. "Obligation *or something* . . . " refers to something directly sensed, and not fully clear yet.

T20: That's closer to it.

C21: Yeah, yeah.

T21: That's what's under the strain?

C22: Yeah. Right. That I owe her something.

T22: That feeling that you owe her something.

C23: Uh huh.

T23: Can you still look at that from the outside, or are you surrounded by that feeling that you owe her something, or . . .

C24: No. I, I've still got it. I'm still looking at it.

T24: Yeah. OK. (*30-second silence*) Can you go beneath that even? That feeling that you owe her something — can you look at that and see what's in that?

C25: Uh huh. I don't know how I got here, but somehow there's a connection. That we're different. Hmm, very different, and I think it's been hard for me to show that with her.

T25: Hmm. So, getting back to the feeling that you owe her something, does that still feel right? Can you check that against your original feeling, when we started? The anxiety. Was there more to it is what I'm saying.

C26: A combination of those two things, of, mmm, hmm. OK. The feeling of owing her something is the feeling that I should carry on the way she did with me, when she was in this position.

T26: I think that's a thought. That's something that you're telling yourself. Now

T20: The therapist helps the client stay with what is as yet unclear, as well as responding to the fact that "obligation" is in the right direction.

T21: The therapist checks if this changed content, "obligation," is actually a step from the previously identified element, "strain," or whether it is simply something different. It is important to see, in this excerpt, that the steps are mutations *of this content*, and not just different things, one after another.

T24: The therapist shows by using the words "beneath that even . . . " that they have already gone several steps, and might not get more steps as quickly as this.

C25: The person is surprised, as happens so often in such content mutation.

T26: We have to assume that the therapist noted a visible change in the manner try and just look at that feeling that you owe her something. You said it was a combination, so it's more than just the feeling you owe her something. There's some other part of it. Can you see what that is?

C27: I keep coming back to the fact that, hmm, I can't stay with that feeling. It's hard.

T27: Maybe it's not right. Maybe it doesn't fit exactly.

C28: God. Boy! It feels like she wants something from me that I don't want to give her.

T28: OK. And what is that? Rather than press on to "what is that" just, just stay with that, OK? She wants something from you that you don't feel you can give her. Just stay with that feeling. Let something come out of that.

C29: I feel real stuck here. Mmm.

T29: OK. Then stay with the stuck. You know. What's stuck?

C30: What she wants.

T30: What she wants.

C31: Uh huh. I think (*chuckles*). She wants affirmation and I can't give her that very easily. It's hard for me to disagree with her.

T31: What's that like, then? First of all, does that check out against that original feeling too?

C32: Uh huh. Uh huh.

T32: That you can't disagree with her. That's part of that original feeling.

C33: That's a lot of it. I'm afraid of something. Yeah. That she will be very rejecting if I disagree with her and don't give her support.

T33: That's what's in the fear?

C34: Yeah. That I will have to say that I'm different from her. (*Laughs*)

T34: So the two parts of that are that you'll have to say you're different and that she'll reject you.

in which this was said. One can often recognize the difference quite distinctly, between someone just thinking about the problem versus speaking from a felt sense of it.

C28: The surprise ("God. Boy!") shows that this has come directly. It is another content mutation.

T28: Here the therapist becomes aware of having pushed a new question at every step — and has left too little time to stay with what is sensed. Now the therapist should wonder whether the C28 comment was in part also about the interaction between the client and therapist right here.

C33: C31 and C33 are further content mutations.

87

C35: (*Silence*)

T35: Does that check out against the original fear too?

T35: Again the therapist checks if this is something else, or if it has genuinely come out of the previous moment.

C36: Yeah, that really fits, Carla.

T36: Hmm. OK. (*Silence, client opens her eyes*) Is that as far as it goes?

C37: Yeah. That's it (*laughs*). That was hard work.

T37: You worked very hard. You really did.

C38: I feel like I've been on another planet and back or something. I mean, I really did. I really did. That was really helpful. I really kept it out there for a long time.

Discussion of Excerpt 3

In this excerpt the therapist seems to push too fast (unless perhaps there were unrecorded silences that gave the session a slower pace than appears in the transcript). It is important to attend a little while, half a minute or a minute, to anything that has just come. The person should not be asked a further question immediately.

Except for its pace, this is a good example of a whole string of steps in which content mutation takes place.

Note how different such steps are from a dead-end feeling with a dynamic interpretation. Even when an interpretation is in some sense exactly right, it lacks the steps of experiential change and resolution, the type of steps that occurred here.

But how does a given content mutate into something else? The answer is that one attends directly not just to that content, but to the bodily sense as a whole (which of course includes it). From the body sense as an implicit whole the further steps come. Without the body sense the content alone would tend to repeat itself.

In the "first movement" of focusing one is asked to set each problem in front of oneself. This enables one to deal with it as a whole; it is the source of the phrases "from the outside" and "I kept it out there." These can easily be confused with something very different, namely, not feeling something at all. Here they are used to describe letting it become *a whole*, rather than component issues being tossed about inside the problem. Instead of going in, as one would usually do, one stays "outside" and lets the whole form "before" oneself.

EXCERPT 4

T1: OK, what I'd like for you to do now is to ask yourself what is the worst of that feeling, what is the most, the main thing in it that makes me feel bad. Now I want you to not answer right away but sit there with that, that question and let, don't let your mind start telling you everything like it was before. Instead let it come from that spot in your stomach that you were talking about. Let your body talk. (*Silence, client sighs.*) It may come to you as an image rather than as words.

(*Silence*)

C2: Do you want to know what the feeling makes me feel like inside?

T2: No, I want to know what is really the worst thing about this problem, that causes this feeling. What's the main thing there, do you get any kind of image or does any word just sort of pop up? It's not an intellectual thing, it's not one of those things that you know you've told yourself over and over.

C3: It's a box.

T3: A box?

C4: Hmm.

T4: Do you see a box?

C5: It's a box with four sides, like a square.

T5: And what about this box?

C6: It has a top and a bottom and it's empty.

T6: OK, now what I want you to do is to take this image of this box and this empty box and check it with that feeling that you've set out there, and ask it, is that right, is this what is the worst of this feeling? This empty box, does that describe it, is that right?

T1: In response to these instructions the client sighs, which usually shows a coming down of attention into the body, an easing, a letting be and letting form whatever will form. Notice the therapist's suggestion: "It *may* come to you as an image . . . " Even though it says "may," it is a little too suggestive. Saying "words or an image" would have left it more free.

T2: The therapist probably should have let the client speak from the feelings. Perhaps the therapist thinks the silence was not long enough, or it may be that this therapist is too oriented toward getting an image, and seems to ask for that *rather than* the direct sensing of the whole. That would be an error.

C6: So, the first content that appears is an emptiness.

T6: This is what one needs to do with an image, so as to get the body sense of the whole, as it will form after the image has emerged. The therapist refers to the whole feeling the client had "set out here" during the "first movement" of focusing.

C7: Yeah.

T7: Does anything else come?

(*Silence*)

C8: The box is isolated, nothing around it.

T8: Again it's like empty.

T8: This is inaccurate. The box has nothing around it, as well as nothing inside.

C9: It's just an empty box.

T9: With nothing around it.

T10: Okay, now try to ask yourself what all of that is, what's all of that feeling of an empty box. What's that all about? And again try to do it in the same way. Let it come from inside, let it come from that spot in your stomach. Let your body talk to you; what is this emptiness? This box?

(*Silence, then client begins to cry.*)

T11: Is your head talking to you?

T11: The therapist perhaps knows her, and knows that she often says mean things to herself. Is that why she is crying? Or has something come from inside?

C12: I don't know.

T12: Whatever, it hurts a lot.

(*Client continues to cry.*)

C13: I'm so scared inside.

C13: She is scared of, or scared of being in, the emptiness.

T13: Are you scared of the box, the emptiness? Or is scared part of the —

C14: I'm scared of being the box.

T14: You think that you might be that box?

C15: Yeah.

C14, C15: She is scared of being empty herself.

T15: Okay. And that's what is scary to check to go in and find that kind of image of an empty box that's isolated? Is that what's scary?

C16: Yeah. It's all alone.

T16: Now, try again to take these feelings, these scary, lonely and empty feelings and take it again and put it out here. Say,

T16, T17: Note exactly how the therapist instructs the client to put the whole agglomeration of feelings down, set it

90

"OK if this weren't with me I'd be fine so I'm going to take it and put it out here. Now I'll look at it while it's out here, but I'm OK I'm going to be OK because these feelings are out here now." Can you try to do that again?

(*Client sighs, silence.*)

slightly aside (not so far that it is not sensed). In this way she can sense the whole. This prevents her being caught inside the feelings. We call it "making a space." The therapist's judgment to do this at this spot is probably right, though the client might have merely been asked for the whole sense, to check the box's being "all alone."

T17: "I feel good. And this feeling, this lonely, empty box I'm taking it and putting it away from me right now. Of course it's a part of me and it's something that I'm afraid of, but right now I'm taking it and setting it out here. And I'm OK."

(*Client sighs.*)

C18: OK.

T18: OK, you have those feelings out here now?

C19: Yeah. (*Inaudible*)

T19: OK, just sit with it for a couple of minutes. You know, get them out there good. Say, "Yeah this is a part of me, and *I want to take care of that part and I will take care of that part, but right now in order to do that I need to set it out here.* And I'll be OK; I'll be better able to work with it."

(*Silence*)

T19: The therapist can see that the whole thing has not yet been set outside. The client has only sighed and said "OK" and "yeah." Also, the therapist tries to engender in her an attitude — how to receive what has just come. "I want to take care of that part . . . " It is a friendly and caring attitude, with which anything that comes should be received.

C20: OK.

T20: OK, you're feeling better?

C21: Yeah. (*Little laugh*)

C21: Here now, with a little laugh, the client is visibly whole again and in better shape. The therapist properly wants her, maximally whole and intact, to process what has come.

T21: But you still, of course, know what this is out here?

C22: Yeah.

T22: This empty box, now ask yourself again with the same bodily sense that we did before, what is so bad about that empty box?

T22: Here it is clear that the therapist asked her to set the problem down outside of herself, not to avoid it, but, in order

91

What's so bad about the loneliness? Being alone? Don't let your head talk to you, just let it come.

(*Silence*)

for her to be able to process it as a whole, rather than being caught inside it. Nor is the therapist avoiding whatever is bad or hard to tolerate about her feelings. The client is asked to sense what precisely the bad aspect is. This means sensing the whole, in response to the question, "What's so bad about _____?"

T23: Maybe if you ask, "What does that empty box need?"

T23: The therapist assumes nothing has budged. Another way of asking for a step is to ask, of the bodily sense of the whole, "What does it need?" It may stir and change as a whole, in response.

C24: It needs to be caressed.

C24: This is a big step and a content mutation. A need to be caressed is a very different thing from being scared and afraid of being empty. Even if you argue that it is not a change, it is surely a different aspect from what was said before. It is not just emptiness as the client feared. It is probably warm and deep, a need for care, for touch.

Discussion of Excerpt 4

There is an issue here: was it right for the therapist to take the person out of the feeling of being isolated and scared, so that she could sense it as a whole? That question does not need to be settled with regard to this particular case, but we can say under what general conditions it would be right or wrong.

Certainly it is important to sense what is there, and not to shy away from fully feeling anything that comes. This applies when the feeling is new, and has not been thoroughly felt. But certain ways of feeling come over and over again; this gets the person stuck. What is the way out of such feelings?

When something has been felt many times, then it is wise to do what this therapist had the person do. It is wise to let the problem become a whole again, set apart. After all, one knows that getting the same old depressed or isolated feeling one more time will not lead anywhere different from where it has led hundreds of other times.

Therefore, when a feeling is old and has been repeated many times, at the first sign of it we can back up from it, and the client should let the sense of the whole come. From the whole new steps can come.

This is especially true of the kind of feeling that is likely to get one stuck — the kind that can be recognized as likely to do so because it has many times before.

But, in this case, because the client was already in a stuck feeling, how did she get out of it?

The first movement of focusing is called "making a space." The whole problem is set at a distance. That is one way of letting it be a whole. "Checking" the handle word is another way; "Does this word express the crux of the whole thing?" There are still other ways. It was in moving from the content to a sensing (and welcoming) of the whole, that the need to be caressed arose in her.

Setting something down or apart allows it to become a whole, "that whole thing." The purpose of this first movement of focusing is not merely to find a tolerable distance for the issue. Even when there is no overwhelming feeling, it is good to begin by trying not to go into the middle of the problem, as people usually do. They go right to their usual dead end spot. Instead, we want to ask them to stand back a little, put the whole thing down, and that will allow it to form as a whole. We should certainly do this if something threatens to be overwhelming. We decide *not* to work on it, but not to run from it either; rather we let it be "a whole thing over there," at just the right distance so the person can breathe more easily. Then the person will not be overwhelmed and after some time can also work on the problem.

In this transcript the client has a way of feeling that "gets a hold of her." When the therapist sees this feeling doing just that again, she moves her to sense the whole, as a whole, by the method of setting it outside, next to her.

This can be a way of working with anything that is too sore or hard to bear (not only, as here, with something that often "gets a hold"). If one has it "at a little distance," it is not placed so far that the person can no longer feel it there, but neither is it so close that the person is totally pulled by it. It is not only more effectively worked with at that distance, but because it is a whole and one's self is that new kind of self which has such a whole, the person can say: "I am here. It is there. Since I am not it, I can relate to it, take an attitude toward it."

Now, what attitude should the person take? The focusing method requires a friendly attitude toward whatever is felt, giving it a friendly hearing. In our excerpt the therapist asks her to "take care of that part."

What happened here is the sort of change that occurs when one lets the whole form while taking a friendly attitude toward it. From a scary emptiness it has become a something inside that wants to be caressed.

EXCERPT 5

The next three examples come from instances when, in order to explain focusing, I turned to doing it. The first was with a man who interviewed me on a radio program. We talked for about half the program time, 15 minutes minus two commercials.

Interviewer: I'm having trouble understanding, and I think our audience probably does too, what this unclear felt sense is, that you talk about.

Gendlin: Well, if you would be willing, choose some problem of your own, for a minute. You need not say what it is, just pick one in your mind.

I: That's easy. I'm right in one. My building is being turned into condominiums, and we have to move. It makes me so angry. That whole way of squeezing people's money out of them — so very much money just for an apartment — and that whole policy is wrong. We're black, of course, and that has something to do with it too. And I *hate* moving. Everything is disrupted. I'm just not ready to move.

G: I know that this is a big issue, about condominiums, and I know we could talk about that for a long time. I can understand that you're angry about it. And the race issue that comes into it is even bigger, I know. But I'll ask you, so I can explain focusing, to do something a little different. Could you just sense the whole of your discomfort, now, about that whole moving business, and — just as if you didn't know about it already — sense how it makes you feel. See if you can get one word or phrase for *the quality* of it.

I: Well I know what I feel. I'm not ready. I'm not prepared for it. It comes as a surprise; I didn't expect it.

G: Just be with the sense of "not prepared." You know a lot of what that means, but just as if you didn't know it, just stay a little while with that uncomfortable sense, that you're calling "not prepared."

(*Silence, . . . it seemed like a long silence because this was on the radio, but it lasted perhaps 15 seconds.*)

G: Probably this is hard to do, right now, you're having to run the program and so forth, but we're only explaining to the audience how this is done, maybe later when you have a quiet minute —

I: (*Laughs*)

G: Why are you laughing?

I: I've got it. It answered me. I know what it is. It came.

G: Now, you don't need to say what it is.

I: Oh I can say it. It's being middle-aged. That's what it is.

G: Oh —

I: I'm not prepared to carry heavy things. What are the women going to say when that comes out? I'm afraid I'll hurt my back. We haven't moved for years, and I haven't done any heavy carrying for 20 years. I am sure going to look foolish. But, of course, that's nothing. It's getting middle-aged, that's what bothers me. We can move.

(*Relief shows on the interviewer's face.*)

Discussion of Excerpt 5

Someone might think that the interviewer has only run into a bigger problem. But he feels that bigger topic in a different way than the moving problem. He sees some humor in it and a sense that there is plenty of time to work on it. Meanwhile the tension about moving has released, and he is laughing at his concern with looking foolish.

Of course, not always does one step release a problem, even a relatively small one. A person might not find release at some particular step. A less developed person might not experience relief and laughter upon discovering that being afraid of looking foolish was the problem. The person might have to go another step and ask what the whole felt sense is, that goes with this looking foolish.

I also want to be clear that I am not trivializing problems about condominiums and certainly not about race. This processing step does not in any way diminish the seriousness that this man feels about social questions. On the contrary, I observe that people are more able to work effectively on social problems when their personal energy has been freed up.

What exactly had this man not known before that he now knows? It is that it was not the well-known disruption of moving that made him feel "not ready, not prepared." It was rather what came there when he let the murky sense give the next step.

EXCERPT 6

My next example also comes from the radio. I was on a call-in show. The caller was complaining bitterly about her husband. He watches TV all the time and says he has to. She and the kids have to bring him things; he cannot leave the TV. Once, when it had to be fixed, he almost went crazy. He will not discuss this with her. What should she do? How can she get him to talk about the problem, get help, or in some way communicate about it?

G: I know there would be much more to say. I am going to ask you to do something a little different. Could you put aside all you already know about this whole thing, and sense how the whole thing makes you feel in your body.

Caller: What do you mean?

G: Well, if you tried to feel fine about it — if you wanted to feel fine about the whole thing, in your body, I bet that just wouldn't work. Try to feel fine about the whole thing. Say, "I feel fine about it" and see what you then feel in your body. Some unclear uncomfortable sense of the whole thing should come.

(*Silence, . . . again, because this is radio I cannot let the silence go on too long.*)

G: Do you get a distinct sense in your body about the whole thing?

C: Yes.

G: Now see if you can find one word, or a phrase, to match just what that sense is. What should it be called? What fits?

(*Silence, then laughter*)

G: Why are you laughing?

C: I got a word that fits. It's "snooty."

Discussion of Excerpt 6

Here she has, to her own surprise, gotten directly in contact with what she is contributing to the problem of lack of communication with her husband. Again there is laughter. Laughter usually indicates that the person is larger and able to see beyond what came. She had been aware only of her husband's unlovely ways. She had thought of herself only as long-suffering. As soon as she has a hold of this handle word, "snooty," she laughs.

Of course, this is only one little step. There was not time on the radio to find out her reaction to this bit of processing. I would like to think that it changed her approach to her husband, and that something improved. But major problems are not usually so simple as to open in one step. This was only one step, and it was not completely verbalized in the short time we spoke.

What is clear is that "snooty" (her own attitude) was not what she had been thinking or talking about at all, and it was not what she or I expected to come. And yet retrospectively it makes a lot of sense.

EXCERPT 7

A reporter called me long distance to inquire about focusing. She wanted to include it in a magazine article on the subject "people helping each other." She told me that she herself felt very hesitant about approaching another woman who obviously needed help. She was going to use this as an example in her article. She asked me, for the sake of the article, what makes people hesitate in that kind of situation. What did I think were the reasons for drawing back from expressing concern about someone's problem and offering to listen. She had obviously thought a lot about this hesitation for her article. She guessed that she felt the woman might not welcome her help, that she might not be able to help, or one of several other reasons.

It puzzled her that there was a past situation in which she had felt fine about asking another woman she barely knew whether she wanted help or someone to talk to. Why was asking *this* woman different?

96

I asked her to put her attention in her body and wait to see what would come there, while saying to herself, "I feel just fine about asking this woman." "Well, I know I don't feel all right about it," she said. I explained that we knew that, of course. But if she would try to feel all right, and tell herself that she did, there would be a physical talking back in her body, and she would be able to sense more sharply the direct sense of not feeling all right.

She tried this, and laughed. "It certainly *isn't* all right!" she said. From her tone I could tell that something had come. I asked her to stay with that body sense and ask it why it was not all right. After a while she had it.

"I might not be the right person, that's what it is." Quite definitely, the body sense had answered. But after a few moments she wondered: "How can I be sure that this, what just came, is what's been bothering me, and not all the stuff I thought before?"

There are ways to check answers that come in this way. The following is one way: I told the reporter to put her attention in her body as before. Then I told her to ask herself, "If I somehow knew for sure that I'm the right person, would I feel OK about approaching the woman?" There was a big sigh and when she spoke again there was a flood of new energy in her voice. "Absolutely! That would feel just fine!"

A little later she had something further: "And I do happen to know that I *was* the right person in that other situation where I felt fine about offering. So it even checks out that way, too."

Discussion of Excerpt 7

This example illustrates especially well how the body "talks back." The reporter could not make her body feel all right about offering help. In working on the article she had tried and could not get her body to feel all right about approaching the woman. Now, with the supposition that she was "the right person," her body felt fine about approaching the woman, even though it was only a supposition. We see how stubbornly and distinctly the body "talks back," very much in its own way.

The body's talking back enables us to double check what comes, if we are in doubt. What is in the way has emerged and we can double check it: If what came as the reason were somehow fixed, how would the situation feel in the body?

The felt shift (the concrete physical change) is often quite small at first. One needs to stay with what comes for half a minute or a minute; then the shift becomes larger. The shift in this example was small at first, and the reporter instantly retreated from it because of her doubt. People often do that. The moment something comes they doubt it, or they become self-critical. Or they turn to some circumstances that cast doubt on what came. Here it was a doubt ("How can I be sure?"). Such quick moves tend to wipe out what has come before it can bring the physical shift. In this example that shift did not fully come in until the "checking" question.

EXCERPT 8

C1: One of the things I try to do is, if I get upset, I try to let it . . . tell me why I'm upset, which has worked! Well, I'm not going to have a heart attack one of these days maybe. I don't know; it seems like it helps.

T1: It eases it.

C2: That's right. And I constantly . . . before I would just get mad, and whoever was within my reach would catch hell. And now I try . . . and I've been successful at it . . . to try to figure out by myself . . . and that works. Now, sometimes, I'm really amazed other people don't do it. I mean I — (*Laughs*)

C3: The other day I thought I was going to die laughing. My lawyer couldn't figure out something and was really frustrated, and he said, you know, "the pressure is too much." And I said, "Let yourself tell you where the pressure is. Why don't you sit down and . . . " I thought, "My God, what are you doing, Martha?" 'Cause . . . it does work. Of course it's a little weird, but it does work.

C1: This excerpt is from the beginning of the fifth interview with a client who is quite unaccustomed to psychology. Here she expresses her surprise at how focusing works. (She has learned quite quickly to use it also between her sessions.) The last line expresses graphically the experience of the physical easing, the tension draining out, which each step of focusing gives.

C2: It seems so simple; why doesn't everyone do it?

C3: Without thinking she began to teach her lawyer focusing, then realized how odd it sounds.

EXCERPT 9

In this excerpt a therapist in training works with a person labeled "schizophrenic." These are his notes on the session in which he first tried to teach focusing.

I had been seeing this client once a week for approximately 3 months following a brief stay at the inpatient unit at our mental health center. This young woman, in her early 20s, has had many difficulties in getting in touch with her feelings in the past. We had been taping the last two sessions and this procedure evoked some anxiety, so at this session we chose not to tape.

Midway through the session the client reported being stuck and was having difficulty getting in touch with what she meant. I suggested that I might have a method which would allow this stuck feeling to be identified and asked if she would like to try this method. She was hesitant, so I suggested that we let her "sample" this method. She agreed.

I suggested that the body often holds knowledge that is not readily apparent to the mind; that at times our bodies are hiding places for knowledge that the mind doesn't want to see. Sometimes we hide this bit of knowledge in our stomach, or our foot, or behind our knee, or in some other out-of-the-way spot that we will forget about.

I asked her to relax her whole body, to stretch and take some deep breaths, and to close her eyes as she felt herself becoming relaxed. She was seated in a comfortable chair and relaxed easily. I asked her to look inside her body for any places that were still uncomfortable or tense and, if she located these spots, to attempt to gently relax them. If we found a spot that resisted she would acknowledge the tension and move around it, knowing it was there and allowing it to be — but to let it be, and after we were finished she could go back to it.

When she was fully relaxed I asked her to try to see what problems were there — not to take them in — only to look at them and allow them to be seen. When she did this I instructed her to put each problem in its own box with her imagination. After she did that I asked that she *label each box; write the name of the problem on the box*. She did this, and then I had her gently move the boxes of problems aside; to allow herself to clear a space, a comfortable distance between her and her problems.

I asked her how it felt to have that space, and she replied that it was relaxing. I gave her a few seconds to experience that feeling and then requested that she look at the problems again and ask herself, "*If all of these were gone would [my] life be OK?*" She responded, "*No.*" I pointed out to her that *sometimes when things are moved we can see other problems. I then had her take the new problems, put them in boxes, label them, and move them aside*. I again asked her how it felt. When she responded positively, I asked if her life would be okay if all these problems were gone. When she nodded yes I then let her acknowledge this feeling and asked her to look at all the problems and allow herself from *inside her body to choose a problem that was special to work on*.

After a while she showed that she had chosen one problem. I told her to focus on that problem, without taking it in, but just to look at it and allow herself *to see how it felt in her body*. She did this, and I asked her if there was a way that she could label how it felt inside. She focused and *sighed (shift), and I said that I thought she might have something*. She said it felt like indecision. I said "indecision." I asked her if that word felt right and suggested that she compare the word to the problem, bounce them off each other, see if they really fit together or if there might be something else there. She did this and after a while *sighed a second time (shift), and I said, "I think some-*

thing else is there." She said it feels more like "frustration." I reflected on that word and then asked her to feel it and see what that was. I asked her to take "frustration" and compare it with the problem, again bouncing each off the other to see how they fit, or seeing if there might be something else. She did this and after a while another shift occurred. *She sighed, and tears ran down both sides of her cheeks. I said I thought something else was there, and she said "guilt."* I reflected on that word and asked her to see how that felt inside. "What was this 'guilt,' what does this really mean inside?"

She was having difficulty at this point and was unable to examine it, so I suggested that the body knows when to stop itself from discovering too much too soon. I said that we had reached an awareness of some new things. This knowledge didn't remove the problem, but allowed us to acknowledge these things. I asked her to allow herself to see what she had discovered. I then asked her if she felt ready to stop, or if she wanted to go on. She said she was ready to stop — so we ended the session.

EXCERPT 10

In the excerpts I have presented so far in this chapter the people were able to use quite easily the kind of bodily sensing necessary for focusing. I selected these excerpts because I wanted first to illustrate this direct sensing of something implicit, but unclear, and how it then shifts and opens.

In the first seven excerpts the individuals had not focused before, and the instructions given were new to them. Even so they were able to attend in this bodily way. In excerpt 8 the individual had already learned focusing. Now let us look at an example of an individual who does not find this easy to do right away.

Excerpt 10 comes from a first interview. (The client said, "I've been in analysis 8 years and I'm quitting I guess because my analyst is retiring.") He had heard about focusing, and one of the reasons he came to this therapist was to learn it. Therefore he had more patience than others who cannot learn focusing right away. I do not recommend this kind of first interview at all. The therapist was trying too hard to meet the client's specific requests. Usually in therapy, instructions like these should be spread out over 10 or 20 interviews if the person has difficulty with them. Otherwise they get in the way.

I chose this excerpt because it exhibits the kind of instructions given in focusing and also the bad results of excessive pushing. I hope you will notice that the interaction here does not have the right quality for therapy.

The client in this case gets as far as finding a "handle." It comes toward the end of a therapy hour in which many other attempts had failed. In those attempts the therapist had simply gone along with what the client said each time. But the client remains willing to try, so the therapist continues to give the client focusing instructions to sense directly the issue he had wanted to work on.

T1: But this that made you tense, come back to it and ask, "Hmm, what is that tension?" But don't ask it until you get it back a little.

(*Short silence*)

C2: (*Takes a deep breath*) I get very knotted up right in here. [T: Um hmm]

T2: Maybe a way to say it is, "Can you be friendly to the 'knotted up'?" Mostly we get mad when we get knotted up.

C3: Yeah. I do. I get very angry.

T3: OK, can you say, "Oh, I see I'm angry at it" and put the anger down?

C4: It feels like I'm too intellectualizing it.

T4: Yeah, it will do that. Can you still feel the "knotted"?

C5: A little.

T5: See if you can be a little bit friendly toward it so you can have a nice conversation with it.

C6: Let's try and go on with it.

T1: The client has been running on, discussing his avoidance of a certain kind of situation because it makes him tense. The therapist hopes he might sense the tension directly instead of going on talking about it.

C2: He has been "knotted up" earlier in the hour. But that alone had not let anything happen because he had not stayed with it.

T2: The therapist hopes the client might create a friendly space for this "knotted up" feeling and guesses that the client is probably not giving it that kind of space.

T3: To make a friendly space when angry, one says: "Oh, . . . I see; I'm angry." This acknowledges the anger ("Yes all this *is* legitimate anger") and then places the anger to one side, or lets the anger through, so that it doesn't land on the new thing that came (the "knotted up" feeling). This should create a safe and friendly space for the "knotted up" feeling.

C4: He means that what the therapist says is not working; it leads him to intellectualize. He does not feel the "knotted up" feeling now.

T4: The therapist admits that intellectualizing might be an effect of his instructions. Then he asks the client to sense directly if the "knotted up" feeling is still there. In this way the client's attention will be turned again toward direct sensing. (One can always do this when everything gets confused: "Can you still feel the . . . ?")

C6: Again he indicates that the therapist's instruction is not working.

101

T6: We would like it to tell us something. So we have to be friendly with it. If we want someone to be a research subject and fill out 2 hours of questionnaire, we have to be friendly. (*Laughs*) Can you take that attitude to the knotted place?

C7: Let's try. I don't know. I just really don't have a good answer to that.

T7: Okay. Go see if you can still touch the knotted place.

C8: I find difficulty with this whole language really.

T8: Yeah. . . . Unclear . . . my words. Might say it a different way too. Can you still feel that "knotted"?

C9: Yeah, I don't know if that's just because of the way I'm sitting or —

T9: Well sit up then.

C10: I feel a knot here. But I don't know if that's just me or —

T10: Well, if it goes away, that's Okay. Let's just ask again, just ask your body, "Is 'confrontation' the right word exactly?"

T6: The therapist tries once more, with an example, to get a friendly attitude toward the "knotted up" feeling.

C7: Again the client says, in effect, "Let's get on with it; I can't do this, what you ask now." Those instructions are too long and do not help him find or stay with "knotted up" feeling, if it is there.

T7: Again, as in T4, the way out of being lost or stuck is, "See if you can still touch the. . . . "

C8: The client says this whole way of talking does not make sense to him. He does not know what the therapist means in T7. He wonders, "touch what?"

T8: Again, first the therapist admits that, yes, this way of talking can be funny, unclear. And again (as in T4), the way out of it is to return to what is there. This time the therapist phrases it not as "touch it" but simply "Can you still feel that 'knotted'?"

C9: Even this issue, by now, is uncertain. The "knotted up" has become vague. Perhaps it is only how the client is sitting.

T9: It is often necessary to ask the person to shift physically in the chair, to let the body loosen, so that what is there can be sensed better. It is amazing how stiff or slumped people remain, unmovingly, sometimes for an hour, if they are not asked to loosen the body occasionally.

T10: If shifting position in the chair makes the knot go away, fine. At last the therapist moves to something simpler, checking the "handle" word from earlier in the hour. (He has for the moment given up on the friendly space. Insisting on that would only keep them stuck.)

C11: Like there's more to it?

C11: The client knows "there is more to it" and could say a lot more that he already knows. (Of course, if he means that he can sense more to it, then that is a direct datum to stay with.)

T11: No, it's more that the body responds to a particular word or phrase or handle.

C12: Yeah, yeah.

T12: Like it will be like "yeah!" There'll be a little breath to it. Like if I said to you, "We have to have one word. We could have a phrase, but let's pretend we have to have one word, should we say confrontation? or should we say pushing?"

C13: Pushing is closer. [T: Ah ha] Pushing is definitely . . . I can feel that!

C13: Here for the first time there is a *direct* response from what the client senses. There is no other reason why "pushing" is closer; it is not more informative and does not make more sense. It is simply sensed as "closer." This "closer" means something directly sensed does stir in response to that word.

T13: There you are.

C14: I can feel a response to that.

C14: The client here shows he has understood what was aimed at and is pleased that now it actually happened.

T14: There you are.

Discussion of Excerpt 10

When the type of bodily attention required by focusing is difficult for someone and the felt sense does not come, then it is quite sufficient at first to work for a small bit of focusing: In this case it is the experience of something directly sensed, which responds to "pushing" and not so much to "confrontation." The client will learn more techniques in subsequent interviews, but much is gained if he can fully have and recognize what it is like to sense directly — and know what it is like to sense an inward response to one way of saying something, and not to another. He is thereby directly sensing something right there, but unclear and unknown, something that responds in its own independent way. He does not control whether "pushing" makes for an inward stirring or whether "confrontation" does. He knows now what it is like to work directly with something sensed but not known, and he can check what he says and thinks against it. Paying such close attention to one tiny sense can show the person the whole focusing mode of working.

CHAPTER 9

Problems of Teaching Focusing during Therapy

WE HAVE SEEN some of what therapists can do to bring about the focusing process, but how can they *teach* focusing during psychotherapy? In the examples we have seen so far some teaching of focusing preceded the excerpt. Therefore the clients recognized and understood the therapist's short bits of focusing instruction, such as (Chapter 4, T13), ". . . the feel quality of it, for a minute you could feel the pull back." Or (Chapter 8, Excerpt 1, T1) "go inside your body. . . . Stay there for a moment and ask your body, 'Is it rage, is that it? Is that the right word?' "

How can one bring people to the point where they understand such brief invitations? Of course the therapist can teach focusing directly for a few minutes, if that is welcome. Elaborate teaching procedures have been developed (See Gendlin, 1981, and other materials available from the Focusing Institute, Chicago.) The problem is that a lengthy teaching process turns the client–therapist interaction into a didactic one in which the therapist is active and the client has to take it all in, has to be "patient," that is to say passive.

The teaching of focusing greatly aids the person's inwardly originating process, but because the teaching comes from outside, it can also obstruct it. This can also happen with anything else the therapist does besides listening and responding exactly to what the person means to convey. For example, interpretations, confrontations, reaching out to the person—anything else—can also be obstructive. Like the teaching of focusing they should happen rarely during a therapy session, and should continue only if it was immediately welcome. If the intrusion was unwelcome, it would be saved for another time. Also, if the therapist tries out something only very tentatively, the client's reaction to it will usually add to and modify the therapist's understanding, without too much disruption. Gypsies use this method. They can tell you all about yourself without knowing you. The gypsy woman says, "You have many friends," and as she sees your face fall, she quickly adds, "but very few good ones." By tentatively trying out little suggestions, a therapist's interpretive ideas can help open an issue without needing to be right about it at the start.

Unlike the gypsy, a therapist does not need the appearance of always being right. Indeed, that appearance should be avoided. It is an unreasonable and unfair demand some therapists put on themselves. I tell my clients constantly, "Of course I don't know. We won't know till you find how it is from inside." Early in therapy, whenever I have said something that turns out to be wrong, I point out my mistake explicitly. I need the client to see that I do not have trouble being wrong, indeed that I expect to be wrong much of the time. Once clients know this, it is easy for them to correct me, and tell me what does come inside them when it is not what I thought. Then my interpretations cannot obstruct the process anymore, and they can help to open things.

Does being wrong sometimes erode the therapist's authority? If I am wrong ten times in a row and right and helpful the eleventh time, then the client gives me credit, and the chain of wrong guesses is forgotten. Indeed the chain of small attempts is hardly noticeable in retrospect, and I still run the risk of seeming magically wise.

But if I as therapist "decide" what I can and cannot know, I can get stuck with something I thought should be right, and there cannot be 11 tries. The client then struggles to resist my impulse or tries to make it seem true to save my feelings, or still worse, becomes confused thinking that it must be true. This results in blockage.

What the literature generally tells us in this regard is quite false. As therapists we are supposed to know what we cannot possibly know. So we are supposed to decide on one interpretation or another, one theory or another. One technique may be recommended by one book and held up as bad by another.

It is better to put the emphasis on feedback from the client, either verbal or implicit. Then the various theories and possible interpretations can alert us to further possibilities. Therefore, tentative bits of interpretation do not obstruct the process.

This is also true with tentative bits of focusing instruction. It is hard for clients when they find themselves unable to do what the therapist asks. If the therapist seems to need the instructions to work, it may be hard for the client to tell the therapist that they do not. It may make the client too shy to tell exactly what does happen instead. ("I get only words going through my head." "I just sank into that old depressed feeling when you said, 'ask your body.'")

Focusing relies on tentativeness on the part of the therapist so that the individual can try out a suggestion, sense inwardly, see what comes in response, and tell about that. Time must be left for this inward trying out. Therefore the therapist should not give the client many steps of instruction at once. Similarly with interpretations, the therapist should not offer a whole analysis all at once. The therapist can offer a part of an interpretation and give the client time to sense inwardly what comes in response to it. The therapist then listens and responds exactly to what the client did find and say. If that leads to a new process in the client, the therapist should save the rest of the original interpretation for some other time. After all, the whole purpose of an interpretation is to generate new inwardly arising processes, so room must be left for them; they should not be obstructed by an interpretation. Clients should always have the space in front of them open so that they can lead where their impulses take them.

If room and time is left open in this way, clients remain in control of their own process. If the therapist does too many things in a row, one right after another, it can be as if the therapist is taking the steering wheel and pushing the client into the passenger's seat for a passive ride. Even if the results are great, the client has not learned to drive, has lost control of the process, and more has been lost than gained. If this happens too often the inwardly originating process will not come forward at all.

This emphasis on the client's control of the process is not a question of democracy, or some abstract desire to let people do it themselves. Rather, it has to do with the kind of change we want, or more exactly, with psychological change as such. Psychological change comes from inside. What the therapist can do deliberately is insignificant compared to the client's inwardly arising change.

At times therapists may want to go back to something that was left behind or stay longer with something; they may interpret, confront, or express feelings of their own. It is proper for therapists to do nearly any of these things, but right afterward they should listen exactly and respond exactly to whatever the client's reaction is. And it is especially important that the therapist not do too many such things in a row. Otherwise there will be no inwardly originating process.

Almost any kind of therapist can be helpful if enough space is left for the client's own process to arise and continue, and can be exactly responded to.

For all these reasons, during a therapy hour we teach focusing only in small increments. Whether such an incremental step was effective or not, we return immediately to listening. The attempt to teach that incremental step of focusing can be renewed later when it seems appropriate. Most clients learn focusing from those incremental steps during therapy, if they are given over a period of time.

SPECIFIC PITFALLS

Now I turn to a more exact description of potential pitfalls, ways in which the teaching of focusing can run into difficulties.

Clients Running Roughshod over Their Own Feelings

Some clients can behave toward themselves like overly pushy therapists. If this occurs the therapist must intercede to help the client make a receptive space inside by asking for a little quiet time in which the space inside can open. The therapist instructs the client to give the inside a hearing, let it breathe, be there, and be felt. It must be protected from criticism, constant superego attacking, inward lecturing, cold rejection, or deliberate engineering of some preconceived outcome. If all these things are coming from the top down, from the outside in, some room must be provided for something to speak from the inside outward.

Here too the therapist intervenes only in small increments and instantly backs off to leave the space and time totally free again. But to provide room for something to arise from the inside out has to be done more actively and insistently than I have described above. The therapist may have to interrupt and defend what is being attacked and criticized by saying that the item has not yet had its hearing. We do not yet know what "it" would say, what "its" reasons are, what "it" knows. It also might be suggested that it is a child and that it should be listened to as if it were a child.

Such interrupting and such insistence could result in the disadvantages we discussed earlier, and it does. But the bad effects will be less if the client knows that the therapist will stop after each interruption and listen. If an interruption has hurt the client's feelings or had some other effect the client wants to express, the therapist's action will be rectified if the client understands that the therapist is quite willing to have been wrong about it.

Overreliance on the Therapist

Some few clients do not learn focusing from the incremental steps even after many months. More elaborate teaching of focusing will succeed with most of these clients. But once they have experienced focusing, they should be allowed to focus slowly for themselves, with, again, only incremental instructions from the therapist. Otherwise they focus only when instructed and helped by the therapist.

The pitfall of overreliance comes if the therapist helps too elaborately to bring about focusing in each hour, near its start. This should not be done.

Some years ago, in several cases, I thought the client and I were doing very well; I was making focusing happen for each client in each hour. I was working hard to help the client find a felt sense and stay with it. But when I tried not to do so much at the beginning, although the previous hour had been wonderful and deep, nothing at all would happen in this hour. Not only had these clients of mine not learned to focus on their own, there was no inwardly propelled therapy process!

The therapist should not always be working to bring the client into the process. After a few experiences of focusing it is well to let the client find focusing on their own with only minimal bits of instruction.

The Therapist Seems Impatient

Another pitfall of teaching focusing is that the client may get the impression (often correctly) that the therapist is impatient. Indeed, once a therapist knows focusing, it is harder to listen to the client going round and round when it seems that a little attention to the implicit felt sense would open what is being talked about and provide a step. If the therapist always follows this urge, the client may feel that nothing but focusing is welcome or interesting to the therapist.

I can see that this has happened when a client tells me what happened during the week and then says, "just one more thing, all right?" as if to say "I know you're waiting for me to stop talking and go into the edge of something." Or, the client may say something like: "I have to talk this out, okay?"

I have certainly not rejected anything overtly, and I believe in receiving anything a client wants to convey. I believe that talking is often necessary. Communication and interaction are vital for therapy. Also, I believe in being able to have simply human conversation. As a therapist I am not a therapy machine. But too much responding in a focusing mode can give that impression.

The therapist should keep in mind that focusing is one way to carry implicit bodily experiencing forward, but there are other ways. Focusing works by direct attention to the body sense. Other ways of working, through interaction, imagery, dreams, changes in habit and in action—though they are made more effective by focusing—can also constitute therapy without it. No one has the right to claim that there is only one way for human beings to grow, in therapy, in personal development, or in anything.

The Interaction Influences Focusing

Focusing is sometimes, quite wrongly, thought to be an exclusively "intrapsychic" therapy. There is no such thing. Interaction is always a vital dimension of therapy, and as I have already said, focusing goes on within the wider context of the ongoing interaction. Depending on the quality of that interaction focusing will generate different contents and have different results.

Therefore, when interpersonal difficulties arise, they must be given immediate priority over focusing instruction or whatever else the therapist was trying to do. Interpersonal interaction is always going on at least implicitly. When it becomes problematic it must be given priority, or everything will go awry.

Although much of what occurs in focusing occurs in silence, silent focusing is still an interaction process when a therapist (or any other person) is present, contributing quiet attention. Everyone finds it much easier to focus with someone's silent company than when alone. Although attending inside, one is alive in the company of the other person. One senses the difference physically. The other person is holding the weight of the world, as it were, contributing energy to the focuser's inward attending. The other person is there each time the focuser looks up. The other person's presence makes all the difference in the manner of the focusing process, even if the content seems to be only about the individual. There is no split between "intrapsychic" and "interactional."

THE BALANCE BETWEEN THE THERAPY FRAME AND OTHER INTERVENTIONS

These difficulties may seem to indicate that therapists should stick to a clearly limited "frame." The frame of therapy is often thought to limit therapists only to interpretation and nothing else, or only to listen but not lead and nothing else. Perhaps, by staying within such a frame, the therapist could avoid all these pitfalls.

I do not think so. The pitfalls will still happen, and no actual human can do "nothing else" anyway. A rigidly formal approach only makes what is going on harder to find and to process.

Great formality of method creates an antiseptic quality which limits therapy more than any of the mentioned pitfalls do. The concept of the therapy frame is to protect the therapy space from being confused with all sorts of other things. But if held too rigidly, the frame would kill what it is supposed to protect and engender.

For example, the therapy frame rightly structures meetings so that clients talk mostly about themselves. The frame protects the client's time and space. It should be the client's hour, not the therapist's. But this can backfire and destroy the mutual contact if the rule becomes so ironclad that the client cannot reach the therapist or is prohibited from finding out about or touching the therapist. For example, suppose the client wants to know or senses something about the therapist. This becomes a need the client has. A real inquiry should get a real response. At times the therapy process requires that the therapist be open on some issue or other.

There is a dilemma in teaching during therapy similar to that of the rigidity of the therapy frame. The focusing process must arise from within the client. So it seems that anything we do as therapists to help this inward arising must actually obstruct it. To try to make an inward arising happen from outside—how can it have anything but the opposite effect?

All personal helping has this dilemma: Whatever is really going to help must be the person's own. What then is the role of the helper? The helper must somehow point out what might help, and yet without taking over and directing the whole thing. Some activity of the helper is involved, and yet the main process is *not* the helping process, but the person's own process, which must arise and continue.

The dilemma is resolved if the helper's activity is brief, so that there is always space and time for the person to move from inside, and so that the person never loses the leading role.

With some clients in focusing these things are not lost even if the therapist says many things and instructs often. With others even one thing every third or fourth hour is too much, and the client's sense of being imposed upon has to be noticed or heard and abided by. Generally, a therapist can only learn this dynamic by doing too much. Therapists can expect to miss the point of balance and must try to learn to correct themselves.

HOW THE PITFALLS CAN BE DEALT WITH

When something gets in the way of focusing the obstacle can itself be focused on. For example, suppose the client's face becomes tight in response to a focusing instruction, and the therapist asks about it. The client is afraid of not being able to carry out the instruction, and then the therapist will be disappointed. If the therapist makes clear that it is fine not to carry out the instruction, the client can be invited to focus on this sense of having to meet expectations.

When the client refuses to follow an instruction, one of the therapist's options is to drop it. It is a very good thing when clients have the strength to push the therapist back, to direct the therapist, to assert their own space against the therapist. This assertion should succeed. The therapist needs to respond in such a way that it does succeed. If asked to stop, the therapist should instantly stop.

Whether a client's move succeeds depends on the therapist's response. If the therapist is told to stop and does stop, the client will have successfully asserted some rights. If the therapist goes on as before, the client may feel weak or perhaps even guilty for having expressed hostility. What one person actually experiences depends in part on the other's response.

There need not be speculation as to whether the client was overly controlling and hostile, or appropriately assertive in a healthy, growth producing way. The therapist can respond so as to make it be the latter.

This does not mean the therapist's influence is easily eliminated, wiped out, or silenced. The client's push must have its effect; it must modify the therapist's behavior, but in such a way that does not damage the therapist.

The way to respond is simple. It is something like discovering that you are standing on someone's toes. You do not argue, you just move your foot off the person's toes. But you do not go home, or sit down and cry, or apologize overly profusely as if what you did is more than you can stand. You just say you did not intend to stand on their toes, and then you do not go right back to standing on their toes again. It is the difference between the other person's rightful space, and your own. You keep your space, and you instantly get out of theirs.

The pitfalls are not in themselves bad—if the client's experience during them is heard, responded to, and cared about. The result can end up being so positive that it is better than if the pitfall had not happened.

This is true with most mistakes a therapist can make. It is not the mistake itself that matters. It is what the therapist does about it afterward. Whether it turns out well or badly depends on how the client's reaction to the mistake is processed. What is important is that clients are heard and their good sense in making the complaint is acknowledged. Although being mistreated is common in ordinary life, a person wanting to understand and rectify it afterward is very rare and special.

Listening is therefore the foundation which makes therapist-aided focusing possible. If a therapist listens, swiftly asks for the client's feeling, and responds exactly to it without arguing, editing, or adding—always returning to this between any two moves—then mistakes will result in an especially good process.

CHAPTER 10

Excerpts from One Client's Psychotherapy

EXCERPT A

THE CLIENT IN THIS CHAPTER had learned focusing the year before these sessions took place in a class taught by a different therapist. Here she is in the fourth interview of psychotherapy with me. She is able to go very deeply very swiftly, both because of the person she is, and because she knows focusing well.

The specific content that emerges in the excerpt is not unusual. It is the sort of material one often gets in therapy, but the swift progression is highly unusual. In one hour you would not usually find movement *from* where this client begins *to* what she senses next, and from that to what she senses after that, and again further, and further.

It is the purpose of this book to show this kind of processing and to point out exactly the means by which clients achieve it and how therapists can help to bring it about. What I want to point out about this client's therapy is the progression, the steps of emergence, and content mutation. That is what needs to be noticed in the excerpts I am about to present.

The question to keep in mind during this excerpt is: Does this kind of opening or next step usually come this easily for a person who was just, a minute ago, where this client was? Trace exactly *how* she got there from the earlier step. Just what intervened, to enable her to get here from there? How did she move? What did she inwardly do? Ask this about each step.

Indeed the number of steps and felt shifts come so fast that I decide she needs a rest in the middle. One cannot do a whole hour of therapy at this pace.

112

The body needs a rest so as not to get worn out. Time is needed for this much bodily change to happen fully.

At the outset she complains of feeling "flat" and "crummy." I ask her to sense where her good energy is inwardly tied up. Now, can we see exactly how a person in her state could just turn inward, and right there, behind a tie-up that she can directly sense, find where the missing energy is?

Naturally I next ask her if the directly sensed tie-up will open and let itself be sensed from inside of itself (rather than sensing it from this side of the barrier behind which the energy is blocked). How likely is it that she would immediately (that is to say in a long silence of some minutes) be able to get that kind of direct opening to happen? How did she do it?

Then comes "a part of me I keep in." What part is that? It is a part of her which, if it were not kept in and not silenced, would say when things are not okay. It would fight back, not give in and go along with people. Of course I hope she can "stay with" that part and not lose it again right away. Having already gone through the steps above, it turns out next that this "part" is very intense; it screams to live!

There are further steps. Each time, please ask yourself by what means each successive opening and physical shift is brought about.

C1: I've been looking forward to coming, much more than I did the other times. I've had a crummy week. My job is really bad, and I'm tired of my house, and everything seems flat like I'm just watching. I'm not in it. And I know it's me.

T1: So everything seems flat and you're not involved in it, just watching. But you know it isn't the job and so on, it's you.

C2: Well, the job really is bad, what they're doing in that place isn't right. But other times I'd be able to do something with it, I know.

T2: So it's true what you feel about them, but also, the way you're being inside you is not OK.

T2: I want to take in *both* that what she says about her job is realistic, *and* I *also* want to refer inside her to that which made her say, "I know it's me." The hour might otherwise be spent discussing her job.

C3: Yes.

T3: So we have to go see where your good energy went to.

T3: This is a direct invitation to attend inwardly, and to sense where the "good energy" is being held back. To be able to issue this invitation, I have to know that

113

such a thing is possible. I know a rather unusual fact here: When one's good energy is missing, one can go inwardly looking for it and come to sense a kind of "where"—a subjectively touchable "place" where it is tied up.

(*Long silence*)

Note the long silence. What is she doing during it? What she says next will show what she did.

C4: I have lots of energy there, but it's tied up.

C4: Here she has found her energy and she senses directly that it is tied up. It is there but tied up.

T4: You can feel your energy right there, but it's tied up.

C5: Yes.

T5: Can you sense what's tying it up?

T5: I invite her to sense directly what is in the way.

(*Long silence*)

The silence seems to indicate that she is actually able to do as I asked, to sense directly what is tying it up. But of course only her next response will show if that is what she is doing in the silence.

C6: It's like a heavy wall in front of it. It's behind that.

C6: This phrasing shows that she is indeed sensing directly an obstacle, a wall, and sensing her energy behind it. However, a therapist should still wonder if this is *only* the visual image of a wall, or if it *also* refers to something directly sensed.

T6: You can feel a heavy wall.

T6: I ask her if she can actually feel it, but in the form of a tentative reflection, "You can feel. . . ." If she hadn't been feeling it, this would invite her to do so.

(*Long silence*)

Note this third long silence. Again it marks the coming of a third step. What she says next shows what came of attending to the heavy wall.

C7: It's a whole part of me that I keep in.

C7: "A whole part of me that I keep in" certainly shows she is directly sensing something there. It is a big step to get from where she began to this.

T7: Did you say a "whole" part? [I thought she might have said "old."]

114

C8: Yes, a whole part of me, like when I say it's OK when it's not. The way I hold everything in.

C8: By "hold in" she means that she says "OK" when she would wish to say "no" to someone, "not OK." She does not get angry, does not fight back. Does she *now* have something that is not OK that she holds in? I am sensitized to this possibility, but wait. Without more evidence I do not want to distract her.

(*Long silence*)

Note the long silence again. What she says next indicates that she has been sensing this "part" directly.

There's a part of me that's dead, and a part that isn't.

Note the content mutation during the silence. Now she has *two* parts, one dead, and one that is not dead. Another step has taken place!

T8: Two parts, one is dead, and one . . . ah —

C9: Survived.

(*Silence*)

C10: It wants to scream.

C10: This shows she is quite directly sensing it. She can sense it wanting to scream.

T10: The dead part wants to scream and be let out.

T10: I am unsure but guess that its wanting to scream is a wanting to be let out. This is an instance of sensing for a positive growth direction. Of course my words here are tentative.

C11: To live.

C11: She confirms it with an even stronger word. It wants "to live."

(*Long silence*)

We have come a long way now, and she is in contact with a wanting to live. If we can keep *this*, it would be quite enough. Hopefully whatever she does in this silence will not lose this part and its desire to live.

C12: And there's also something vague. I can't get what that is.

C12: Still another step, something new came.

T12: Make a space for that vague thing. You don't know what it is yet. There's something vague there, but it isn't clear what it is.

T12: I want to help her to hold on to the new "vague" thing that came. "Make a space for" means to say, all right, the vague thing is, as it were, "here," and the other parts are "there," and "there." She knows how to make this space from earlier times of focusing.

C13: I feel a lot of tension.

T13: Okay, take a break. Just step back a little bit. There's the vague thing, and then also there's the tension. Let's talk a little. You've come a lot of steps.

(Client relaxes, then shifts in her chair.)

T14: Yes, that's right. Let the body get whole again, when we come a long way there have to be little breaks.

C15: It's hard to take a break.

T15: That's why I'm talking, I'm just saying anything so you can have a break.

C16: Yes, I'm getting a break because I'm listening to what you're saying.

(She shifts in the chair again.)

C17: Now I'm going back.

T17: There was a vague thing, and tension.

C18: It's like I want to run.

T18: Step back just a little step, and be next to the wanting to run.

(Long silence)

C19: Someone will be *mad at me if I let that part live*, and that's very uncomfortable.

C13: She shows strain. She has come so many steps so quickly; a break would help. When one's body is strained in focusing it is good to take at least a short break, to let the body feel whole again.

T13: I am aiming at a short rest that would let her body ease. If she actually takes a break, it will be visible.

I can see, visually, that her body has eased.

C15: She means she has been pulled very strongly toward what she sensed, and it is difficult for her to let go and take a break.

T15: I talk to keep her break going, and tell her exactly what I am doing.

T17: I remind her of the last two things that came.

T18: This is a typical focusing instruction. She says, "I want to run." My response turns it into a something, a wanting to run, a something that she can be next to.

C19: Apparently she has stayed next to the feeling, because another step has occurred. The "wanting to run" has opened, and she can sense what it is. Again this is a big step, an opening. With someone else, it might have taken a long time for this step to come because "wanting to run" is a difficult thing to stay with long enough so that it can open, and let one sense what is implicit in it.

T19: If you let that live, someone will be mad at you, and that's hard to stand.

C20: Yes.

(*Long silence*)

C21: I want to run and never look back, and just be free.

C21: After the long silence she is still speaking from the same spot. It is not a new step, but she was able to stay with it through the silence.

T21: You want to run, just not look back, go free.

T21: I cannot know if this running and being free is good or bad. Being free sounds good. Running sounds bad. But I do not need to know, and I should not decide. I reflect it as she said it.

(*Silence*)

C22: Then that's sad.

C22: Now it is clear that running and being free in just this way is not so good; it is sad.

T22: Somehow it feels sad, if you run and don't look back.

C23: Yes. Running from the vague thing is sad.

C23: Here it becomes clear. Running and not looking back would leave the "vague thing" behind.

(*Long silence*)

C24: Some of me wants to find out what the vague thing is. Some of me doesn't.

T24: You can feel a part of you that doesn't want to find out, and a part that does.

(*She looks angry.*)

T25: Be friendly to this place, just step back a little bit, like, "OK, this could take a while; it's OK if it takes a week to find out, slowly." Make room for a part that doesn't want to find out, a part that does.

C26: I don't feel friendly. I want to . . . jump on it.

C26: Here is the typical case. She does not feel friendly towards it, as I had asked her to feel.

T26: Yes, that's what I thought. Well, make a space for the anger too. The anger

T26: There is a way of "making separate spaces" for the various currents that con-

117

gets to be here too. Just don't let it get on this thing. Let the anger flow through.

flict with each other. One can make room for one's anger, and still also save a space for something (such as "the vague thing") that has not opened yet, so that the anger does not push it away.

(*Long silence*)

C27: I'm very angry.

C27: She senses her anger now, not just in order to make room for the vague thing. The anger is here now in its own right.

T27: Lots of anger.

(*Long silence*)

C28: It's a big loss, something missing. That's what the vague thing was.

C28: Another step. The vague thing is a big loss, something big is missing. Often a step of physical opening up reveals a whole new layer, and yet, in terms of information, one might not seem to know that much more. Still there is a whole step from "something vague" to "a big loss, something missing."

T28: A big loss, something big missing.

(*Long silence*)

C29: And my energy is right there too.

C29: This is quite a change. She feels a flow of energy released, and she feels much better.

T29: So that's also where your energy is. It is there with the vague thing that turned out to be a big loss of something big, missing.

C30: Yes, I feel lighter!

T30: It feels better.

C31: Yes, I don't know what that is yet that's missing, but even though I don't know what it is, I feel lighter. I feel all right inside myself again.

C31: She will mark and keep the spot at which the "vague thing" is and the energy was freed. That spot is her new frontier. During the rest of the day and the next few days she will sense it there, again and again; if she can. Sometimes a client can do that only with the therapist.

This segment with silences had taken the better part of the hour. Both the client and I knew that it was enough having taken so many steps, and having reached an especially good stopping point. The rest of such an hour would be spent talking about something else, perhaps, or as in this instance, going into the kitchen to have tea.

Because the client had spent such a large portion of this session in silence, and because she knew of my strong beliefs in focusing, I felt I must ask her:

T: You're not mostly doing focusing because it's my thing, are you? I'm glad to *talk* things out too.

C: Hell no. I don't do anything I don't want to. I mostly *can't* say anything when I'm quiet. It's too sore. If I had to talk I couldn't stay with it.

T: That's fine, I didn't mean you should talk. Just making sure you're doing it as it feels right.

There were times when I asked her if we should stop — when I sensed that too many steps were happening in one session, that her body needed a rest. For me, having spent so many years developing how to deepen therapy, it was ironic that I would be the one to suggest having small talk or tea! Over tea our small talk was generally animated and enjoyable.

Discussion of Excerpt A

We are now accustomed to the fact that people can sense different parts of the self. We should not fixate on the parts. Sometimes they seem stable; at other times they change rather quickly.

For example, here she first senses (behind that wall) *a part* of her that holds everything in. Then she soon says, "There's a part of me that's dead, and a part that isn't." Now we do not need to know whether one of these two parts is still the same as the part from before that holds everything in. It may still be one of those two; or perhaps not. The inner geography of such parts may remain, or it may change in the process. We want to allow the parts to be as they are found and sensed in each moment. It might stop the process if either client or therapist were to try artificially to stabilize the parts, or to merge them. Notice how the process moves *on its own*, from inside, as she simply senses what is there.

Soon she says that the dead part wants to scream and live. After the silence, when she says, "And there's also something vague," we need not ascertain whether this is yet a third part, in addition to the alive and dead ones, or whether the geography has changed somewhat. Now there is also a wanting to run. As it turns out, the running would leave the vague part behind. So one might say that again there are two; the vague part and the one that wants to run. But we do not need to stop the process in order to find out if these two are the same or different from the earlier two.

119

It would only get in the way if we attempted to make a cognitive map of these parts, and tried to keep them stable, or to merge them. If the client or I had made a conceptual map at any point, the next step would have altered it. I hope the reader can observe that each time her next step could not have been derived logically from the previous point. What emerges at each of her steps is different and also much finer and more intricate than what one could derive from any conceptual map.

EXCERPT B

This and the remainder of the excerpts come from sessions that took place one year after the first. There were times when suicide seemed very possible; the client was dealing with an early feeling of unwantedness, and later on, on top of that, some very bad childhood experiences. She often experienced states of intense anger and moods in which "then" felt like now.

It was all I could do, at the end of each session, to extract a promise from her that she would call if the suicide urge got too bad. She would deliberate each time before making this promise. This is a vitally important agreement.

I also would say, "If the process gives you a rest, that's good; don't push. If it opens, call." But such a wide invitation to call should be extended only if the therapist can expect to be able to welcome calls over the long haul.

Sometimes she had a very angry feeling and a voice in her head that told her just to leave, that she did not belong anywhere, that it was no use. She knew that this feeling came from the past, but the knowing got very thin and did not help her make it through the days.

During small talk between us it would be evident to me that she was all right for the time being. Several times when that did not seem so, I would interrupt the small talk: "It's not OK yet. Right?" She would sigh and say, "No." Then we would go back into the therapy room for a while longer.

Early in therapy I may tell a client that it is all right to do something like scream into a pillow, or pound on the couch. I do this when I sense a lot of pent-up emotion that is not coming out. I demonstrate it myself, kneeling in front of the couch with my arms over my head, making fists, then pounding on it a few times. I say "You might want to do this some time. If you feel that way, you can just do this." It is a generalized invitation, to be taken up whenever it fits.

Twice this client pounded and kicked for some 10 minutes or more, and then she felt better. Each time it concerned a different experience from the past. You can therefore assume, throughout these excerpts, that she knows she can do this. I do not decide when it should be done once a client knows it is an option. At times I may suggest it when I see that the client's feet are already tapping. In the following segments she does not look that way except where I indicate it.

C1: I've been very heavy all week.

T1: Mmm.

C2: It felt like . . . like . . . last week I got in touch all right, that unwantedness was very heavy with me all week.

T2: That whole experience . . . of . . . unwelcomeness . . . was very heavy for you.

C3: Feel like I'm crumbling. That shakiness inside, and . . . I felt real shaky about coming here.

T3: It would be nice if we could first ease it. Let's make a little space and stand back a little from it . . . and say, "Oh yes . . . that's right to be there . . . It feels like . . . it feels at least like there's going to be a lot of stuff crumbling, and it's going to be very . . . shakymaking." . . . It feels like that now at least . . . do you know, like if a building were going to crumble, you would stand back half a block.

C4: Hmm. We don't know how much crumbling it needs, but —

(Long silence)

C5: Yes, I feel a little bit back, but —

T5: Hmm, spend a few minutes until you can have a nice feeling about this, like, there's going to be a big change, and —

C6: I think I have that, I got in touch with that, but it's not a bad feeling. And for a while there was a place inside me (. . . *inaudible* . . .) but now there is a *scary* feeling.

T6: So you *are* to one side. . . . [C: Hmm.] So let's be with the "scary" for a minute; perhaps we can be with the "scary" first. I'm in favor of always feeling very comfortably situated about something *un*comfortable, very securely placed about something *insecure*. . . . You have that mostly. . . . Let's hear from the scary part. You feel good . . . but scary.

T3: It is early in therapy. I am teaching focusing. She feels a "crumbling." I think it means that a lot will crumble. Whatever it means, before going into it, I try to generate the focusing type of space, in which a pretty solid "I" stands over against whatever comes. This is the first movement of focusing, called "making a space."

C4: She modifies what I said. Then she tries to make the space of "standing back" as I suggested.

C6: She says she has that place to stand already, and the big change I am talking about is *not* a bad feeling. It does not require standing back. But there is also a scary feeling.

T6: I move with her to the scary feeling, still trying to establish a good standpoint from which to feel it. This is a little too much teaching/guiding. Whether it helps or not, I will surely drop it for now, after all this.

121

(*Silence — 80 seconds*)

C7: The scary part, . . . that's the crumbling feeling. . . . (*Silence — 30 seconds*) The scary part is that I'd be alone, and if I crumble how will I (*inaudible*)?

T7: How will you build?

C8: How will I rebuild?

T8: How will I rebuild. Right, right. So there are really two things. . . . There may be more. . . . There are questions in the "scary." And one of them is about being alone.

T8: Note her correction. Having already responded to the "rebuild" part, I say the "alone" part here. I forgot before.

C9: Mmm. (*Silence — 10 seconds*) Yes, that's different. . . . I'm usually real willing to be alone, but now it feels different.

T10: There is an "alone" you know, and —

C10: Right now it's different, and I touched on, uh, not to be alone is a good feeling. . . . [T: Hmm] But now, somehow I'm in between the two. [T: Hmm]

C10: She means she has always been able to be alone in a good way. Now, newly, it feels good *not* to be alone. But this minute she feels neither alone in the old way, nor really in contact either.

T10: So it's real scary to know the "*un*alone," and maybe it changes how well you can be alone. . . . There's some difference; you're not in your . . . solid place, you're —

C11: Definitely, definitely, . . . it's more of an insecurity, like a feeling of, . . . (*silence — 15 seconds*) that I couldn't feel that comfortable. (. . . *inaudible*)

T11: This in between place is not as comfortable.

C12: No.

T12: And it has something to do with experiencing some closeness . . . or connected . . . or something . . . or *not* alone.

T12: I know it probably has to do with the client's relation to me, but I add nothing to what she says because just touching it this far is hard for her. The simple reflection response also *keeps*, *makes*, and *is* the closeness I spoke of.

(*Silence — 50 seconds*)

122

C13: ... (*Inaudible words*) I feel really vulnerable.

T13: Mmm.

(*Silence — 1 minute*)

C14: My defenses are gone. . . . There's some different strength. I'm vulnerable, and also there's something new there.

T14: You still feel the vulnerable, and something new also came, a strength.

C14: Here having sat nearly a minute with the insecurity and the "not alone," something new arose, a strength.

Discussion of Excerpt B

This is how process steps come. No one could manufacture "a different strength" out of the pieces that were present before. We can speculate that such new contents come because the process in this situation is interactional and personally close — or it could have been otherwise. But the contents came because both people gave time, room, and received what inwardly came.

Between C12 and C14 something very important has come. Prior to and at C12 she finds a sense of being related or connected (to someone), and she no longer feels that old solidly alone feeling to which she is accustomed. This makes her anxious. I only reflect back what she conveyed. At C14 the anxious feeling is still there, but she also finds "some different strength . . . something new there."

A new strength in wanting to be related to others is just what we would hope a person might find when the old isolation breaks. But if this sense of new strength did not *come* somehow of its own accord, we would not know how to provide it.

We must ask: Why did I not mention our relationship, so that it could be worked on? There are certainly times when a client speaks indirectly about the relationship, and it is right for the therapist to bring this out in the open, or at least to ask: "You mean you and me, right here?"

I was nearly certain that the relatedness which she found threatening was the ongoing one, with me. Had she said that, I was ready to talk about it. She might then have said more about just what felt threatening about it. I would have affirmed the safety of the relationship *in words*. She might have gone into her history to explore why any relatedness felt threatening to her. This sort of exploration is frequently helpful in therapy. But what is *more* helpful is *a concrete experience* of safety in the actual happening of relating.

I say absolutely nothing additonal here that would further threaten this hard-to-bear feeling. In refraining from anything more than saying it back, I am letting the relationship *actually be safe*, rather than centering on why it feels unsafe.

A moment of actual safe relating is worth much more than focusing on feeling unsafe.

The next moment she senses the new strength along with the anxious feeling. At that moment she *is* in relation. What she senses just then is herself in this ongoing interaction, and although she did not expect it, she senses a strength.

We see the role of the interpersonal relationship in determining what content one will find inside. *What* one finds inside is made directly from *how* one is concretely living just then. And our living *is* interactional. Therefore the quality of the interaction determines what one will find when one senses what is there just then.

A therapist must be conscious of the quality of the actual interaction, and must make that very safe at all times, but especially while the client focuses on feeling unsafe. If the *experience* of safety can concretely happen, the old threat will be experienced within a wider new experience of safe relating. Then, if the client focuses, new steps (such as her new strength) can come.

EXCERPT C

May 27

C1: I don't feel very good today.

(*Silence — 1 minute*)

C2: It's like I want to run or something again.

T2: The "wanting to run" is back.

C3: But now a yellow light goes on and says, "wait!"

T3: Yeah, now we have something that keeps you from running, that says wait, wait, wait a minute —

C4: And it's like I feel so shaky inside; all day I couldn't function.

T4: Hmm, that "shaky" too is there, that "shaky" that says something is about to open up there.

T4: At other times "shaky" has turned out to be a sense of something coming or opening, so I assume that. It is very often helpful to say the edge that seems to be there.

(*Silence — 15 seconds*)

C5: I don't know what it says.

C5: Note that she corrects me: "I don't know what it says." It is clear that she knows that I am interested only in what *is*

124

there; I do not care about being right or wrong. She wastes no time on what I said, or on being careful about correcting me. She stays trying to sense what *is* there.

T5: We don't know yet.

T5: I accept her correction with as little interruption of the process as possible.

(*Silence — 150 seconds*)

C6: It feels like a river that's dammed up.

C6: During the silence something new has come from focusing on the "shaky."

T6: Something real powerful that needs to flow and it's stopped, it needs to break the dam.

T6: I am all for letting it out. At the very next step, however, it becomes clear why this is not easy to do.

(*Silence — 40 seconds*)

C7: But it's poisoned.

T7: Okay, let's go gently. . . . (*Silence — 15 seconds*) Something about it is poisoned, or there's a feeling that it's poisoned.

T7: Now I am glad not to have pushed for something at T6. Whatever "poisoned" will turn out to be, it needs to be processed first. But again, no such decision is made by me. At the most, I add a focusing attitude, such as being gentle.

Discussion of Excerpt C

Should the client have been encouraged to pound the couch or to ride out on this dammed up "river"? Can we sense that "poisoned" says, all in one word, that merely going forward on the "river" urge and rolling past the "dammed up" feeling might not be the right thing to do? Please reread C6 and C7. C6 might make one want to encourage a catharsis, a "letting it out." Many therapists would think so. But C7 indicates that the quality is not quite right. Some things must first be processed, probably in small experiential steps, before a "rolling out" would be advisable. Regardless, it is not the therapist who should decide, either to push people or to hold them back. She knows she can pound on the couch if she wants to.

When very sensitive or problematic feelings first come, my immediate response is very often something like: "Go gently now," or "Now go easy," or "Let's go very slowly now. . . ." Such a feeling needs an extra gentle space, so that it can be further sensed without pushing into it too fast, or too crudely.

She had begun with the image of a yellow (traffic) light, a caution light. Then her sense of "something dammed up" conveys life-energy trying to move forward. Hearing of this we are glad. Life wants to move forward! Then it is painful to hear her say, "But it's poisoned." Whatever *that* is, we must not just push into it. We want to stay close to it, without big sudden movements. We want to give it a slow and gentle space to be in.

Notice that neither of us directs the process here in any way. Neither of us tries to foist anything onto it, or avoid anything that comes. Aside from receiving each thing, I only offer instructions concerning *how* to receive, sense and hold on to what comes of its own accord from her direct sensing.

EXCERPT D

June 11

(*Hour begins with a 70-second silence.*)

C1: I feel real restless inside like —

T1: Mmm.

C2: Like I just don't want to sit; I don't want to stand. . . . I even felt like crying at work.

T2: So, hello! Something wants to come through, and we better have contact, right? Hello, hello! hello? (*Moves chair closer.*)

(*Silence — 150 seconds*)

C3: It's like something inside me is going to blow.

(*Silence — 50 seconds*)

C4: I should be alone.

C4: In the 50 seconds of silence, this is what has come. It is that angry voice that often tells her negatives, such as "Why are you here anyway if you won't talk . . . ?" or "Go home."

T4: Is this the thing that says you shouldn't be here?

C5: Hmm.

T5: Hello. It says you shouldn't be here, you should be alone. (*Silence — 25 seconds*) So something in there is about to blow, or it feels like that, and it's tremendously shaky, right?

T5: Note the "it." Without long lectures or arguments, I set the superego off as, "it tells you. . . ." After a silence I want to help her return to where she was before the negative voice interrupted. Very often such a "voice" interrupts the person's contact with something. But my judgment is tentative, and leads only to a reflection of what had just been there. The reflection is a little out of phase (it refers to C3). Her next steps are free to come in whatever way they will. If I am wrong the steps can show it.

126

C6: Right.

T6: And it's like you can't stand or sit or nothing, . . . and that's one thing that's there, and the other thing says you shouldn't be here, right?

C7: Right.

T7: You should be alone. That's that unfriendly one that says, "If you're not going to say anything, why are you here?"

C8: No.

T8: Different, different thing.

C9: No, it's not that, 'cause if I don't want to say anything I'm not gonna say a God-damned thing.

T9: Yeah. Good.

(*Silence — 120 seconds*)

C10: Like a push–pull . . . inside me.

(*Silence — 10 seconds*)

T10: Mmm.

C11: It's like I can just stand so much closeness right now.

T11: Mmm.

C12: Like I was feeling I'd like you to sit beside me and not hold me.

T12: Mmm . . . it's in both directions. . . . Something really wants some closeness, . . . and something else . . . (*inaudible*). Can

---

C6: She corroborates that what T5 referred to is still there, and she is glad to have it responded to.

T6: With that corroboration, I respond more fully to what was there before the interruption. I make my characterization of the two issues neutral: a step might come from the part that I do not like, the "you shouldn't be here" part.

T7: Because she said "right," I go on to deprecate the negative voice.

C8: She shows I am wrong somehow.

T8: As simply as possible, I retract, so as to leave room for whatever *is* there.

C9: Even so, she has to spend time explaining to me that the negative voice does not bother her. If *she* does not want to talk, she will not; it does not matter what the voice says. But she would not have to digress into that, had I not brought up the "unfriendly" (T7) assumption about the voice telling her to go home if she will not talk.

T9: I want to get out of the way as fast as possible, so she can get back to her own track.

C10: This comes after a very long silence.

C12: In previous hours she has sometimes asked to be held when she wanted more closeness. Here she is saying that she wants more closeness but not to be held.

T12: I want to respond to both sides of the "push–pull," and in such a way that each side has its own separate space. Of we do that? (We move to the couch to sit beside each other without holding.)

T13: It knows just exactly what feels right just now.

course the response in action is the main response.

T13: Here I indicate that the request is welcome, and express some joy at the fact that she could sense so finely what would feel right.

Discussion of Excerpt D

It is generally important to encourage clients to sense for what would be right, at the moment, to let the process direct both of us. When that happens, I often express gladness about it.

At T12 her process produces a solution that is very characteristic of the focusing process. She wants more closeness and also cannot stand more.

Throughout she has been one of those clients who needs some physical contact to feel that the connection is real, indeed sometimes in order to feel that anything is still real. When directly asked for, I gladly provide some moments of clearly nonsexual physical contact.

But right now the childhood experiences that are coming back to her are too painful for her to have them in the presence of another person. And yet, just because they are so painful, she needs the contact all the more. What comes to her to do is characteristically more intricate than the two sides of that dilemma.

I give nonsexual hugs or holding when asked. I do not offer them. Therapists must refrain from sexual or sexually confusing actions of any kind, but physical touch is often asked for to make the contact real.

"Sit beside me and not hold me" in one sense brings me closer, but with the assurance that there will not be any holding or touching. And since I will not be sitting opposite her, I will not be looking at her. In that respect the contact will be less direct.

Of course I am willing for that finely shaped solution, but, even so, I *ask*, "Can we do that?" as I make an initial move toward the empty seat on the couch. I give her a chance to say, "No . . . wait . . ." in case she had not meant for me actually to do it immediately.

Again here, if discussions of all this were needed, either of us could begin them. Such discussions could also instance a relating that would be both close and safe. The actual relating always counts more than the relationship as a topic of discussion.

EXCERPT E

June 16

C1: I just feel really shitty.

C1: During this period the client began each hour very depressed. Other clients might spend the whole hour remaining depressed. Notice how she moves out of this and what I do to engender the steps that move her out of it.

T1: Mmm, mmm.

C2: I just can't go on like this.

(*Silence — 50 seconds*)

T2: Are they bad feelings from that . . . same . . . part of the past?

C3: It feels like . . . shipwrecked or something . . . I can't . . . (*inaudible*).

T3: They're all on this . . . (*inaudible*).

C4: Yeah, it feels like *now*, but —

T4: It feels like now but it is that theme, or that time, but it feels like now.

(*Silence — 40 seconds*)

C5: It feels like now but it isn't. It feels like it doesn't matter.

T5: *Now* it feels like that.

C6: And that's the only . . .

T6: The only thing there is, is *then*.

> **T6:** I acknowledge that merely knowing it comes from then does not help much. The "then" seems here now.

(*Silence — 30 seconds*)

C7: Like the only thing I feel all right about is (*inaudible*) The rest is —

T7: It really *does* feel like that, *now*.

(*Silence — 120 seconds*)

C8: It feels like . . . (*inaudible*) pain inside me, and I can't, it just gets —

T8: More pain in there than you can . . . feel or . . . stand? It just gets . . . what, did you say?

C9: It gets worse.

T9: It gets worse, uh huh. . . . So the way we have it right now, the way we have it con-stellated, getting into it makes it worse. . . . (*silence — 15 seconds*) We need to come at it some other way or from some other angle.

> **T9:** It might have been this way: There are times when it is clear that one cannot go into something. Then the idea that "we need to come at it some other way" can be helpful.

(*Silence — 12 seconds*)

129

C10: No, it's like . . . *feels* worse. It's always been there . . . it's not . . . it's that it's uncovered.

C10: She indicates that this is not how it is. It is not an issue of coming at it from a different angle. Rather it "feels worse" because now it is open.

T10: It's like?

C11: Uncovered.

T11: Uncovered. Oh, it's not that *we're* making it worse, that wasn't right what I said. It's always been there.

T11: Now I understand.

(*Silence — 5 minutes*)

C12: It's like . . . it doesn't feel dead anymore . . . 'cause it's throbbing.

T12: Mmm (*takes a breath*) . . . so in another deeper way we're glad it's alive. . . .

T12: I think that she might be glad, but in case she is not glad, I want to introduce that possibility. Of course such "gladness" would not cancel out the pain. The breath is my own relief that "worse" did not have to do with our interaction. Nonverbally such inadvertent natural expressions on my part make for more presence without anything being imposed. She can say she is not glad, and I am prepared to respond to that.

(*Silence — 5 minutes*)

T13: Hello.

T13: After 5 minutes of silence I make contact.

C14: Hi —

C14: She responds, then continues the silence.

C15: It's real (*inaudible*).

T15: It's real . . .?

C16: Real cutting.

T16: Oh (*sighs*).

(*Silence — 30 seconds*)

C17: Lying there and it's like I'm lying around bleeding.

C17: The old experience is vividly relived.

T17: Mmm . . . real cutting and like you're bleeding.

(*Silence — 150 seconds*)

C18: (*inaudible*)

T18: Bleeding and all exposed.

C19: (*inaudible*)

C19: We assume she said something like what I respond to in T19. The past

130

feels like now and I seem like the people in her past experience, who hurt her.

T19: Mmm mmm, it's like I'm going to hurt you.

C20: It feels like it's now. I get anxious.

T20: Mmm. It makes you anxious that . . . *I'm* going to hurt you, *now*.

C21: It's like whatever you *say* right now, it would hurt me.

T21: Mmm mmm . . . I couldn't say hardly anything without hurting.

(*Silence — 10 seconds*)

C22: It's like . . . I have a sudden sense that there is something that isn't exactly (*inaudible*), almost like an underneath message that (*inaudible*).

T22: Mmm. You can sense yourself . . . and you don't like it. You can sense yourself expecting, or looking for . . . some kind of bad message from me.

(*Silence — 10 seconds*)

C23: (*Inaudible*) . . . And the reason I said, "When are you going away" was because and you said, "I'm *only* going away Friday and Saturday. . . ."

C23: She refers to an earlier time. She took the word "only" as a criticism, as if I had said, "How can you be upset about that?" Note how in the midst of this painful reliving of her past there is a need to straighten a very fine-tuned aspect of her present relationship with me.

T23: It's an example of how oversore it is. Mmm.

(*Silence — 50 seconds*)

C24: (*Inaudible*)

T24: Mmm, you mean that's how you felt, so it's how you felt. Why . . . criticize it? . . . Did I understand what you meant? I'm not sure.

C25: There seemed to be a message, like (*inaudible*).

T25: It seemed as if what I was saying duplicated an old place, "Why is she so sensitive?"

C26: Not real bad, like I wasn't —

T26: I understand, I didn't mean that anyway.

C27: I know.

T27: I know you're saying it brings home how sore it is right now.

T27: I understand that she knows my real attitude. *Both* the actual present and the reinstanced past are here and real. But a lot of talking would get in the way. A moment of interaction with the right quality is all that is needed, in addition to listening.

(*Silence — 90 seconds*)

T28: Hi.

T28: A moment of contact helps the silent struggle, without necessarily interrupting. She can go on being silent. Also, I still feel the need to interact warmly after my seeming criticism which she just mentioned.

C29: There are so many (*inaudible*) in that thing (*inaudible*).

T29: There are more feelings there than you can stand . . . all at once. It's like . . . more than we can sort out. . . . (*Silence — 10 seconds*) And there is at least the unwantedness, . . . and it feels like . . . abused on top of it.

(*Silence — 5 minutes*)

C30: (*Inaudible*) I need to feel you're connected.

(*Silence — 20 seconds*)

T30: That should not be hard. . . . (*Moves chair closer*) I guess you can't quite feel it.

C31: I feel your presence, sure — if you don't preach at me.

C31: She says this with much warmth and a sparkle in the eyes, teasing.

T31: (*Laughs*) How nice!

C32: Anyone preaches at me —

T32: Did I do that?

C33: No, not very often . . . few times . . . not too often.

T33: Not too often —

(*Silence — 60 seconds*)

C34: (*Makes some noise, looks up a certain way*)

T34: Some tea, is that the right time?

C35: Yeah, I think so.

Discussion of Excerpt E

In efforts to help, I had previously often told her to try to distinguish then and now. I said that if she could really feel the experience in its context then, it would free up the situation now. It did not help here, and she called it "preaching." Here I already know not to do that anymore.

She is reliving very painful experiences. She says "it's like I'm lying around bleeding" as though it were a metaphor. Much later she could say much more about these experiences. One horrendous experience did involve bleeding. But I know that she is uncovering and reliving some whole experience as if it were now, although she verbalizes only small bits of it.

With another person I might have been asked to explore why I had been defensive about going away "*only*" Friday and Saturday. Inside myself I would have found something along the lines of: "Yes, I was trying to fix it. I was worried you would find it hard. Yes, I was avoiding your feeling instead of asking about it. I avoided it unconsciously." Showing her some of what really went on inside myself would let her experience that I had not meant it as a criticism of her, as if to say, "Shame on you. How can you feel bad about just two days?" But here no such discussion was needed. She already knew that I did not mean it as a criticism, and she already felt how the events of her childhood had made for this sense of being criticized. Had we not understood each other so easily at each turn here, more would have been said. As it was, once again the concretely healthy interaction is worth more than all the discussion.

Having expressed her sense of being criticized, and felt our fresh interaction, she can now return to her childhood experiences in another long silence (1½ minutes). Then she turns to the relationship again, asking for more closeness. I move my chair forward. She teases me about "preaching" (about "then and now" being different).

During this whole period, of approximately a year, she would arrive heavily depressed, feeling "its no use," her energy backed up into her as if she were under a heavy weight. She would leave (as she does here) visibly better, with her energy moving forward. But the regularity of this was characteristic of her. (I have often had to let other clients go home as depressed as they came.) But the interaction in this hour was special for her, as she says in the next excerpt.

EXCERPT F

The session this excerpt records consisted of a dream told and worked with.

June 18

C1: My brother, we used to skate a lot together and really have fun doing that.

T1: Someone [in the dream] wanted to know if you could skate on your toes. Can you?

C2: Yes.

T2: You can?

C3: Yes, you stand straight up, and you go round and round.

T3: What's it mean to you?

(*Silence — 10 seconds*)

C4: It doesn't mean that much except a fun thing. . . . I used to do it sometimes just for fun or to show off.

T4: So how would you translate that: "Can you skate on your toes?" means "Can you have fun? Can you show off?"

(*Silence — 10 seconds*)

C5: It's like can you take time to have fun?

T5: Mmm.

C6: 'Cause it's a fun thing to me.

T6: There's some fresh air in that!

C1: She has just told a long dream with many disturbing family events. In midst of them she goes out to skate on her toes with her brother.

T6: I sense that there *could be* something positive and important in what she said, and that she does not sense it as important. "Fresh air" is a metaphor for something that feels like it brings life forward. Play and taking time to play, these can be major, vital themes that bring life forward.

C7: Mmm, like everything's not *that* serious, sort of. Can I let the other part of me —

T7: So that's important. Let's keep that, yes?

C8: And it was said in fun. Like it wasn't . . . almost like the person in the dream who said it was someone that I felt OK about.

C8: Here she corroborates my impression.

T8: So that really is an invitation to have fun . . . at the same time that this family stuff is . . . worked through. Is that right? I could parlay that into a good thing if you let me, but you have to see.

C9: OK, go ahead.

T9: Well, it's like, can you have fun while this family drama is worked out?

T9: Because she acquiesced I go further with it, then ask her to sense if what I said is right.

(Silence — 30 seconds)

C10: I think that fits! Yeah. (*Silence — 5 seconds*) Some contrast with the seriousness, like there are many different parts to the dream (*silence — 10 seconds*), like it moves from serious to not serious. It's not all —

C10: Here she does spend the silent time sensing if that is right—if some positive energy comes in response to it.

T10: It's not all serious.

T10: This is using her word from C7.

C11: No.

T11: There's some part that could have fun while the other part happens. Someone was going to be hanged, was that it?

T11: This refers to her dream, and follows her sense in C10 of a contrast. Applying that, I recall what was also happening in the dream, just before the skating.

(Later in the session, we are discussing the same dream.)

C12: I don't like the color gray.

T12: Why not?

C13: It's too drab, I like brighter things.

T13: Does that fit the gray?

T13: I mean, "Does that fit the way gray felt in the dream?"

(Silence — 10 seconds)

C14: Well . . . if I look at it another way, I sometimes feel, . . . but after the last day I was here —

T14: Yeah?

C15: I remember feeling . . . and thinking . . . like from how everything was so black? . . . I don't know what happened but I felt a hell of a lot better, the first time in a long time, after the other day, here. . . . I think I told you at the door —

T15: Mmm.

C16: It's like something lifted, something really got OK inside. I could *feel* it, and I remember thinking, "Well, now it's just gray, kind of. It's not all better; it's not all black; . . . it's more of a grayish.

C16: But how did such a positive thing come? The previous session to this was mostly silence.

T16: Oh, right!

C17: And that felt OK.

T17: Yes, sure —

C18: It was more of a . . . deep place saying, "Yeah, it's still gray, . . . but that feels OK; it changed from black to gray for me. It really did, the other day here.

T18: That's wonderful, . . . and gray is a kind of in-between thing that's —

C19: Mmm . . . I felt too it was like . . . I felt so much lighter after the other day but also knew, . . . like I didn't want to stop there. . . . Just continue to feel this, but it's quite OK; it'll keep moving as it needs to move, that was the gray.

C19: "It'll keep moving as it needs to move." That is my credo. But now, after a long time, it is also the client's own, experienced sense of it. It comes not from my saying so, but from "it" having often "moved as it needs to move."

T19: It's not a final gray, it's a gray that's not black anymore.

C20: It won't stay.

T20: And she respects it. Somebody respects it [in the dream].

C21: I think *I* do. And it was different too, like . . . you said to me on the way out, "If your process wants to open further in two hours, or tonight, or whatever." And you told me, and you told me . . . it was really a deep place like, "Yeah, I'm open there, Gene," and I really meant it. It was really different, like, before I said, "Yeah, I'm open," but . . . I always know I will, but this time it was from a really deep place.

C21: Here she quotes one of my earlier statements. During this crisis period I had urged her to call if she needed to or felt the pull toward suicide. I often asked her to promise to do so. Also, I told her to let it be, not push it. If the process did not open, if it were to give her a rest, she should let it be.

Like yeah, "I'm not gonna fight it, OK." I think that's part of it.

T21: Yes, yeah . . . OK. . . . So your own rigid part is respecting it.

C22: My own rigid part? . . . Yes, that's a good way of putting it.

T22: If there is one. . . . (*Laughs*)

C23: Well, there is.

T23: I'm just being careful.

C24: You don't have to be so careful now, because . . . I'm connected, feeling connected with you, . . . but when I'm not, watch out. (*Laughs*)

C24: This is similar to the teasing sparkle at the end of the last excerpt.

Discussion of Excerpt F

My interpretive statements are always questions, and I try them out a little bit at a time. Only if they "take" do I expand on them. T1–T5 are such small questions about her dream, her skating, and play. Because they are all confirmed, I can state something more at T6.

Therapists need to watch for anything positive or life-advancing, especially in the midst of terrible material. In Chapter 14, on dreams, I discuss this further. Play can be trivial, but it can also bring infinity and freedom from the triviality of much that we consider important.

Thurber said that tears of laughter are the most precious kind.

EXCERPT G

June 21

T1: Hello!

(*Silence — 18 seconds*)

C2: It's going to be hard for me to sit here.

T2: Are you saying you want to sit somewhere else or that it's hard to sit?

C3: It's hard to sit with this restless feeling.

T3: It's hard to . . . sit still with this jumpy restlessness inside.

(*Silence — 45 seconds*)

C4: It's like nervous.

T4: Mmm . . . mmm . . . it's nervous.

(*Silence — 45 seconds*)

C5: It's like I *need* to stand still, though. I'm just keeping myself busy or something since Monday.

T5: You do need to stand still and see how you feel —

C6: Yeah.

T6: Not keep yourself running so you won't feel?

T6: I think this is what she means by "keeping myself busy." Otherwise I would not say something like, "so you won't feel." This is not usually a helpful interpretation because people attribute enough negative motivation to themselves as it is.

(*Silence — 65 seconds*)

C7: It's like all I can feel is anxious.

T7: Mmm . . . so it's hard to be with that because as you . . . pay attention to what's there, all you get is anxious, and anxious is hard to sit with. Is that right?

T7: This is a response not just to "anxious" but also to her whole inner process and to her trying to sense.

C8: Mmm.

T8: Yeah, anxious is hard to sit with. . . . Hello! Thought I'd say hello, give you a break for a second. I'd like to.

T8: Again my "hello" is making contact. Also, because she finds it hard to be with the anxious feeling (and what goes with it), contact will help, and also give a moment's respite. Perhaps it will help to give the right distance to it.

C9: You got there and back? [This refers to trip I took.]

C9: She accepts the idea of a break. Had she not, I would have kept quiet.

T9: Yes.

C10: Looks like I won't.

T10: Oh, because of the airplanes going on strike —

C11: Yeah.

(*We talk for a minute about her planned trip. This is followed by a 15-second silence.*)

T11: Are you tapping it again?

C12: What came to me right now was . . . like I know what it's about . . . because it started when I was typing my dream, the one I did with you the other day. And, uh, I did active daydream with images, and I cried all the way through it; I couldn't stop crying, 'cause I really got into it. . . . it was awful, and since then I've been walking, and I couldn't —

T12: It's where that went, that went real deep and then it got stuck, isn't that right? And since then it's been jumpy.

C13: The part where it really got stuck was, . . . it was all okay about the people on the platform. It felt like a grieving there, and that was okay, but the other part, my father walking out and all that, I just wasn't ready to deal with it.

T13: Mmm mmm. Wait. There was a part of the active imagination you did that was all right.

C14: Yeah.

T14: But there was another part that had to do with him walking out, that part.

C15: Mmm.

T15: Did you go a ways with it and then got stuck in the middle of it being bad, or was it that you could sense it was going to be that way.

C16: When I started out it was fine; then I really got into it . . . um . . . it was sad. It was real different, trying to process it alone. There's a change there, because I could before. It felt real lonely, it felt awful!

T16: (*Laughs*) I have a part to play after all. It's different being able to relate to people. Used to be your way to do it was alone (*silence — 8 seconds*), but you can do more with other people, than you can do alone.

T16: Now her need for relating is not sore and bearly touchable. I can happily make overt that our relationship is being talked about, and affirm it.

C17: Well, the desire is there now, to be with other people. It's different.

T17: Here we are!

C18: I knew you would say that!

T18: All 4 billions of us, and me. (*Silence — 25 seconds*) Um, where'd you go?

C19: What?

T19: Did I interrupt? It's OK.

C20: (*Looks up.*)

T20: Where did you come from?

C21: I just touched the pain.

T21: Mmm.

C22: And then I started playing around again.

T22: So you know where it is, and you . . . *can* touch it, but it's pretty bad.

C23: Mmm.

(*Silence — 10 seconds*)

T23: It's all right to just touch it and then back away from it. Can you say that's all right? (*Silence — 10 seconds*) Then you don't have to play around. You can just know you're doing that . . . and take a break. (*Silence — 10 seconds*) That's a right way to do, just touch it and take a break.

(*Silence — 110 seconds*)

C24: I'd say that there is something in my way.

T24: Mmm.

(*Silence — 125 seconds*)

T25: There is something in the way?

C26: Yes.

T26: At the painful spot? [C: Yes.] Between you and it.

T18: I sense a change during the silence, away from the easy way we were just together.

C19: She was far away and did not hear me.

T19: I would like to manifest being present, but without getting in the way or interrupting. Though I know I did interrupt, contact at this point is vitally important.

C22: Indeed she was not able to stay long with the pain, and she means here that when I interrupted her she had already veered away from it.

T23: I wish she would just deliberately touch it, and then give herself a rest until she can touch it again. This is an example of the teaching of focusing.

T26: First I reflect (T25 and the first part of T26). When that is corroborated, then I am sure enough to say it as I think of it, "between you and it."

140

C27: Mmm . . . like I'm trying to climb a mountain or something and, uh, can't do it.

T27: Mmm, mmm, makes me think of climbing the mountain with the truck [an image from her dream].

C28: Mmm.

T28: You're trying to climb the mountain and you can't do it.

T28: Now I reflect what she has said. She did not pick up on the dream and, since I brought it up, I want it out of the way.

C29: Mmm.

T29: And do we know what the mountain is?

T29: This is a typical focusing reflection.

(*Silence — 104 seconds*)

C30: Mmm . . . it's like . . . I want to get to the top of the mountain so I can see everything clearly, but I don't think I want to go through the pain of getting there.

C30: She takes me up on sensing what the mountain is (i.e., what she can get from sensing it as a felt sense). But she probably would have done it without being prompted.

T30: Mmm. So from the top of *that* mountain you'll be able to see it all clearly, but there is a lot of pain still, . . . between you and . . . seeing it clearly, something that feels like it doesn't *want* the pain. . . . Is that right?

(*Silence — 10 seconds*)

C31: Yeah, I'm going to get hurt getting up there. (*Silence — 10 seconds*) I think I'm still looking at the routes how to get there.

T31: Still looking for the routes?

T31: I have no idea what she means. When that happens, I ask. I want to grasp and keep her company with every bit of experience.

C32: Other ways.

T32: Oh, I see. You'd like to find some other ways of getting there, than the pain?

C33: Mmm.

T33: Yeah, I got you.

(*Silence — 10 seconds*)

C34: Then something comes and says "Haven't you tried that long enough?"

T34: Mmm (*laughs*).

C35: It isn't working.

T35: I see. Uh-huh.

(*Silence — 155 seconds*)

C36: Let's have some tea.

T36: Mmm . . .

(*We retire to the kitchen, make small talk, and have tea. Later, still in the kitchen, she is quiet.*)

T37: Are you tapping it again?

C38: Yes. It's restless again when I don't feel the pain.

T38: Maybe there is a place where you can be *closer* to the painful spot but not be in it.

(*Silence — 4 minutes*)

C39: It's okay now. I put the restlessness down, and I put the pain far away, and you know what made it okay? It was imagining *playing*!

C35: She means there will not be a way around the pain.

C36: Note the long silence. It was a long time to be with the pain, or to be trying to touch it.

T36: I am glad she wants to take a break. The capacity to stay with what is there takes time to develop. Tapping, then resting makes one stronger. Except for the few exchanges recorded here, she had been doing that for most of an hour. It is time for a break.

C38: She means that the restlessness comes when she loses direct contact with the pain. That is characteristic. As painful as something is, directly sensing it eases the rest of the organism. When it is lost touch with, the diffuse discomfort returns.

T38: This is another standard focusing instruction.

C39: Note the long silence. This client knows focusing. "I put _____ down" is focusing terminology. She reports three separate active focusing moves: She put the restlessness down; she put the pain far away; and she let the "playing" in that she spoke of in Excerpt F. Note that such focusing moves are active. They require energy on the part of the person in relation to the "what is there." Performing such acts also strengthens the person in relation to experiences.

We can speculate that the "playing" came as she moved to "put down" the other two. When one "puts something down" the organism eases, and other energies *can* then come forward.

142

Discussion of Excerpt G

Later in these sessions there will be dramatic breakthroughs and more interesting content, but I am concerned with showing how the therapeutic process first develops.

We go forward on the assumption that it helps to let oneself feel one's pain and painful experience, but it does not always. We say it will help, but we rarely say how or why. It has to do with the manner of the process and the manner of the interaction. It is not just a question of being aware or unaware of some otherwise fixed content. It is how one is aware that brings steps of change in the content of one's difficulties.

Notice that the way focusing "taps it" and "puts it down" feels much better in the body than having to run and avoid it. When this client loses contact with the pain it makes her "restless" (C38). So this type of processing is neither the usual way of avoiding pain nor the usual way of feeling pain.

It is an active process. *She* taps the pain and *she* puts the pain far away again (C21 and C39). But it is not this "putting down" and its resultant loss of contact with the pain that makes her restless. Rather, it frees her body but still relates to the pain.

In focusing we say the "putting down" happens only when the whole body feels distinctly released. Otherwise we say "it has not been put down yet." This client put the pain far away. She acted upon it. And in the resulting space, which she made, a good feeling came in: the playfulness.

As an example of the focusing process, this has been an enormously eventful hour. But in terms of content nothing new emerged.

The client's dispersed "restlessness" returns as soon as she loses hold of the felt sense. While the felt sense is right there, the rest of her whole body eases because the acute feeling collects itself and becomes *a direct referent*. Without the felt sense, it disperses again and makes her whole body "restless."

The last interchange illustrates the focusing procedure of "making a space," neither bullying the problem, nor running away from it.

She uses the play place to enable her to put *both* down.

EXCERPT H

July 21

C1: Barrier is like . . . many different things.

T1: Oh . . . it's a lot of things, OK.

(*Silence — 20 seconds*)

C2: OK, this isn't going to make a bit of sense. . . . OK?

C1: She is saying what she had been sensing during a long silence that preceded this discussion.

C2: People are so used to others telling them that their own experience and imag-

143

ery does not make sense. They expect such a reaction.

T2: All right.

C3: What came to me was like, the image I have, when I got it I had an image of a fence, and part of it is really treacherous. It's like . . . barbed wire. . . . You don't touch that; you can't go through or get past it, but another part of it has a little hole, and that part I could slip through —

C3: This is an image that gives us exact instructions. One section is too tough to handle right now, but another part can be handled. There is also a hole in the fence through which, immediately, we can get to the other side. So of course we should go through to it, if that is possible.

She may know what is represented by these parts, or she may not. Probably she does. I do *not* need to know what they are. I can guess, but should not. If she had to say what the part is, which should *not* now be handled, she would be handling it. She does not. If she had tried to say what should not be handled now, I would have stopped her. Had she gone on anyway, I would have stopped her again and demanded that she sense if it really feels right to go on.

This client knows, without any doubt, to obey her process. I need to say nothing of all this.

T3: Ah, yeah.

C4: A part of it is . . . just poles and a little barbed wire, and I could really crawl over it if I wanted to. There's one part like, the far end that would be dangerous.

T4: That's the barbed wire part.

T4: I try to say back exactly what she meant.

C5: Yes.

T5: Yeah, yeah. There is a part that you could easily go across, and a part that is really dangerous.

T5: Again I am saying it back exactly.

C6: The part that felt the best right now was to crawl through that little hole, that felt —

T6: Yes.

C7: . . . like . . . felt like saying, "Here I am; I'm coming through," a really neat part coming through, and looking back to see

C7: Now it turns out she had a visual image of some part of her going through the hole, and obviously the felt sense of

144

the reaction, at the same time feeling, I don't care what the reaction is.

T7: Yeah!

T8: You're saying for right now what's important is for you to go through there on this good lead, to go through there —

C9: Yeah, that's right. Right now I need that . . . more than I need to deal with the barbed wire.

T9: Yup, that makes sense. Sounds like you can look at that later. Right now it's important that you go through.

(*Silence — 20 seconds*)

C10: Mmm. It's like there's a really good (*inaudible*) in that, that part coming through. . . . There's also a confidence that the other part will get there, but if that part can't get through, forget about looking at the other (*both laugh*).

T10: I can feel that. If this part can come through, we'll be fine!

C11: Yes, because that's the all right part of me . . . yeah (*silence — 10 seconds*) I feel good. (*Takes a deep breath*)

T11: (*Laughs*) . . . Mmm . . . (*We both laugh.*) . . . Mmm.

C12: Now I'm not hot. I was real hot!

T12: (*We both laugh.*) . . . Mmm . . . that makes me so happy when it gives us such exact instructions —

(*We make small talk.*)

(*Silence — 2 minutes, we hug.*)

doing so was marvelous. It looked back to see what the reaction was, and at the same time, did not care what the reaction was! There is a life-affirming, playful quality to this; it is also an independent sureness. If it is related to the playfulness in Excerpts F and G we do not need to know. Perhaps it is.

T8: This responds to C6, but certainly communicates that I agree.

T9: Again I only reflect, but tone and words also show that I very much agree.

T10: Again this reflects what she said, and adds that I also feel it.

T11: Here she expresses sheer gladness.

T12: This expresses what I feel. It also communicates my strong need for her to obey her process, to go by what is sensed as the right thing to do. It is usually (not here) hard for people to go by what the process needs next, or even to sense for it.

Discussion of Excerpt H

How to judge what to go into, what to just tap, what to put down? The therapist usually cannot decide. A therapist can only tentatively guess in a manner that invites the client to sense what is right. Here I did not need to invite her to do that. The client had learned it long ago.

This segment demonstrates perfectly why one should not just go pushing into anything in just any order. We depend for therapeutic change on a process that comes, but that also may not come. We do not fully understand that process or what causes it. We cannot therefore simply push and assume that going into something, in any arbitrary order or manner, will have good results.

When the process steps are allowed to unfold, they have their own order. One sits before something intolerable, as this client had done for some hours, and very little change of content, if any, may occur. Yet the whole territory is processed; as a whole it changes. As one stays, applying that sort of attention, the whole rearranges itself. Over the last few excerpts and therapy hours the words were few. There seemed to be little change in content. It was all about just being as close to the pain as the client could stand to be, but not so close as to cause her to want to run from it. Contact was important during those hours. Being able to "put _____ down" and "make space" is a different way to live with the pain. In this kind of living more implicit edges appear.

Now, quite of its own accord, the pain has two "parts." Also, quite of its own accord, one of the parts is clearly marked: *Not Now*. Another opening may be possible in the future, but right now the second part has already opened, and she feels it as very life-affirming.

She feels physically very different, "not hot" as in the first part of the hour. Relief shows all over her face and in her body posture.

Is she actually through the barrier, and on the other side? Yes, partially she is. If many steps of this kind can come, we will get across, of this we can be sure.

A bit of experience like this will stand as an instruction for the client and myself during subsequent sessions. There will be times when I will say: "Now wait. Is this the barbed wire part?" "Yes." "We aren't supposed to do that part until after we get through this part, remember?"

Of course I will not stop her endlessly if she feels it is right to go further into that topic, but certainly I will ask her to check, sense, and see, three or four times, if that is really the right thing to do.

The same bit of experience stands also as a positive promise: If she says, "It's useless," I can say, "Can you still find that little hole? It said you are able to get through, there."

Is this putting too much trust in a little image? It is not the image, but the message, that is so trustworthy. Consider the following: The message says that part of the pain is too tough to handle at first. What can be lost by believing

146

that? It says that another part is more right to take up first. What is the risk of believing that? It says that there is a way, right now, to get the positive energy of moving through the barrier and being all right. Who would want to oppose that?

So it is not a question of believing in an image. If it had been an image of hopelessness, I would have encouraged her not to believe it. I would say "Right now, the way it is constellated, there is no way, but that can change."

When change is happening how can we see it? How can we catch it? How can we understand it? Note that the change in this excerpt was not one of content. It is therefore easier to see. Even if the content had also changed, what is still most important is the change in the manner of being alive, the manner of process, the quality of energy, the life-affirming direction.

For example, the client in Chapters 4 and 5 had a sense of pulling back from challenges, and this sense opened up. What it really "was," emerged. There too I tried to call your attention to the change in manner of the sense. From being a hated obstacle, the "pulling back" revealed itself as "an all-good part" of her that would rather be dead than have her be wrongly judged. I tried to say that the important aspect of the change is not so much one of content, but rather a new manner of process, of ongoing living: She could feel as loving and protective something she had previously felt as stifling and frustrating.

New and more positive contents emerge from a new and more positive manner of process. I am not proposing false optimism. There are too many deeply ingrained psychological demons for it to be the case that if we do nothing, but with a positive attitude, everything will turn out all right. But *if* we enable ourselves to institute a positive manner of process, then it will not be mere optimism to look forward to more positive contents and blockages that resolve and wounds that heal. Without content it is easier to examine the manner of the process, and the process is changing.

What is changing is that some good energy is coming in. Playfulness comes in. But "playfulness" is just a word. If playfulness is thought of as content, the point will be missed. In playfulness is a different way of being alive, a willingness to engage the tough issues with an appetite for living, an ability to recall good times and a joy of life.

As the playful energy enters, what happens to the painful content and all its ramifications? Superficially nothing happens to it; it remains the same. It is "put" at some distance, in the focusing sense of "put." It remains unchanged, we think. It will be there to be dealt with later on. But in a deep way things are happening to it that need to happen. Before the content gets worked through explicitly, the whole thing will have changed implicitly in the ways it needs to change. That is why it will work through successfully by the time we take it up.

Without the preparatory change in attitude that is now happening the client might very well relive the content of her pain, perhaps cathart and cry, but the content would still be there afterward in the same way, with the same ramifications for her present life. Therefore we definitely want to let this kind of process come first.

The body works its own changes on the content implicitly even while we do not work with it explicitly. By tapping it, letting it in, and putting it down it is being related to, lived, sensed, seen, backed away from, tapped again, and kept where it is not lost sight of. All this is the opposite of suppressing or losing contact with it (and when she does lose contact, a generalized restlessness comes).

The pain would be made worse if tackled head-on, but avoiding it is also not tolerable. In contrast to both, alternately tapping and putting it down is less painful than the restlessness. There are therefore three different states: the loss of contact and its "restlessness"; the pain dealt with directly, which is too much; and the focusing-approach of tapping and backing away, which puts the pain in a certain space, a place that feels much better than where it would be in the other two states.

Contact with the therapist is vital throughout this kind of development, these minutes of touching, tapping, and putting down. Theories of therapy tend to simplify the model of how this development takes place: It is all "the relationship." Or, it is all an "intrapsychic" process. But what is the relationship if it does not involve the individual's intrapsychic responses to the relationship, especially those aspects of an individual's psyche that develop as a direct result of interpersonal interactions (of which the therapeutic interaction is a subset and an analogue)? Therefore these are not two different things, the relationship and what one lives within oneself in the relationship.

Many living processes are interactional; they cannot be ongoing when one is alone. Another person is essential for part of the process I am describing. The need for companionship and issues of dependence are a separate matter. One cannot live relational processes alone. The client in these excerpts has always prided herself in being able to function quite well without close relations. But it is not dependence. It is rather inherent in human nature, that certain processes are relational and cannot happen without someone. Focusing can be done very deeply alone, but it is always still deeper and different and generates different changes and contents within a relational context.

The image of the fence is not just an instruction for the *future*. It is that. But in a way, she had already *gone through* the kind of living, now, which the going through is! From the new present interactional living, such images can come.

Every item of "content" is also a living process. The concrete bodily living process is always more important than what seems to be the content. A new and positive living process will soon conform its contents positively, even though right now the contents may still be the old ones.

Contents are made by the living, of course. So everything depends on the manner, the kind of living according to which a given content is experienced.

Only superficially is there such a thing as a "content." A "content" ("I hate my job.") can be written down. But to be lived, it always consists of an experiencing, a living. As an "ing" it is not this or that thingish thing, but an implicitly intricate mesh that is moving. Implicitly it is always a million separable aspects that are not separate and have never been. Living is organismic, lived implicitly, and not just in its explicit little manifestations.

Therefore the kind of energy, the kind of interaction, the manner of being alive will tell much more about what "it" is now, than its explicit form which may still be unchanged.

That is why I say that the seemingly unchanged painful content is changing all the while in this example, although we hear nothing about it. For the client, I would guess, there are still no explicit content changes. She just taps "it" and backs off again when it gets to be too much. Many specific memories may be coming in, but they are as they were, and are not going through any change of content-changing.

By the time the implicit change in content and all the mysterious and dramatic results do become visible, the real change will have already happened. If we saw only those dramatic events, we might say that we do not understand how and why they happened.

Of course, even though we are seeing much of the how and the why here, we can still say that we do not understand the process. It is much too big and deep and arises of its own accord; we cannot encapsulate it in our concepts or even in our intuition. It belongs to itself. It is a healing that comes from underneath. With this kind of relational and inward attention the whole intricate mesh reorganizes itself. All we understand is that this happens if we enter in a certain way, if we let a felt sense form, if we "make a space for it," if we "stay with it" with our attention, and if we honor the little steps that take place.

We do very little. Notice how little! But that little seems to be crucial, and it is understandable and teachable. We can conceptualize and isolate what the process needs to be engendered and maintained. Given that, the process does the rest from underneath much like a cut heals from inside, from its deepest spot upward if we keep it clean.

EXCERPT I

July 23

T1: Hello.

C1: Hi. (*Silence — 30 seconds*) I've been feeling like I'm afraid all the time, and I don't know —

T2: Somewhere fear is coming in.

T2: This is a typical focusing response. She said, "I'm afraid." My response *points* to the fear. Without actually asking, the response invites her to sense just how and where the fear is coming in.

C2: Yeah, it's like I . . . don't know what I'm afraid of.

(Silence — 20 seconds)

C2: She does not immediately go to sense that; she has more to say.

T3: You're scared and you don't know what of.

(Silence — 25 seconds)

T3: I wait, to leave time for her to attend inwardly, then respond exactly to what she said. Such a response is aimed at contact. A therapist wants contact with each bit of experience that is there. Here I did not talk right away because she seemed to attend inwardly, and I did not want to stop her. But also, I did not want to leave that bit unresponded to. After such waiting the response is out of phase, but it is worth it.

C3: Being alone is part of it, and I never was [afraid of being alone], but I am —

C3: The "alone" theme has just emerged from what was only fear before.

T4: Being alone is part of it, and . . . that's new, it just came. It's not like you.

(Silence — 120 seconds)

C4: *(Looks up)* Painful.

T5: It's pretty hard to stand it.

C5: Mmm. *(Silence — 110 seconds)* Same thing, scared.

T6: It's just there, and nothing moves. Talk a little bit.

T6: Note the two previous long silences. I guess that her body could use a rest. Of course my suggestion is only tentative, even though I put it as if it were a request. She knows not to do it if it does not fit. Also, I need to know more exactly what process events are happening. I do not want to leave her alone for too long. Talking and interacting can help.

C6: *(No response)*

T7: Talk a little bit. Let me listen. It feels painful . . . and "scared" . . . in the same place —

C7: Afraid.

T8: Mmm, afraid.

C8: Like something's gonna get me —

T9: Something's gonna get you —

C9: Like I have to sleep with my light on.

T10: Oh, yeah, especially while you're sleeping it will get you.

C10: At night it's worse, when it's dark. I keep the lights on.

T11: Mmm, mmm . . . it has a "from-then" feeling to it, to me. Does it to you?

(*Silence — 10 seconds*)

T11: It often helps to ask a person to sense whether something belongs in the past, or now. Here, however, her response says that this qualification does not help now.

C11: That's with my head, something's going to get me, I can't feel that [that it comes from "then"].

T12: Mmm . . . it feels like you're scared *now*, with your head you can say, well, . . . but it feels like just being scared something will come and get you, . . . attack you?

C12: Hurt me.

(*Silence — 20 seconds*)

T13: Hurt you, something will come and hurt you.

(*Silence — 70 seconds*)

C13: (*Inaudible*)

T14: In your feelings nothing comes except "afraid."

C14: And tense.

T15: Tense.

C15: Mmm.

T16: Afraid and tense.

(*Silence — 60 seconds*)

C16: It feels in my body like I would run, but I'm too tense, . . . paralyzed-tense and also like real scared, as if you'd heard somebody coming in the night or something, . . . stiff with tension —

EXCERPT J

August 4

T1: You don't need to do anything, I'll just keep you company.

C1: Hello.

T2: Hey . . . if you're tired we can just sit here for a while.

T2: I do not want her to push or force the process if it does not come on its own. Therefore we institute a possible mode of "just coming for tea, only." If during such a meeting something does come, we can of course process it.

C2: I'm not tired at all, but my own crummy place came back. (*Silence — 20 seconds*) If I could separate. . . . I'm real bad at that.

C2: This is enough to indicate that she is not taking up the offer just to chat. I simply wait.

T3: If you could separate then and now, it would be so much easier.

C3: Yes.

(*Silence — 30 seconds*)

T4: So that lets me say it really is "then," and you know it. But it sure feels like now, so that it does not really separate.

C4: . . . It feels sometimes, . . . when you say that. . . . It feels like there's very little "I" to separate the "it."

C4: Notice that she says it requires an "I" to do this separating between then and now. Also, she hints that, when I mention the separating, she *can* feel the separation a little, but cannot do the separation alone. It is as if my response strengthens her "I," or provides something to let there be a little separation between then and now.

T5: Little "I."

C5: Yes, it's difficult to do that.

T6: It makes sense, that particular "it" is taking up most of your space.

C6: That's true what you're saying, but . . . there's no separation there; I'm too little.

C6: This says "that's not the point." She says "That's true . . . but." She wants to emphasize her littleness.

T7: Do you feel little?

C7: Do I feel little? Yeah.

T8: Are you there, as little?

C8: Yeah, and I'm in a really bad place. When I come out of it I feel bigger.

T9: When you're in that bad place, you're there, but you're little. When you come out of it you feel bigger. But you *are* there, and little.

C9: . . . It keeps saying in my head "It's now. You're an adult now."

T10: Right. You can say that, but you're really feeling little.

C10: Yeah.

T11: And you are there. It's just that you're little. . . . Somehow it isn't right to say that.

C11: . . . What came there, when you said that — I'm being churned or something, . . . twisted this way and that.

T12: Twisted, you're being churned around.

(*Silence — 40 seconds*)

C12: It says in my head, "You can breathe; you can breathe," but I can't.

T13: You can breathe *now*, but —

C13: Yeah, but I'm afraid I can't breathe. (*Silence — 30 seconds*) It's real uncomfortable. I'm in the womb?

T14: It fits, as an image at least, and probably it's true. You're getting churned around like in the womb.

(*Silence — 20 seconds*)

C14: Like I'm being snuffed out, or going to be.

T8: I briefly respond, to see if I understand it correctly.

T9: Now that she has corroborated me, I say it fully. I want to keep her company *there*. And I am also glad that she can come out of there and feel big.

C9: It turns out here that in her head her superego has been telling her to be adult, which has probably gotten in the way.

T10: Both sides need responding to equally. I lean a little here—I do not like superego messages.

T11: Verbally nothing further is needed, but I want to keep her company, be with her there, make the process interactional. Where the ellipses appear, I see some expression on her face, indicating that what I am saying or doing does not fit.

C11: It was not that I said something wrong—rather, something new came.

T14: I want to respect the meaning of the experience, and I hope she does, without getting hung up on whether it is literal or not.

153

T15: Any second.

C15: Yeah. (*Silence — 90 seconds*) Feels like an urgency.

T16: Something is really urgent, right now.

C16: (*Silence — 40 seconds*) Can I hold your hand?

T17: Yeah, sure, both of them you can. (*I move my chair closer to studio couch.*)

C17: I have no control.

T18: Oh I see. You can't, in that situation, say something or breathe.

(*Silence — 80 seconds*)

C18: I need to be picked up, but I can't explain that to them.

C18: If we take the birth experience literally, then this need to be picked up comes from a later time. But all times are implicit in any experience, or at least many different times.

T19: You need to be picked up but you can't tell them, or there's nobody there.

T19: Nonverbally I am squeezing her hands more tightly as part of this response.

(*Silence — 150 seconds*)

C19: It's worse. (*She feels nausea.*)

T20: Open your eyes and look at something.

C20: (*She does this.*)

T21: It's better to open your eyes. . . . It's the churning around?

C21: Mmm.

T22: Back and forth or in one direction?

C22: Round and round and up and down.

T23: Round and round and up and down. (*Silence — 100 seconds*) Maybe you're about to be born.

C23: When you said that the image I had was something around my neck.

C23: Did T23 help, give energy to enable this new specific to come? There had been more than a minute's silence before I said it.

154

T24: (*inaudible*)

(*Silence — 20 seconds*)

C24: So tense, my whole body's really rigid or something.

T25: (*Takes a long breath.*)

T25: Sometimes one's presence can be manifested just by a loud breath, if it happens to come.

C25: I need you to hold me. (*Breathes*)

T26: Mmm. (*I do so.*)

C26: It's like I'll choke.

T27: Mmm. Keep your eyes open.

C27: It's like everything is frozen inside me.

T28: So tense.

C28: Stiff.

T29: Stiff.

C29: (*Groans.*)

C30: I'll get a drink of water. (*Goes to the bathroom*)

(*Silence — 60 seconds*)

C31: (*Inaudible*) Cord was around my neck.

T32: Mmm . . . mmm. . . .

C32: (*Cries and sobs continuously for 9 minutes, then sighs, cries for another minute, then breathes with relief.*)

C33: That's better

T33: Mmm.

(*Silence — 3 minutes*)

C34: (*Yawns*)

T35: (*Laughs*)

C35: It changed, I was born then.

T36: Mmm. If it's literal, it's welcome, and if it's not literal, it's also welcome. Do you know what I mean?

155

C36: I know what you mean. It feels right.

T37: That's great.

C37: (*She rubs her neck.*)

T38: You still feel it around your neck.

C38: Yeah. Hold me like this. It feels like I'm falling. (*Shows me how to hold her*)

T39: We're getting beautiful directions here.

C39: (*Laughs.*) . . . Halfway through it felt like I *wasn't* going to smother. Not at first, it was like I was choking.

T40: Mmm.

C40: But then (*inaudible*) I was kicking free down there. . . . I was (*inaudible*). . . . That felt good.

T41: (*Breathes*) Yeah.

C41: You're still breathing. (*Laughs*)

C41: She sees that I am still recovering from the experience. Note the "still." She has been aware of my breathing all along.

T42: (*Laughs*) Yeah.

EXCERPT K

August 8

C1: I felt real sleepy all day, fatigued, and I laid down and my chest felt like it was caving in and I was real scared. I was going to sit down and try to see what was so scary, but my body just reacted, like it wouldn't let me.

T1: It said "Go to sleep." . . . No?

T1: I am worried that she was pushing into things when her body wanted to go to sleep. Especially after the birth experience I expect her body to be tired.

156

C2: No, it didn't say go to sleep. That's what my head was saying, "Just go to bed; you've done enough; just leave it." But there was something about my lying down that was still scary. . . .

T2: Oh, I see.

C3: And I was up, and down, making tea, trying to just feel, . . . let that scare go away. . . . But yet my body was saying, "I don't." . . . Then I took a walk and while I was walking I asked what it needed to feel OK, and that didn't come, at first, and then it said like, "have to feel safe." "Feel safe" kept like resonating in me, and felt better.

T3: To feel safe, it was right some way, to *feel safe.*

C4: At the beginning my head said, "Well, what is it you're not safe about?" and again it said "Nope, don't touch it," and it was just kind of a letting it be for the time. . . . It was nice.

T4: (*Deep breath*) Yeah. . . .

T4: I am happy that she could sense when "it" said "Don't touch it," and that she obeyed this instruction.

(*Silence — 20 seconds*)

C5: Okay, there's two things: one is a really good place; it's real soft; it's like, . . . remember I said I got to something underneath that I couldn't reach?

T5: Yeah, yeah.

C6: Well, I reached it. It was that stuff with the cord and all that.

T6: Fantastic!

T6: I had no investment in whether the birth experience was or was not specifically something that had long been there, waiting. As long as what comes next is taken up, sooner or later it will be what was needed. It is good to hear that this birth experience is what she now senses as having been "that," underneath, which she had previously felt and alluded to.

C7: I was always putting the cart before the horse, something always underneath

157

that I could never get to because I never knew what it was.

T7: Yeah. . . .

C8: Feels nice.

T8: Yeah. (*Both laugh. I sigh some more.*) That's wonderful.

C9: That is! Now I can move forward . . . (*Silence — 20 seconds*), an optimism. . . . And the other part said "yes, but time." The word "time" came, like to respect my body, to recuperate now.

T9: Yes!

C10: If I listen, my body really tells me . . . when it's ready to go, . . . but I don't always listen.

T10: Beautiful. It has time to grow now; it's here.

T10: I am willing to say that I favor this, not only here but throughout.

C11: Right now . . . I really want to live. I really do. . . . It's different . . . okay. I may go through a time of not wanting to live, but underneath there, now, I know I'll live.

C11: Who knows in advance just what will make just what difference?

T11: You feel now, that you can. The sense that you can't *was in that thing.*

T11: Of course I join her in stating this.

C12: . . . I need some time (*Silence — 40 seconds*) and I need you to hold me.

C12: What I said went a little too far, perhaps. As she senses she finds again that she should let time go by. She needs time *and* contact.

T12: (*I hold her.*)

EXCERPT L

August 19

T1: Somewhere on the other side of all that anger . . . that really felt like hate and anger . . . you could directly touch your, . . . how you have a lot of loving there too, . . . and that's something you've known.

C2: Yes, that's something I knew in my head, but I've touched it now. It's like . . . that part is sort of like . . . the anger and hate is not all of me anymore. I can also

touch that, for the amount, there's probably more love

T2: Yeah, yeah, which you always knew.

C3: But now I can touch that part. Yesterday, too, I touched this — I was half
awake I think — that as long as I can hold
on to my anger and hate it's like I don't
really have to touch that loneliness that's
there.

T3: Mmm.

C4: Not relating, the anger prevents me
from relating. When I feel that anger I say,
"Well, I don't need anybody." I don't feel
the "lonely," whereas the truth is that that
keeps me from feeling the need to relate
in a different way from what I had before.

T4: Yeah.

C4: And I need to touch that loneliness
and live that first, and then there'll be fresh
air coming through there — that's the way
it feels.

T5: Yeah, that's related to what you
said: "Maybe I'm not an island."

C5: Yeah, that's what I was feeling. . . .
It's not, "Maybe I'm not an island." I know
by what I feel that I'm not an island.

T6: (*Laughs*)

C6: Whereas I like to put up that front
that I'm self-sufficient, and I didn't need
anybody.

T7: Yeah.

C7: But geez, I've learned otherwise
(*laughs*).

T8: Yeah.

C8: With you (*both laugh*), also with
Martin, . . . if I commit myself . . . I could
pull back whenever I want to. . . . It's hard
to explain. I need to live not on the fringe
of relationships.

T9: You had yourself really fundamen-
tally alone.

C9: Right!

T10: And just on the edge of relationships, if you needed to, you could pull out.

C10: Yes. What I'm feeling more is a relationship, is two different things, not just me.

T11: Yeah.

C11: It's more I've lived on the fringe of life, and lived alone, . . . and I'm tired of that.

T12: (*Laughs*) "I'm tired of that."

C12: Yes! And it's real different with me, it's real different, I don't understand it all.

(*A little later in the hour*)

T14: You've been in the doorway.

C14: Yeah, like, . . . or I need to control the relationships.

T15: You have had to control.

C15: Yes. I don't know if control is the right word, something isn't free in me, and it has to be cared for, not used or —

T16: Something is cautious, careful, not letting things in all the way.

C16: Yeah, real hard for me to believe that . . . an adult could love me just for being me and not use me, or for what I can do, or not. . . . Somehow that can't reach me. . . . That's different with you now, like I can feel you'd care for me if I didn't do a God-damned thing!

T17: (*Laughs*)

C17: That's true! That's really new for me. So maybe then . . . I'll be able to feel that more with other people.

T18: Mmm, something is careful, still there, like, "Oh, they only want to use me, or they only want what I can do."

T18: Twice she talked about being "used," and I had not yet responded to it.

C18: And yet I know that's not right.

T19: It's a feeling.

160

C19: I think too it's part of, . . . I'm not going to set myself up to be hurt again.

T20: Mmm.

C20: Like I'm, . . . I know what it's like to feel alone; that's the part I know.

T21: That you've had.

C21: It almost feels better to be that than to be . . . let down again or something, there's something —

T22: It's better to be alone than to have *that* happen again.

C22: Yeah, it's (*silence — 50 seconds*) like nothing is lasting or something.

T23: Mmm, any moment it could break down.

C23: This whole thing is different now.

C23: Note: "This whole thing is different now." Relating with me has changed it, but of course it is also still there. As the implicit whole changed as she describes it here, the old experience will soon go through the process, too. The change is described next, which will then make the reexperiencing come out well.

T24: Mmm. A fear of being betrayed or something.

T24: This is surmised from other things she has said.

C24: I think this whole thing has to do with my father; I really do. (*Silence — 5 minutes*) It's real screwed up there.

T25: There's something about him, how he related to you. We don't know what it is yet, that made for this "any moment he could betray" you or "any moment, any time, I could get betrayed."

C25: More like intruding.

C25: Note that I got it wrong, and/or it is changing, opening before us.

T26: He could intrude on you?

C26: Yeah, . . . somewhere I lost the balance about my space, like an extreme, like wanting that space for my own, being real sure about that space. Unless I, . . . and some way I haven't come back yet, from that, to a balance between —

T27: Yeah, like you've got so sore about being intruded on completely that you went all the way to being not at all intruded upon. You had to have control of the door and not let *anybody* in.

C27: Yeah.

T28: And you're sensing that there is a . . . middle place somewhere, where you can let people in . . . and still not . . . feel. To have them all the way there, I can't say it just right but I get the difference.

C28: Yeah, that touches anger in me.

T29: Mmm, there's real live anger about being intruded upon.

(*Silence — 30 seconds*)

C29: (*Inaudible*)

T30: That connects then with where you don't feel . . . cared about.

(*Silence — 30 seconds*)

C30: It's like I became an island . . . but an island only he could use whenever he wanted to —

T31: It was more, you were an island when he wasn't using it.

C31: Yeah. (*Silence — 40 seconds*) I can really touch it, that's the loneliness in me.

T32: Yeah.

C32: (*Inaudible*)

T33: Yes, that is not the way it was meant to be.

C33: Yes, and now I . . . (*silence — 40 seconds*), . . . (*inaudible*). That wasn't right, there's hate and all that, but another part came through. . . . It is . . . (*silence — 30 seconds*) the part of me that I like . . . said . . . um that old shit is only part of it. . . . It won't get the good part of me lost. . . . It was to the extreme for a long time, but, . . . but it's like that part is scared; I'm going to keep that part.

C33: "It won't get the good part of me lost." Note her direct sensing of something more than the bad experience and the ways of feeling that go with it. This is not just knowing better, just having positive thoughts of oneself. Rather, it is a directly felt "part," and an energy. As long as we have that, working through the bad parts will succeed. When did this come? We saw it developing in the previous hours.

T34: Oh . . . yes, . . . that right part you don't want to lose and you won't lose, oh sure.

C34: Yes, so that part is separate from the other, like my love for nature. . . . All that is a nice part that I learned because I had to.

C34: Love of nature and her sense of infinity are *old* good "parts." But there is a *new* good "part," and energy. But of course the old aspects she had before go along with the new. What is good and right never gets lost when experiential change occurs. Even if these old capacities were misused before, now that she is moving toward relating to people she will not lose them.

T35: The infinity part.

C35: Yes.

T36: Came to you because you had to be alone so much, but that, you are not going to lose.

C36: Like I don't need people to entertain me (*laughs*). That's the good part.

T37: (*Laughs*)

C37: The idea for the boxing gloves came right after . . . I kept saying, "I have to deal with my anger!" And I was really preoccupied with, "When are you going to deal with your anger?" And then I lay down to see if I was feeling tense and uptight because I thought I have to deal with this anger. "When are you gonna, how much longer are you gonna stall," all those critical things, you know? And I thought of all sorts of ways, a padded room I need, where I can't break things, and I just don't have it. . . . And then I lay down, and half asleep and half awake, and it was like when I woke up I wasn't asleep very much. It was like, "Gee, I want to deal with my anger" . . . and "Oh yeah . . . that's it; I need boxing gloves." And I could wait and let it be and let it come in its own time. As long as I was forcing it, it couldn't come.

T38: We hadn't known the way you would express your anger. You didn't want to break things and hurt yourself, . . . and what came through —

C38: I could feel . . . if I wanted to. . . . What came through was, "As long as my attitude is that I have to deal with it, I block it from coming." So then that went, and . . . then what came through was, "Gee, I need a pair of boxing gloves and those things on your feet, like kids use, to kick," because I really feel I need to kick.

T39: The thing about the boxing gloves came as a result of, . . . once you got the *"have to* express my anger" out of the way, then came . . . the way.

C39: Exactly *(laughs)*. And I can arrange, . . . feeling so much anger and hate inside me it was like . . . a well full of water that's just all polluted. And I felt I could beat the walls and all that, and I could empty it and feel a void. I'd feel space here like I described the other day, but then it would just fill back up with the polluted water.

T40: Yeah.

C40: And what it felt like was, uh . . . it needs to . . . do that, because I haven't done that enough.

T41: Right, right.

C41: But then it needs the little spring from way underneath coming in trickling, . . . that there's less polluted water, and, and . . . the fresh water will keep coming, coming, coming, and I'll clean out. . . . That's what it felt like.

T42: Yeah.

C42: And that happens like when you hold me, . . . and when I feel related and connected.

C38: When she put aside the pressure about having to release her anger, then a way came to her for how to do it. She would buy boxing gloves. (Pounding pillows and the couch had not been enough to keep her from hurting her hand.)

C39: She describes how kicking and pounding the wall had felt to her, two times before. The space it freed up was filled again by the same thing.

C40: And she does feel clearly that she needs to do more kicking and pounding, but

C41: Something new and different comes in from underneath, slowly. A trickle is her image of it. This is directly sensed as being different.

C42: The "trickling" is linked with contact.

Discussion of Excerpt L

Her imagery probably contains the key to whether catharsis helps or not. It depends on whether the same old "polluted water" refills the space, which catharsis temporarily empties, or whether some new "fresh water" comes in. From where does the fresh water come? "From underneath," it comes from inside her, but it seems to come when there is contact.

Please note her answers: First, she pushes away the pressure, the "I have to [get my anger out]." Then the way she can get the anger out comes. Next she senses that just kicking and pounding will not fix it. She can sense the need for kicking and pounding, but the space these actions empty will fill up again with the same thing. Something slower, a "trickle," is bringing a different result.

EXCERPT M

C1: Real distinct this morning for me, that I, it was like I'm angry with my father but he wasn't inside me. I was able to put him against the wall and I smacked him with the gloves. Otherwise I'd be beating myself, or I'd soon turn it inward again, but I didn't this morning. I felt I let the tip off, but then it was important to fill that space with fresh water so that that much is really gone, and I can process the rest. It's real important that I fill it up with fresh water, water coming in from underneath. It's that itchy feeling — I get an itchy feeling. I know I need you to hold me then; that's the healing for me — like when a wound heals, it itches, that's real deep down. And that's so exact for me, I had to have you hold me until I could feel that whole space filled from underneath. I call that my "spring" coming in, and it feels too like I can feel that little trickle of warm fresh water. It's uh, . . . there's room for it in there now; I can let it in and it trickles in — that's tied in with that longing to get filled with love and caring so that the other can get out. Because if it came in at the top it would all get polluted again together, whereas if it comes in from my core —

C1: The client did some pounding, on her own, in her room. She can feel ("I let the tip off") that there is much more to come. What occurs here also occurs later in major cathartic experiences she has in 2 later hours: She has to "put" her father out of herself, in a space outside her. Only then does the desire to pound him arise naturally in her. Otherwise her urge would be to hit herself. Also, this will enable some "fresh water" to come into the little bit of space she has just made.

The client's therapy continued with many touchy moments for 3 more years and ended very successfully. At this writing 10 years later it is clear that she was successful by any standard.

PART 2

INTEGRATING OTHER THERAPEUTIC METHODS

CHAPTER 11

A Unified View
of the Field through
Focusing and the
Experiential Method

MANY ORIENTATIONS to the practice of psychotherapy exist today; for example, there is Freudian and Jungian Psychoanalysis, Gestalt Therapy, Client-Centered Therapy, Primal Therapy, Behavior Therapy, Psychosynthesis, Hakomi, Transpersonal Methods, and so on. Orientations like these are vital because they function as social and training organizations. Each involves a certain spirit, a kind of culture. Fruitful discussions go on among the practitioners of each of them, which would not happen if they/we were atomized individuals. Therefore we need to belong to orientations and also be able to value our differences and what we have in common. But orientations and methods can confuse what we need to know in order to practice therapy. There are now said to be several hundred. Our field presents a chaotic array of radically different practices, theories, and aims.

WHAT ARE THE REAL DIFFERENCES
AMONG ORIENTATIONS?

If we look more closely, we see that different orientations have many procedures in common, although they use different vocabularies to describe them. Freudians and Jungians both interpret what takes place in "transference," Kohutian and Client-Centered therapists both use reflective listening, and many Jungians use Gestalt's "two chair" procedure. Each orientation seems to consist of a certain cluster of procedures. If we add all these together they form a very large pool of procedures.

1. Our first move is to *unpack* the orientations. Doing so we find that many procedures with different names are really much alike. If we free them from their vocabulary, they reduce to a much smaller pool of specific procedures that a therapist of any school could use. In the following chapters I will speak not of orientations but of this smaller pool of procedures.

2. A second move is also necessary. We must consider how a procedure is used. Different schools may not use the same procedure in the same spirit. There are great differences also among therapists of the same school.

Theories and vocabularies of psychotherapy do not define exactly how a procedure is to be used. When practitioners of the same school discuss their cases, they find that they practice very differently. Therapists of different orientations often resemble each other much more than they resemble some members of their own school.

How we use a procedure involves a host of specifics for which there are often no established terms. In case consultations we invent new phraseology for the vital practical discriminations we must make. We can therefore conclude that what we actually practice is not the orientation nor the procedure. What we practice is much more specific.

We cannot hope to integrate the overlapping orientations or the unspecified procedures.

Having said this we seem to be adrift in a sea of specifics that are not organized by orientation or procedure. Are there then no meaningful groupings of the procedures at all? There are, but we must make a third move and divide the field in another way.

3. If we set orientations and their current descriptions aside, large real differences among procedures do appear: Therapy can consist of totally different *kinds of experience*. I call these therapeutic "avenues." A given therapeutic event can consist of images, role play, words, cognitive beliefs, memories, feelings, emotional catharsis, interpersonal interactions, dreams, dance moves, muscle movement, and habitual behavior. These different avenues are *genuine differences* in the very stuff of which the therapy consists.

Orientations are not organized by avenue. For example, Jungians use several avenues. Imagery is the therapeutic avenue of the Jungian "Active Daydream" procedure. No other orientation uses that procedure, but Autogenic Training, Systematic Desensitization, and others do employ procedures of their own on the imagery avenue. *We can, therefore, group procedures by avenue, despite the fact that they may be part of different orientations with different theories.*

Dividing the field this way has great advantages. There are more procedures than we can learn, but their number becomes manageable if we group

170

them by avenue. Learning two or three procedures on an avenue can give us a familiarity and skill *with that avenue*!

How well we use a procedure depends partly on our familiarity and skill with the avenue. For example, an imagery procedure depends on our familiarity *with the nature of images*. If we used only one fixed procedure with images, we might not develop enough of a familiarity, but if we used two or three imagery procedures, we probably would.

Currently the different procedures on one avenue are taught in different orientations. To learn several, one would have to seek them out. But once we have learned three procedures on one avenue, we know not just three separate things, but the characteristics of that avenue. For example, when we use three different imagery procedures, then, quite naturally, we employ each procedure so as to take account of what the other two have taught us about imagery. We modify each in very specific ways that constitute a sensitivity to the characteristics of imagery.

In this way we unpack not only the orientations but also the fixed procedures on any given avenue. Gradually we develop skill with the practical characteristics of each avenue.

But how well we work on any one avenue also depends on the other avenues, because some others are bound to be involved as well. When we have become familar with many avenues, we notice when something begins to happen on one of them. We automatically modulate what we do on one avenue by what we know of the others.

So our third move is to think of ourselves as working on avenues, rather than with fixed procedures.

4. Focusing and the experiential method enable us to use each avenue in an experiential way and to move between the avenues. This is our fourth move.

Steps of change, as I have described them, come not just from images as such, or emotions as such, but from their felt sense. If we think of ourselves as working with the client's felt sense, then each avenue becomes a way to lead to a felt sense. And, once there is a felt sense, all avenues are ways to carry it forward. From a felt sense the next step can come as words, an image, an emotion, or an interpersonal interaction.

Since any avenue can lead to a felt sense, and any other avenue can carry it forward, the felt sense provides a juncture between avenues. Our sensitivity to many avenues enables us to modulate what we do on any one, so as to respond uniquely to the intricacy of each situation with each client.

The felt sense that arises from inside the client enables us to work, not within orientations (although we belong to them), not with fixed procedures (although we may learn two or three on each avenue), not with avenues (although we become familiar with each avenue *as such*), and not with the felt sense (though it brings change steps and junctures among the avenues), but always with the person in front of us.

THE ADVANTAGES OF UNDOING THE ORIENTATIONS

Currently students of clinical psychology learn the approaches of several orientations. Each of these is effective and helpful in a different way. Then the student is asked to choose one to practice. A choice among professional communities with which to associate oneself makes sense, but it should not be a choice of how to practice. The students should not be expected to forgo so much of what they have already found to be effective just because it does not fit their chosen orientation. Rather than relating to clients and doing what might help, the students are expected to practice the orientation.

All orientations and procedures interfere with psychotherapy insofar as they are held to tightly. Priority must always be given to the person and to the therapist's ongoing connection with the person.

Like procedures, all theories can be destructive, if we think that a person is what a theory says. A person is a who, not a what. *This* person is always this living one, in front of us. The person is always freshly there again, always more than ideas and procedures.

Another way theories can be misused is that they can lead one to miss the unpredictability of the next bit of experiential differentiation. I have tried to show that a step or two into the felt edge can bring something new and surprising from seemingly well-known experiences and events.

Procedures and theories are vital, but they need to be used in relation to our contact with the person. Then they can lead to something we can try, without imposing on the person or losing our immediate contact with the person. What we do on any avenue or take from various methods must be fitted into the relational conditions I have described so far.

When therapy has become stuck, we need a large repertory of procedures to try out, and we cannot invent them all ourselves. But if something makes sense to us it becomes our own, and we employ it out of our own sensitivity, and modify it specifically and creatively.

To become able to do this, we will be greatly helped if we organize our understanding of the field of psychotherapy in terms of avenues; then we can arrange to learn several procedures on one avenue. For example, one procedure on the interactional avenue teaches us that we must sometimes let the client interact with us as if we were a person in the client's past. Another procedure shows us that we can sometimes transcend the past by responding in a new and positive way to the client's present behavior toward us in the therapy hour. Another procedure is to confront the client, another that we be implicitly accepting, and still another that we respond by remaining neutral. Once we have experienced several of these interactional procedures, we will no longer be frozen in whatever mode we would normally use. Even if we use one of them most of the time, we will no longer be able to practice it as a fixed routine. We will now have become familiar with the interactional avenue as such, and our responses will automatically take account of our sensitivity to the possibilities and characteristics of therapeutic movement on that avenue.

Every therapist finds that colleagues trained in other methods are upsettingly insensitive to certain things. The practitioners of each method are sensitized to a certain range of observations. Imagine a therapist who has experience in two methods, but now practices only one. Orthodox practitioners of the chosen method might notice nothing else. But observers from the discarded method will find this therapist not as bad as they expected. Such a therapist will not grossly override sensitivities and observations which the other method features.

Because any moment of therapy involves a multitude of specifics, *how* one actually employs a procedure can vary greatly. How the procedure is performed naturally will be modified so as not to violate the observations and sensitivities we have gained from knowing another procedure. *Rather than combining contradictory procedures, we combine specific sensitivities.* They are not contradictory! If we have sensitivities, we find ourselves quite naturally behaving so as to take account of them.

One way to learn two or three procedures on one avenue is to experience them for ourselves in the client's role. We can easily obtain such experience in a few hours with colleagues of another orientation. Once we have become familiar with two or three of these other methods, we cease to use any one of them as fixed. We acquire the capacity to innovate flexibly on that avenue.

A bright person expressed her dissatisfaction with a rigid lawyer; she said, "In *my* field if someone doesn't want me to work by the book, I can find eight other ways."

Say we learn Systematic Desensitization, a complex sequence of instructions in which images of specific situations are deliberately invoked. We also learn the Jungian Active Daydream technique in which an image must be allowed to come of its own accord, so that the client can then actively respond to it as if it were reality. We also learn Simonton's imagery sequence. Once we have experienced the function served by each part of these procedures, they break up into a useful repertory of small-scale moves. These familiarize us with the imagery avenue and make innovation natural and inevitable. We devise new small-scale moves to fit each unique juncture. Then it seems artificial to use always the same procedure.

There are good reasons for working on all the avenues. Currently most therapists work only on a few of them. Some therapists employ only talk, others reject talk and insist on imagery, or role play. Some work mainly with interactional events in the present therapeutic relationship. Some spend most of the time on dreams, examining how the new dream "comments" on the dream work of the previous hour. Their therapy is largely a "conversation with dreams." Some massage therapists work on muscles, ignoring the life-meanings implicit in bodily experience. Some therapists spend the hour planning what I call action steps for the client to do during the week (for example, in Operant Behavior Therapy) in order to reshape habits. They don't pay attention to the therapeutic interaction as a source of therapeutic success. Some therapists employ cognitions rather than feelings; others consider only feelings and call cognitions "mere intellectualization."

One reason for making a choice is that the different avenues seem not to go together: How could cognitive therapy be combined with feelings or muscle therapy? They use different parts of the person.

We would do well to remember that *these avenues are already together in every person*. Everyone thinks and feels; has dreams and comes from a family; has imagery, memories, and muscles; and has habits and interacts with others. In a human being these functions *do* already go together. So their use as therapeutic avenues can and must go together also.

THE LINK BETWEEN THE AVENUES

The theories of the various orientations cannot tell us how the avenues go together. The felt sense provides this crucial link.

Experience is often thought of as if it consisted only of feelings, interactions, cognitions, memories, actions, images, and so on. But is it really divided into these neat little packages?

These kinds of experience appear to be separate from each other. An action seems to be a movement in outside space. Feelings seem to take place inside the individual. Interpersonal events seem to happen outside, with other people. Memories contain events from the past. We define the packages separately. But are they all there is to experience?

The felt sense is an experiential mesh that is not divided. At the conscious–unconscious border zone one senses the ongoing experiential process, and it is always *implicitly intricate*. That means it includes a whole range of images, feelings, actions, and so on that have never happened as such, but *could* come.

Starting from any of the different kinds of experience one can seek *the felt sense of that experience*. One can seek the felt sense of what one has just said, felt, or done; the felt sense of how one just responded to another person; the felt sense of some part of a dream, an image, a memory, or a pressure in some part of the body. So it turns out that these "packages" are never alone, never only the defined experiences they seem to be.

Let us make a fundamental change in our understanding: *Human situations and experiences do not consist of only separate, defined packages.* We usually attend to these, but there is always *also an intricate experiential mesh that is greater than any of them*. (It is as yet unformed, or let us say that it is more than formed, because it includes many forms from the past and yet it is implicitly more intricate). Each therapeutic avenue can lead to and emerge from this central experiential process, which is none of them, but which involves each of them.

I must emphasize again that a felt sense is not simply there, underneath, before it *comes*. The central process is always ongoing, but only if one turns one's attention to it — and waits — does a felt sense form and come. It comes *from* (it is the felt sense *of*) what was there before, but one can feel its coming and feel that it was not already there as such. *Its coming is a bodily change.*

The coming of a felt sense is a physical change, and there is a further change when formed experiences emerge from it. The words or images that arise are often unique, creative, and more intricate than common experiences are.

The new words, images, or emotions were not already part of the felt sense. They arise from it and yet they change it. We say that the felt sense is *"carried forward"* by them.

A felt sense is amazingly fussy about which words will carry it forward. It holds out for certain words. It refuses other words that have the same meaning in the dictionary. This is because different words have different connotations, and it is those we feel.

In the absence of a felt sense, the client may move from a dream image directly to a thought, then to an emotion, and then to an action. All four, however, will usually express the same state. They provide no road to new experiences. The emotion does not lead *from itself* to a changed emotion, nor to images that would spark different emotions. Emotions, actions, images, thoughts, and interactions can lead to each other, but the transitions do not change them.

Change doesn't usually happen as a result of these defined experiences. Therefore we would not want to try to combine them, even if we could. We would miss the experiential change process.

Just as we cannot integrate the orientations or the fixed procedures by using them unchanged, so also we cannot integrate the different kinds of experiences that are the different avenues. But how do these kinds of experiences go together and coexist in each person?

To integrate the avenues we call attention to where they join, which is in the ongoing, implicit experiencing process; it is always greater and is not cut up.

Each avenue can be used in relation to the mesh of experiencing which it is implicitly part of. So used, it becomes greater than the formed experience it is. Each is sensed as leading to the edge where a felt sense comes. In turn, the new and wider felt sense that comes can give rise to *new* experiences on each avenue.

We will examine procedures in terms of what happens in the client's experiencing during each element of a procedure. For example, rather than working only with action, as in Behavior Therapy, we can also work with the sources of actions in the client's experience, and their effects on it. We come to know the experiential changes that actions can bring about. Then we are able to achieve behavioral aims more effectively because we know the role of actions in the broader therapeutic process.

Through the linkage a felt sense provides, every kind of therapy can become experiential. Once it has become experiential, we can articulate what, beyond formed experiences, is involved in a given problem.

From here there are two possible applications of the experiential method. I will first discuss how the specialized forms of therapy can use a felt sense, thereby becoming experiential on their own avenues. Then I will show how a focusing-based therapy can work on all of the avenues.

THERAPEUTIC OPTIONS

Staying on One Avenue

Unfortunately no one can be an expert on all avenues. The avenues make different demands on the personality of a therapist, and they involve different kinds of therapeutic approaches. Each specialization draws on valuable accumulations of knowledge. Would it be possible for one therapist to learn the skills of interpersonal interaction, empathy, and focusing; absorb the vast material Jung amassed to correlate myth with dreams; and then still also acquire a massage therapist's years of experience with muscles? No. Therefore we must sometimes refer clients to a specialized therapist for some therapy hours.

But specialized methods can become experiential on their own avenues. For instance, in imagery, clients can move from an image to a felt sense, and from that to a new image. The therapist works not only with the images but also with their experiential sources and effects. Or, during hands-on body work, the client is invited to let a felt sense come. Its coming is found to change the state of the muscles. Further work on muscles then changes the felt sense. The specialist works not only with the muscles but also with the experiential sources and effects of muscle tensions.

Instead of working only with images, the experiential method works by looking at the whole experiential process that takes place between one image and the next. In most orientations something like this already does happen. Every method depends on a wider context than the formed experiences with which it deals, but the nature of its contribution has not been articulated. Procedures often neglect the wider context. With deliberate attention to the bodily felt edge and its systematic use, any method can become more effective on its own avenue.

Experiential Therapy on All Avenues

Now let us discuss how we can work on all avenues. There are good reasons to use the full range. The objection might be raised that the whole person changes on one avenue; why are the others needed? Shouldn't the same change arise from the felt sense, no matter the avenue on which the felt sense comes, or on which it is carried forward? The answer is no.

A theory is beginning to develop (Gendlin, 1996a) that says that the avenues carry experiencing forward in *different* ways. An image can show us wild new possibilities that cannot be represented in movement or action. There are different human ways of living, and it follows that these make different changes possible.

The avenues do affect each other. The coming of a felt sense from an emotion will pave the way for further changes in emotions but also for changes in dreams. But the change it makes will be different. Similarly, working with dreams will change behavior, but it will not provide *that* change which an action step would bring. Each avenue can bring something irreplaceable.

Is one therapist capable of performing therapeutic work on all the avenues? Not as specializations, of course, and without specialization we lose certain advantages. But there are also great advantages to be gained by using the avenues together. It allows us to discover what is essential on each avenue, what no other avenue provides. We learn when an avenue's special power is needed. We change how we work on an avenue so as to include what we know from the other avenues. Even if we do not happen to be working with the therapeutic interaction, we work with an image in such a way that does not violate the therapeutic possibilities of the present interaction. And when we are working with the interaction we can notice that an image has arisen that could be of help. All avenues that are familiar to us affect how we work on each one, and makes our work more effective.

HOW THE AVENUES ALL FIT INTO THE FRAME
OF ONE THERAPY HOUR

There is another great advantage to *not* being specialized. When we let each avenue modify the others, they no longer require totally different temperaments and circumstances. Now the avenues all fit within one psychotherapeutic context.

We can work with the body without becoming body therapists with massage tables. We can utilize role play without directing the client to get up and perform a drama as in Gestalt therapy, and without using the personal style of Fritz Perls. We can learn from operant behavior therapy without taking the whole hour for it, and without becoming Skinnerians.

Deciding not to fill the whole hour with a single procedure involves a change in how we think about our profession. Psychotherapy is often thought of in terms of the therapist's procedure. Clients who go to a Gestalt therapist expect Gestalt therapy.

On the other hand, if we think of psychotherapy as the client's process, rather than as a type of procedure, then psychotherapy is whatever helps the client. We don't know — and we don't have to know — in advance what that will be for different clients and at different times. Therapist and client are free to change and modulate what they do, and to move between avenues.

Procedures on different avenues do not remain separate, as if we could try them only one after another. If the essence of each avenue is grasped, they modify each other so that it becomes natural to include the others when we work on one of them.

Moving between avenues happens naturally, because, for example, we are not trying to work with actions as such, but rather with actions that could carry a felt sense forward. These are the kind we naturally look for, because there is already a felt sense from some other avenue. What we know about Skinnerian principles tells us when one of them could contribute something essential, and we offer it only in that way. Similarly we do not work with images as such, but with how an image could bring a new felt sense, or carry one forward, so as to make a special contribution.

There is an imagery procedure that employs prearranged sequences of instructions that require the whole hour; there may be some interpersonal relating during this, but the work is chiefly with images. It seems that the therapist must choose: work *either* with deep imagery *or* through interactive relating. Of course something is lost if the hour-long context of an imagery method is set aside. But much more is gained than lost if we can find a way to use the power of images without filling the whole hour. In the following excerpt the therapist asks the client a small image-oriented question. Nothing is risked; such a small question does not alter the client's ownership of the hour. Yet, the question begins a powerful image sequence, one that simultaneously employs a special client–therapist interaction. The client is exploring a felt sense.

C: That [child] part of me is *so* hurt.

T: You can feel the hurt in this child part.

C: Yes. (*Silence*)

T: *Can you see her?*

C: Yes.

T: What is she doing?

C: I see her (*cries softly*). She's all rolled up in fetal position with her arms over her head.

T: Can you and I just sit by her, quietly? We won't say or push anything. We'll just be here. You and I will keep her quiet company. That way she has time.

(*Silence*)

(In Chapter 15, on imagery, I will describe in detail how one would continue from here.)

This therapist's familiarity with the imagery avenue has added an image to the usual experiential practice of staying with a feeling and creating safety around it. Conversely, the therapist's familiarity with the interactional avenue led to a new imagery procedure.

Please notice that the question "Can you see her?" does not violate the client-centered spirit of the interaction. Without forcing or directing, without taking control of the hour, the therapist recognizes the possibility that there is or could be an image.

DIFFERENCES AMONG THE THEORIES

It seems that there are basic conflicts, for example, between Freudian and Jungian interpretations. And even the same theory can generate conflicting hypotheses about any situation. All "interpretations" are really only hypotheses. Current theories are so broad and general that they seldom give us only one plausible hypothesis to explain an intricate situation. However, there is a touchstone. The coming of a step arising from the felt sense decides among hypotheses at any juncture. All theories therefore can be used to generate hypotheses. Only when one of them opens the felt sense and carries it forward, is it then more than a mere hypothesis. By the time the felt sense opens and a flood of detail spills out, there can no longer be any doubt. But what comes also alters and augments the hypothesis. The result could not have been deduced from the hypothesis that helped to bring it about.

In a course I teach called "Theory Construction" students learn to use many theories and devise new concepts in relation to a felt sense. The students have backgrounds in many different fields and work on topics from their own field. I ask them to begin with something they know and want to work on but that they cannot yet articulate — a felt sense. In this way they have a touchstone against which to evaluate the conceptual moves they make. I tell them: "If it doesn't resonate with the felt sense, discard it quickly, before the felt sense leaves or shrivels."

At first, a new idea cannot be expressed because the available words mean something else. The felt sense of something new is more precise. This greater precision is then articulated, but clumsily, in odd new phrases. Gradually new concepts develop. Their detailed structure is derived from those verbalizations that carry the felt sense forward.

Most students in this class are not in psychology. Therapy is rarely mentioned. I was therefore surprised one year when, at the end, one student said: "Well, thank you. Now I can be a therapist." I did not immediately understand what she meant. Her topic had not been in psychology. She explained that she was now graduating as a clincial psychologist, but had thought that she could not practice, because she found herself unable to choose a method. She said it gave her "the willies" to think that she would work to change human beings in some arbitrarily chosen way.

My course had solved that problem. It showed her that people can check each move they make, to see if it carries the felt sense forward or not. In this way we can safely use all methods and theories, and choosing among them becomes a false problem.

In each of the following chapters I will show first how each *specialized* method can be made experiential by a systematic relationship to focusing. Then I will present new procedures that allow us to use the essential power of each avenue within the usual frame of psychotherapy. Because we work on all avenues, what we do on each is modifed by our awareness of the others. Therefore the content of each of the following chapters will be brought along into the next one.

CHAPTER 12

Working with the Body: A New and Freeing Energy

WE HAVE ALREADY SEEN that focusing involves the body. But the body also provides an avenue of therapy. The type of procedure I am adding seems quite modest, but it is very important, and we also need it to understand and use the other avenues. Therefore I take it up before the others.

Please permit me to use the word "body" as the body sensed *from inside*. Of course, it is the same body that can be observed from outside. And it is more than sensations and observations. Your body feels the complexity of each situation, and enacts much of what you do all day without your needing to think about each move. What you think is of course important, but you can think only a few things at one time. It is your body that totals up the whole situation and comes up with appropriate actions most of the time. Human bodies live immediately and directly in each situation.

Dr. Kulka, a well-known gynecologist with 50 years of experience once told me: "I know a lot about a patient's personality from her vagina. From periodic examinations I can tell how a patient is doing in therapy. I have checked my impression with the therapists many times." Certain foot specialists tell us that everything about a person is mirrored in tensions in the muscles on the soles of the feet. Perhaps it is possible to recognize what is happening with a person from any part of the body if one is enough of a "specialist" in that part to know its variations.

People live life with their whole bodies, not just with their nervous systems. This is also borne out by recent findings on "chemical messengers" that rapidly connect all parts of the body. Therapists who work with muscles find that past experiences, emotions, and imagery can emerge, seemingly as a result of release of tension in the muscles.

I have often helped a client work with physical symptoms from the inside, concurrently with a physician or a body therapist working with them from outside. Like Dr. Kulka did, I found the correlations striking.

For example, a shy newly emerging "part" of a person I worked with needed to hide and not be approached too directly. The part brought a pain in the client's side. A few days later the client went for medical testing concerning the same pain. During the ultrasound test she felt that this part of her wanted to hide and avoid the equipment's probing. Soon the technician said, "I'm having trouble getting at it."

Some of my clients have been helped by a few hours with a body therapist at the same time they were in therapy with me. Sometimes I suggest it and I often see the correlation I'm talking about.

There are a great many different body therapies. Some work with muscles, some with quite a number of other systems in the body. Focusing is being added to many of these kinds of body work. For example, Hakomi (Johanson & Taylor, 1988) is a body therapy in which focusing is regularly used and taught. Another is Ernst Jüchli's (1995) "GFK" in Switzerland. It is also being used in a more interactional mode of body work and healing, in which energy flows from one person to the other.

One massage therapist I know teaches her patients focusing and, during a massage, asks them to focus, giving them time to do so. When she resumes her work with their muscles, she finds an easing of tension that is a result of the focusing.

We need not ask whether a symptom is physical or psychological; any human experience is actually both. But, unlike a felt sense, mere bodily sensations are not intricate; they do not usually have what I call a life situation implicit in them, but they can lead to the felt sense of a life situation. Then we experience that what is happening in our life is generating those bodily sensations.

A felt sense is most easily found in the middle of the body. Therefore it helps to move a physical tension to the body's center. There are two ways to move it. In the following example I tried both ways. First I ask what the client feels in the middle of his body *about* the pain in the original location. When that fails and nothing comes in the center, I try the second way: "try and make the pain move into the middle of the body."[1]

C: I have this pain right here (*touches the center of his forehead just above the point between his eyes*). I just can't get anything from it, what it is.

I listened for a while, then I said:

T: How do you feel in your stomach and chest?

C: Fine.

T: Really pay attention, for a moment, in your stomach and chest and see what is there.

C: . . . I feel fine there . . . relaxed.

T: OK, wait there, keep your attention there, and see what you feel *there*, *about the pain in your forehead.*

C: (*Looking puzzled*) I don't know what you mean.

T: Be in your stomach and chest and *see if, maybe, the pain will come down from your forehead, into your stomach.*

C: (*Looks puzzled*) [But, before he can speak,] Oof . . . yeah, it's fear.

T: Stay with that. Now, gently, sense the whole of what goes with that fear.

It seems odd that a bodily sensation can move. Yet this capacity is familiar. For example, when you feel anxious in your stomach, you may start to tap your foot. It makes your stomach feel better because the discomfort moves to your foot. You can test to see whether this is really the same feeling of anxiety, transferred: As soon as you stop tapping your foot, the discomfort moves back into your stomach. It does move!

Another problem: to find the felt sense of a physical sensation, we may need to attend to a place in the body *just next to*, or the feeling *just before*, the mere sensation happens. Here is an example:

C: I am getting one of my headaches.

T: Oh, let's see what is making it.

C: I don't know.

T: What's in the middle of your body?

C: I feel nauseous, sort of like throwing up.

T: Try pulling back a little from the nausea, and then coming back. But when you get close to it again, don't go all the way into it this time. Stop just before the place where the nausea comes; see if there is a sense of meaning there, just before the nausea.

C: (*silence*) I would cry. That's what is there.

T: Oh, yes. Let it cry.

C: I can't.

T: Right. I didn't mean you could just do it. Just let the crying place be.

C: (*long silence*) If I'm there, my headache is less! (*long silence*) I'm scared of those headaches. What do I do if the headache comes and I can't find the crying?

T: When I said, "just before the nausea," did that help, or did you find the crying place in spite of what I said?

C: It's a little further up than the nausea, a little away from it.

In this example we see the difference between the nausea, which is *only* bodily, and the implicitly complex sense of a whole problem; it comes in "a little away from it." With a body sensation anywhere but the center of the body we ask, "What would come in the middle, *about* that pain?" But in this case, nausea is already in the middle of the body. Still, a felt sense can come there also, *near* it.

The middle of the body "speaks" more easily, but sometimes we can sense this type of complex situational meaning in other locations. Take for example your facial expression. It has an implicit significance which you can feel in your face. You can best pursue it further by attending to what it becomes when it transfers to your gut and chest. But if a sensation won't move, you can sometimes focus on it where it is.

A NEW AND FREEING BODILY ENERGY

Now I come to the main kind of body work procedure I want to add here. Therapy is greatly augmented if a new step develops further in such a way that a new and freeing physical energy actually flows in the client's body. When a bit of therapeutic change has already come, it can lead to a larger change if the client spends an additional moment, deliberately letting that bit of change come *as an energy flow in the body*.

For example, say there have been some small steps, and now there is a large one. By focusing, the client has experienced a change-step which brought a new and better way of being.

C: Yes! (*short silence*) [The client nods several times, as one tends to do in focusing when something checks.] Yes, I do feel [some new way]. That's all right now. The other thing I wanted to bring up . . .

T: Wait. Can you let that good new thing come in your body?

C: (*Short silence, smiles*)

The client's step had been quite genuine as it was. It was not merely an idea, but an experiential sense of a new and better way of being. It had come from his bodily felt sense. The new step felt complete. And yet, a much fuller change happens when he is asked to *"let that good new thing come in your body."*

It is not easy to adopt hands-on procedures in psychotherapy. However, once we have become sensitive to the whole dimension of bodily energy, we will not be able to help noticing energy changes when they happen. We see the client's body change. The posture alters and the face comes alive. We will also notice when such an energy is *missing*, even though a therapeutic step may have come.

It is not inevitable that a new physical energy will come from simply focusing. Having a felt sense is a quiet process. *From* a felt sense many stormy emotions and energies may arise, and lead to further rounds of focusing. But when at last a new and good way of being *has* come, we often see that the client's body has remained in that quiet, receptive mode that is typical when a person attends to a felt sense. In that posture the body cannot yet be filled with the new way of being.

When a new way of being is allowed to let its energy flow in the body, clients find their bodies changing. They may find their shoulders squaring themselves, or they may feel as if they were striding unstoppably, or they may feel new energy as if they were inhaling fresh air. Or, the whole body might ease, like letting oneself just be, lying on the ground in the sun, being fully supported. The new energy will manifest itself as whatever comes in the body of its own accord.

Every focusing step is of course a bodily change, but we often notice that not enough of the whole body has as yet participated in the change. Therapeutic change is in part an actual change in the body's tissue. When a new way of being comes during therapy, clients often have it only minimally. Asking them to let it come more fully in their bodies can produce a great deal of physical change.

Of course we ask for a moment to let bodily energy flow only very occasionally in therapy, when a change step seems too good to pass by without having it come in a full-bodied way. New steps are often much too sensitive to be interrupted with this kind of request. But a therapist who is aware of the bodily avenue can sometimes find ways to move further on it. Here is another example:

A long-time client begins the hour by hurriedly mentioning a seemingly small event. A child she takes care of has baked a cake for her in a very creative way. The therapist knows that the client has been worried about the child and that it means a lot to her that the child has been creative, rather than seeming inwardly damaged and shut down. But the client only mentions the cake as an off-handed aside, before the session begins. As the session begins she hurries on to the main problem she wants to work on, and the therapist says,

T: Wait. That's a joy, that she did that! *Let that come through a little more, please.*

C: (*Short silence, breathes*) Yeah!

The therapist believes that the next bit of therapeutic work is going to be more successful if this good news becomes a physically felt flow of energy. Then the client will have a stronger, more fully alive, body with which to work on any issue.

Notice that here the therapist did not mention the body, but the response has the same effect, and it comes from the therapist's seeing and hearing that the good thing was not flowing in her body.

The response may also create an interaction in which therapist and client feel the joy together. Implicitly he shares her joy. If his joy was not evident to her, he might have said, "Lets celebrate that for a moment."

Here is a similar example, again without any actual mention of the body. A client has long talked about "waiting" (forever) for her father to notice her, to hear her. Now she says:

C: I told him [the man she dates], and I am telling you: I am making my own decisions. I am not waiting anymore.

T: You are saying *on all levels*: You are not waiting anymore.

C: Yes. [She appreciates that the therapist's phrase, "on all levels," means the man she dates, the therapist, and her father.] And when I called, he was busy, and . . .

T: [Interrupting] Wait, you told me a big thing. *You aren't waiting anymore!*

C: (*Silence, cries*) *And that's a lot.*

What came forward here was well worth the therapist's interruption of her. The therapist expected a visibly assertive energy. What came instead was that the client was deeply moved, more fully experiencing what her step forward meant to her.

Sometimes a new bodily energy is already fully there, but only for a moment. For example:

C: I could just do it for no other reason than that I want the freedom. Yes! I'll do it *just because I want to*. I am not going to be so h-e-a-v-y anymore, about e-v-e-r-y little thing, the way I've always been.

A therapist who sees and hears the bodily dimension will notice an energy change like the one in this instance. A bit of new and freeing energy flashed for a moment ("I'll do it *just because I want to*"). But was it long enough to last? The client here had probably already lost the energy a moment later, when he used his body to dramatize how he used to be ("heavy . . . the way I've always been"). We need clients to regain that *new* physical energy flow, and let it fill the body longer. Since the energy *did* come, it *can* come again, but a split second of being alive in a new way is not enough to change a person.

We can ask: *"Can you let that come again in your body?"* This question is so simple, yet it supplements the process with a whole avenue of therapeutic change.

When a new step has come, the therapist can often notice that the client's body has been sitting *quite immobile* the whole time, totally left out of the action. If so, a change in posture is required if new energy is to come in. The client needs first to loosen the body, to release it from the frozen position in which it has been.

T: Could you let that come in more? Please sit forward for a moment, like this (*the therapist models, sitting forward on the edge of the chair*), and just loosen your body a little. Then let that come in whatever way it comes. Sense what comes *in your body* when I say it back to you.

Of course we don't want clients merely to mimic how they *think* a new step *should* make their bodies feel and look, and we don't want clients to have to perform or show us something. Therefore we might add:

T: I don't need to see anything. Just inside, let yourself feel what comes in your body.

A small invitation is enough. Strongly suggesting something to a client pushes the client's energy back; that would be the opposite of the energy we want. We only ask the client to let a bodily energy flow come. We do not need proof that it came.

We might ask for this type of pause when something wells up and is instantly gone again. Take the following example:

C: (*After he has talked unemotionally for some time, there is a break in the client's voice.*) I'm so tired of my depression, and other people also get very tired of it. My friend Nick got tired of it and he doesn't want to see me now, much. If I go to his place I try not to complain and ask for care. And in my group they said I'm passive and all I do is complain. I do say to myself: "I can take care of myself. I can do that myself."

T: You can sense that the depressed feeling *is* wanting care, and you do kind of give it to yourself. It scares you, though, that the people are getting tired of you.

C: And I'm worried you will too.

T: And that includes me. You're scared I'll get tired of you being depressed and asking for care.

C: Yes. (*Silence*)

T: I notice *something welling up in you* when we talk about your needing care.

C: Yes, it loosened things in my throat. Mostly I don't feel anything.

T: Saying you need care loosens your throat, *and you do really feel that wanting, wanting care.*

C: It loosens that locked place. (*Eyes tear up*)

T: *Do sense that now as clearly as you can in your body;* the stuck depressed place is really this need-for-care place. Is that right? Can you sense that?

C: It loosens when I say "I need care," and *if somebody is there to say it to.* And it's also the connection with all that stuff with my mother that we talked about.

What has felt stuck and tight moves into a flow. It was there before, but it was stuck and tight in the client's throat.

In the next interview the client said,

C: It has worked some, to turn the locked place into tears, if I think of asking for care . . . and my mother.

When all seems dead and numb, if a feeling does well up it needs to be pursued. A therapist can hear when the client's voice breaks, or there may be a glistening in the client's eyes.

In our example the therapist certainly responds to the relational side ("You're scared I'll get tired of you being depressed and asking for care"). This had been talked about before. Here, being *concretely* nonrejecting and caring will do more to respond to the client's fear and need for care than simply talking *about* them.

The flow that welled up was new. It could be heard for a moment in the client's voice. Although he went on in a very meaningful way, what had stirred was gone. Could it be invited to come in more fully so that it could really be here? Before attempting to get it to come forward, however, we must recognize that because the client's feeling comes in response, partially, to the presence of another person, our pushing him could violate the relational side of our interaction. With that in mind we realize that inviting his need for care to be here more fully was *concretely* accepting and welcoming of it, rather than our being tired of it. The example shows that the other avenues of therapy were deepened when the client was asked to "sense . . . *in your body.*"

Depending on the relationship, sensitive interpersonal moments risk being destroyed if the bodily dimension is overtly mentioned. There are other ways to affirm the client's move so that it can come fully in a bodily way. Therapists who are sensitive to the bodily dimension will notice changes in the client's bodily energy. They can be responded to without some jarringly unusual response.

What sort of changes might be noticeable? New forward energy certainly, but also if the client's energy seems suddenly sapped. The therapist can then ask, "Wait, what did that mean to you?", "What happened?", or "Something just changed?" If a response like this is corroborated by the client, we can then pursue what just arose inside and is getting in the way. Or the therapist can try to bring the good energy back: "Is this right? You were moving forward when you were saying . . ."

A sudden loss of energy is often due to a superego attack (see Chapter 19). If the concept of a super-ego attack is familiar to the client the therapist can help bring the good energy back: "Wait, that's *that* voice again. You were just saying. . . ."

But the most important role of the bodily dimension concerns new and freeing energy. What is a new and freeing energy? It differs from individual to individual. The content could have been the opposite of "I'll do it just because I want to." For example, it might have been something like:

C: I think I could study that book the way I am supposed to do. Hmm. (*Silence*) In the past I have always refused and I've always had to do something else. But just now it felt almost like a privilege if I don't *have to* do something else, if I can let myself do what I'm supposed to do.

From here the therapist reflects the client's new freedom, the client relates some incidents, and there is some discussion. The moment when the feeling was real to the client seems long gone. Yet he is still talking about it.

T: Can you still feel that *in your body*? Could you sit a little forward like this, and see what comes in your body when I say it back to you. What comes there if I say, "Now you have your permission to do just what you're supposed to do.

C: (*Silence, his posture eases.*) Feels grounded.

T: Ah, it feels grounded.

C: Yes.

T: Is it still there?

C: Well, it *was*.

T: If we repeat how you came, does that new energy come again? You got to it from that book and from your saying that you could study it just the way you are supposed to do it. (*Waits*)

Clients can get the new energy back if they remember one or two of the steps that led up to it. But remembering is not enough. If the client can vividly go over the steps again, up to the original spot, then — aha! — the energy might *physically* come again.

Between therapy sessions, a client can let such a new energy come again and again by repeating the steps that led up to its coming. But it is all right if the new energy comes only when the therapist is present.

For some clients a new and freeing energy is self-assertive. But for active and restless workaholics a new and freeing energy might be more like a peaceful stretch of time. We don't know in advance what it will be. The client can evaluate it once it physically comes.

Letting something come in the body is useful in a number of ways aside from maximizing a step that has already come. For example, many clients lack a grounded way of being. We might ask such a client to imagine lying in the grass, on the earth, to see what comes. It might be a bodily release, a deep exhale perhaps, or something else that comes in the body.

Of course, it is also possible that nothing will come, but these invitations take only a few moments. We can ask clients to sense what comes in their bodies whenever we see the possibility of a new and freeing energy. It doesn't take long to recognize likely sources for such an energy.

I had a client who had worked through events in his past with much success, but now no longer seemed to move in therapy. I usually do not interrupt silences, even if a client does not know what to say, but with this client I said,

T: Can I ask you to do something for a minute? Suppose you had behind you just the childhood that you really should have had? Sit forward just a little [I sit forward myself] so your body knows it has a fresh start. Put your attention in the middle of your body and wait. What *would* come there if you had had the kind of past that fits with your being all OK now?

The client had a definite physical experience, resulting in a large smile. I cannot be sure how much this session contributed to it, but thereafter he began many interviews by saying, "I feel good. I don't know why, since my situation hasn't changed." Then we would work on steps he would take to change his job and his lack of relationships, which he had not done earlier, although I had suggested such steps.

Another client had been coming to therapy for 2 years. Despite much progress, a part of him that was like a hurt child never seemed to recover from all the defeats he said his father imposed on him.

C: He *always* had to have *his* way. I had to lose *every time.*

T: Can we try something?

C: OK.

T: Sit forward for a moment like this. Put your attention in the middle of your body. What would come if you were whatever way you *would* be if you *had* won some of those battles?

C: (*Sighs*) It would be nice to have won some of them. (*Silence, his body straightens, with evident new energy.*) Maybe *all of them!*

When therapists gain experience with bodily energy, in clients and in their own bodies, they become able to invite it, and respond to it in a variety of ways.

The quality of bodily energy is also a guide for working on other avenues. In the following chapters we will see that every other therapeutic avenue contributes not only the characteristics of its own dimension, it also provides unique ways to engender a new and freeing bodily energy. Therefore this topic will develop further as we take up the other avenues.

NOTE

1. Examples in this chapter are written from memory. They are not as accurate and detailed as transcripts from tape.

CHAPTER 13

Role Play

THE ROLE-PLAY METHOD of therapy developed by Moreno, Psychodrama, employs an actual stage; the client acts in a drama. Many French psychoanalysts have a "stage" in their offices. Other people may be brought in to portray characters from the client's life. An assistant, the "alter ego," stands behind the client and expresses more directly feelings the client expresses or implies. Role play can bring a great deal of important experience that the client may never have felt before.

Gestalt therapy employs a "two chair" technique in which the client pretends to remain in one chair and in fact gets up and sits down in the other chair. The client is asked to *be* (to play the role of) a significant person, dream figure, or feeling. In that role the client speaks and acts toward "the client," who is imagined as still sitting in the first chair.

Role play has the potential to change *the direction* of a bodily energy. For example, if a client feels sluggish, discouraged, or oppressed, the Gestalt therapist would say: "*Be* that feeling, charade it, act it out as if you were an actor in a play." The client gets up and acts the sluggishness *at* "the client" in the chair.

To experientialize the technique of role play, we examine how it arises and also how it affects the client's experience. This enables us to see what role play *does*. From this we can recognize which of role play's effects are not provided by the other avenues. Let me state, and then show, its unique contribution:

From the example above, instead of being a passive figure who is *made* sluggish by the sluggishness, now the client *is* the sluggishness and *makes* "the client" in the chair feel sluggish. This is actually enjoyable because the client is *in the active position* rather than being the victim. Being the heavy feeling *at someone* is very different from having the feeling. It is the same experience (of sluggishness) from the other side, but what comes in the client's body is an entirely

192

different energy, for example, a maliciousness: "I'm going to weigh you down and press you into the ground!" This may be accompanied by a gleam in the eyes, a flow of hostility, and a laugh. Such an energy may be quite new and unusual for a shy and gentle person. Yet it can come alive in a moment's role playing.

Is such an energy a totally new formation? Yes and no. It is the client's own inwardly directed aggression; the client has been chronically the victim of it, but it is now experienced from the active side. Therefore it is old, but as a bodily energy and a way of being alive it may be very new indeed.

Experiencing something from the opposite side changes the direction of the energy. Before, the energy *came at* the client; now it moves *outward from* the client.

When something "splits off" like this it not only separates from us, it also turns around and comes back at us. For example, depression is said to be anger turned inward. This poses the question: How do we reverse the direction? By playing the role of the depression, a client may find a great change in energy in which the depression says and feels this: "You can't budge me. I'm staying put! I'm solid, strong. I will not be moved!" The client's energy is suddenly strong and active.

The essential irreplaceable contribution of role play is this role reversal, living and feeling something from the other side. No other avenue of therapy provides this. Clients can talk about and focus on a problem indefinitely without ever experiencing it from the other side.

The aggressive energy which has long been split off can now become integrated because it has changed direction. No longer turned against the client the energy becomes a part of the person because now it flows from the person.

Let me explain what the word "integration" really means: In a class I teach on therapy a student complained that her extended family criticized her all the time. I was teaching the class to employ two chair technique (which I use only rarely in its fixed form). The student stood up and faced "herself." Now she *was* the criticism. After some shouting and gestures she bent down over her imaginary self in the first chair and sucked blood out of her imaginary neck. (This scared the class.)

As one does in Gestalt therapy, I then asked her to sit in her own chair again, and see what reaction she would have to this blood-sucking werewolf. She was silent for a few moments, and then she calmly and firmly said to it, "*Get* off my neck."

This example shows that we need not be afraid of something that is flamboyant and vile in its split-off and turned form. Here it transformed into a quiet, adaptive strength when the energy flowed through her body and joined with all the rest of her; it became integrated and owned.

Let us now unpack the fixed procedures of role play and adapt them to our therapy frame and to the other avenues. First I want to explain why I don't use two chairs and don't ask clients to return to their own chair, as in the example. As I said in the last chapter, clients return to their usual role far too quickly anyway. I prefer to keep them with the new energy flowing as long as I can.

Clients do not change (for example, they remain sensitive and caring) during role play, even while being the aggressor. This is why they often laugh as they feel both sides at once. Because both sides are lived in the same body, an integration results. In our example the quality of the student's energy was already very good even while she was sucking blood. It only looked awful from the outside. In role play the energy that is generated feels positive and life-enhancing however negative the "other side" may have seemed before it became enacted. As the student's critic it was negative indeed, but when it flowed from her body outward it did not have the ugly quality it had when she felt it directed at her.

The experiential method solves a problem that sometimes causes Gestalt therapy to fail. It happens when clients *think up* the lines for a feeling or a character to say. Role play is intended to be "spontaneous," but what this means is not well specified. "Spontaneity" sometimes only means not taking time before speaking. Clients may role play, off the top of their heads, without making a connection to their bodies.

With focusing and our emphasis on bodily energy flow, this difference can be identified quite clearly. The suppressed side is meant to well up, that is, to come from the body. Gestalt therapists agree that role play must come from the body. But only some Gestalt therapists know how to insure that it will. When focusing is added to role play clients attend within their bodies and wait until an impetus to say or do something comes from *there*.

Focusing also makes a contribution after role play has brought something new. When role play generates something spontaneously, clients who know focusing can stop, and go directly to the source of what came. For example, let us say tearful words came. The client can be asked to sense *the crying place*, inside. That inside "place" is a felt sense and will lead to further steps of therapeutic change.

Role play is not necessarily spontaneously physical. To prevent merely inventing or imagining, we give focusing instructions to attend within the body, and do not require the client to get up and act the role. The emphasis is on *waiting* for what to say or do to come from within the body. Stanislavsky had to teach actors to immerse themselves in their roles in this bodily way. He had to train them to play a role in this way.

The experiential method contributes a whole vocabulary of specific instructions for bodily role play. We ask for role play specifically *in bodily terms*. We say, "Put your attention in the middle of your body and wait. What would come there if you . . .?" From experience with focusing we can recognize when clients cannot attend inside the body, and can teach them this bodily attention. We are able to insure that clients discover that role play can well up from the body.

Not only do we emphasize the bodily dimension but we modify role play in such a way that it does not fill the whole therapy hour. The client needs most of that time for other avenues. We do not want role play to violate those. For example, the avenue of interaction must not be violated. We want no more than a few minutes of the kind of interaction in which the client is told what to do.

Let me present our modified version of role play in the context of one special use. Role play is indispensable when working with dreams. We ask the client to "be" a figure or an object from a dream. Anything in a dream is likely to represent a part of us we may eventually enter into, but without role play it might take years to gain access to it. With role play we can enter anything in a dream and experience it bodily from its own side. We know instantly what it is.

The parts of ourselves that appear in our dreams do not always require a change in the direction of energy flow, but they do need to be experienced from their side. We have no idea what they are when we see them only from the outside, as pictured in a dream. With role reversal, when we enter the images of a dream and act as them, we quickly feel them and discover what they are.

Clients who are not used to constant role play often have stage fright. They become tense and worry about how they will *look* and how well they will play the role. These concerns are irrelevant to the purpose of role play; the observer doesn't need to see anything. Performing visibly is good but is not essential. What is essential is the role reversal, to feel oneself physically in the other role so that the new energy comes in the body.

Successful role reversal must happen spontaneously, and that means it must be allowed to well up from the body. It is not necessarily by having to perform that the client can best let *that* happen.

If role play is done experientially, the emphasis shifts to the time before the actual performance. It is while people peacefully *prepare* to play the role, that they best let bodily impulses arise inside themselves uncensored. They then have time and privacy to feel their way physically into the role.

This resembles what Stanislavsky taught his actors: They were told to spend time feeling themselves living inside the character. They were to ask themselves, "How would I walk? How would I stand?" They spent time letting such impulses come, weeks *before* the play.

We give surer, more physical role play instructions when we let clients know that they don't *have to* stand up and do anything visible. I say, "I'm pretending that I am putting on a play. *The play is next week.* It's a children's play; everything is exaggerated, overacted. We have great villains and witches with big hats, and wild colorful dragons. In my play—next week—we need you to act—to overact—this character from your dream." Or I might say, "You know, there were medieval plays in which the characters were different virtues and vices, and various feelings. One character was envy, another jealousy, and so on. I am putting on a play like that—next week, not now. *In my play one character is this figure from your dream. Would you be willing to play that part?* Right now you don't need to do anything I can see. Just feel your way into the role. Put your attention in your body. Sit forward a little [I demonstrate this]. Loosen your body. Now, imagine being this figure.

Wait till your body wants to say or do something. How would you come on stage? Would you walk, jump, sneak, or how? How would you stand? You need not *do* it now. Just inside you, see how it comes to you to do it—next week. Don't make it up. Put your attention in the middle of your body, and—wait."

It is welcome if the client does wish to act the role outwardly. Some clients do stand up to move and act, but no outward activity is necessary. They do need to loosen their body, as I have already explained. Then, when a new bodily energy comes in the client's body the client's color and appearance change. When this happens we can nearly always see it. It will also usually be accompanied by a laugh.

When clients merely describe how they might act the role, I interrupt and say: "Wait. Let it come in your body. Put your attention in your body, and see what impulse comes *there* if you are this figure."

If the energy does not come in the body and there is no laugh, what is probably needed is for the client to overact. For example, if an obnoxious character is being acted, I may encourage the client by saying: "Please ham it up. Overact: Be *so* obnoxious it's unbelievable. Try sitting on the other actors, or maybe even walk on them. Maybe make them fall off the stage; they can't stand it. But these are my projections. What comes up in *your* body to do? See what comes if you vastly overdo it. Let it go all the way."

With role play we can enter anything in a dream, especially the most extreme or opposite figure, perhaps an aggressive, obnoxious, contemptible, threatening, or evil figure. In the following example, the client has engaged in this kind of role play many times before. This was the image from the client's dream:

C: There was a *huge* dinosaur and it threatened me with its head.

T: *Be* the dinosaur. How would you move?

C: I thought you'd say that. (*Silence, laughs*) I *stride*!

Sometimes a client cannot play such a figure but playing the role opposite that figure can bring a similar new energy. After giving instruction in a workshop to play such a figure, one person said she could not do it. Asked further, she explained: "I dreamt of the man who abused me as a child." I said, "Oh, of course you don't want to play him. Play opposite him in my play. To confront him, what would you need? You can have anything you want, a lance, a flame thrower, a tank?" Her body changed. She took a deep breath and said, "A tank would be j-u-s-t right."

Playing the role opposite the one in question is not quite the same, but it can bring a good step.

Of course we would not override a client's obviously negative or fearful reaction to a suggestion. We might suggest focusing on it. We would be responsive to the reaction in some way.

Role playing an aggressive character is not advisable for people who have impulse control problems and act out aggression involuntarily.

Some clients who are unfamiliar with role play may be uncomfortable at first, needing an explanation or a brief demonstration by the therapist. ("Would you come on stage like this . . . ? Or like this . . . ? See what comes in *your* body.)

Overly controlled clients may utterly refuse to pretend to "be" an evil or ugly figure, because they have always avoided feeling anything of that kind. I remind such a client that the exercise is a play, a pretense. "Could you *enjoy* playing that role?" I ask. After a few moments a large smile may break out on the client's face, "Oh, yes!" In that moment the client's body has changed. The new energy has arrived.

The new energy always feels very positive, even if the words that describe it are quite negative ("sloppy," "obnoxious," "evil," "hostile"). While it is still split off, this part does not feel positive, but it becomes positive when its energy comes physically in the client's body.

Energy must be distinguished from action. Actions have consequences. "One ought not to harm any living creature," I say, "but in terms of energy it can be very good to role play the act of smashing someone over the head. A murder a day keeps the psychoanalyst away." Of course no action is intended, only a freeing flow of bodily energy.

There are many times in therapy when it may help to point out the difference between energy and action, for example, if a client blocks his fury at his father because he would not want to hurt an old man. "He would have a heart attack," the client says. I answer, "Of course I leave it to you what you actually say and do. It might be nothing like this. But *the energy* of your anger needs to move forward. Since your father isn't here now, you could *imagine* doing or saying anything to him. You can do it here, now. Energy and action are two different things."

If this suggestion isn't taken up, I simply listen and follow the client.

This method can be tried at any juncture in therapy. It requires only a minute, and if it fails nothing is lost. Once clients have learned it, the therapist needs only to say, "Do you want to *be* that figure?"

Role play can be used to deal with things other than dream images. For example:

C: I can't use the room because his [a friend's] boxes are still there. He's been promising to move them out for months and months. I would tell him to move them but that would be mean.

T: Play someone *mean*, in my play, you know, that I'm putting on next week.

C: Hmm. (*There is visible bodily energy change.*) I'd put them out in the snow *on the street!*

As I said in the chapter on working on the body's energy, clients often lose a new energy almost instantly. For example:

T: In the dream, Mike [the client's young son] rescues the baby. What part of you is Mike? Can you *be* him with your body?

C: He's courageous. (*She expands her chest, smiles, and clearly has the energy she is describing.*) He'll meet anything.

T: Let that come, more, in your body, just as you have it.

C: (*Slumps*) Oh, that's so far from me. I'm always hanging back, mousy (*makes an infantile face*).

T: Wait, go back and have Mike in there for a little longer. How was that again?

C: (*Silence, breathes*)

Here the client did spend a while, being the new way physically. What she then said showed that she had:

C: I wouldn't have to hide so much.

If a whole hour of therapy is spent in role play, many other vital dimensions of therapy would be neglected. The therapist can turn into a stage director, which can make the client passive in the relationship. But the client's ownership of the hour is not disturbed by an occasional "What would come in your body if you . . . ?" And this provides an irreplaceable resource for therapy.

Once role play has given a therapist sensitivity to *the direction of energy*, the therapist will notice it all the time on all other avenues of therapy. We notice when a response of ours has made the client's energy collapse or back up, and we quickly respond so as to let the energy move forward and outward from the client. If the client slumps, if all the animation drains from the client's face, we would ask if "Something went wrong just now? Something I said or did wasn't right?"

Role play gives clients the opportunity to be spontaneous, move around, shout, or roll around on the floor. This is an important addition, since so much of therapy is quiet and inwardly attentive.

Therapists familiar with role play have a similar advantage. Most forms of therapy seem to need a quiet, overcontrolled therapist. In suggesting and demonstrating role play it is okay to become noisy and open up spontaneously. It provides a balance for those of us who are most familiar with quiet inward attending. Clients don't need us to be only quiet and inward. They need to see us become animated and roll out. We can always back up quickly, and listen again.

CHAPTER 14

Experiential Dream
Interpretation

DREAMS ARE AN IRREPLACEABLE avenue of therapy for two reasons: (1) what is far from the client's awareness cannot be processed, but if it comes up in a dream, it can immediately be processed; (2) dreams translate a person's problem into images that implicitly contain an energy that moves toward a solution.

To experientialize the usual procedures that therapists use in dream analysis, we examine the source of dreams and their effects on the client's experiencing. The last chapter showed how the method of role playing a dream figure can be understood and used experientially. Let us now examine other methods of dream interpretation to see exactly when and how they bring experiential change.

Let me explain 1, why distant unconscious material is not helpful, and why it helps if it is a dream that brings it up.

Dreams come from deep in the "unconscious" (experientially we mean by this, that which exceeds a person's awareness and deliberate control). If drugs or a therapist forced something to come up from the client's unconscious, it would probably be disorganizing to the client. At the least it would be out of order because it would not be *what is next* in the process that arises naturally from inside.

Experience does not consist of fixed facts that can be "dug up" separately. There are no separate contents. Experience is a mesh. Any one memory, event, or feeling is part of an experiencing process that implicitly contains many others.

Throughout this book we have seen that the next step is always finely implied and demanded, before it comes. Each moment of experience *is* not only what it seems to be; it also *is-for* further steps. The process of therapy always moves from what is now implicit. Each step carries the process further, so that something new becomes implicit. Only so does a further step become possible. Therefore there is no way to use "unconscious material" that arises very far away from the client's present edge of experience. It would skip too many steps that ought to happen first. Steps come at the edge of the client's experiencing, and they should come in their own order.

But a dream by its nature is not dug up out of order. It has come through the client's organism this very night. So it does arise at the client's present edge. It contains something that can come next, if we can generate the *process from inside* that the dream implicitly contains.

But the phrase "from inside" states a vital condition. What is next in a dream is not what an interpretive system sees in the dream. *What is next is only what the client's body makes of the dream.* I will present a number of procedures by which the body can make therapeutic steps from a dream.

Let me now explain 2, how it is that the dream's version of a problem implicitly contains clues to and energy for the steps to a solution.

In Freud's theory all dreams are wish fulfillment. This is not so, unless we read it *this* way: A wish is of course always for something we lack. It indicates an energy that cannot continue into living because something is missing. We might not wish it to be the way it is pictured in the dream, or to have the dream's consequences in actual life, but we *would* wish the energy unblocked, if there is a safe and right way to live it forward. So Freud's theory can be read as saying that dream images contain an energy that moves toward continuation.

In Jung's theory life creates "opposites." (Some theories call them "conflicts.") What we develop in our consciousness involves the *not-being* of the other way, and that one becomes unconscious. Thus our original animal wholeness is divided. Two opposites form one *issue*. A single tear in a cloth creates two separate sides. If something is an issue, it has two sides. Last night's dream comes from an unresolved issue that *is* being experienced in the dream. The dream is exactly at the client's present edge of experience. It shows two factors, how the aware person now lives, and how the rejected part of the organism reacts to that way of living. The dreamer's actions are one side, the others and the events express the other side. Jung thought that a dream should lead to a kind of negotiation between the two.

If we experientialize Freud's and Jung's approaches, we try to capture the actual experience of an energy that wants to continue, and will bring the other side (the organismic side) of an issue. Through eliciting the felt sense of various parts of a dream we will soon find that energy. *We find it in the body.* And, it does not remain static. When it comes from a felt sense, it generates a therapeutic step toward a solution.

Except in rare cases, the step forward is not actually in the dream. It comes from the energy that the dream's images imply and create. What this means will be apparent in specific examples.

To experientialize the usual dream-analysis, let me present our procedures in roughly the order in which we might use them. The central issues in a dream are usually approached a little later.

PREPARATORY PROCEDURES

Loving the Dream

In the beginning it is important to help clients to form a good relationship with their dreams. People often feel that their dreams are bizarre and this scares them. We can help a client to love a dream, if we turn it this way and that, admiring its creativity. If we admire some intricacy in a client's dream, we can express our wonder. I exclaim, "Aren't dreams wonderful?" when I feel that type of amazement. "You could never invent something like that on purpose!"

When what I call "the manner of relating" to dreams changes from fear to interest and welcome, it changes the way the client lives inside.

A client's dreams *need* not be interpreted. No specific dream ever needs to be interpreted, because dreams happen every night. If we work too long and hard on a dream early in therapy, the client might be reluctant to bring up another dream. Enjoying the process of telling and working on the dream is implicitly much more responsive to the dream than a forced effort.

A Private Space

If a client has decided to say everything as soon as it comes, very little will come. As we work with dreams in an experiential way, we notice that meaningful associations and steps require a private space. We say to clients, "When something comes just give me a signal and stay with it a while. After a minute or so you can see what, if anything, you want to say about it."

Dream work happens in the client's body, not in verbal conversation because only what comes in the body counts. We do not conclude anything from a dream without its involvement with the client's body, and the client is the first to know what comes. This total freedom in a private space maintains the crucial relational conditions, and enables much more to come up inside the client.

THE PROCEDURE OF ASKING QUESTIONS

Different theories of what dreams are and how they function lead to different interpretations. Why must we choose among them? Rather than choosing an idea as an interpretation, in experiential therapy we look for actually experienced steps. Any of the competing interpretations could lead to a step from the dream.

Then again it might not lead to a step. With this as a touchstone we can employ any of the theories we know. Instead of saying what a dream means, or what some part of it means, we ask, "Does something come if we suppose such and such?" Experientially speaking, different interpretations are simply hypotheses. Hypotheses are best expressed as questions. We can therefore use all the theoretical systems to generate small-scale questions, until the dream is interpreted in terms of concretely experienced steps arising in the client's body.

Therapists can use all theories as a source of questions (see Gendlin, 1986a, for the particular set of questions I have derived from all the theories I know).

Many clients answer questions of this nature very quickly, saying, "No, nothing comes." Or they may make an interpretation of their own and believe it. If we work experientially, we do not address our questions *to the client*. Instead, we ask the client to take the question down inside, to ask it of the felt sense.

Before clients can do this however, they need to have found a felt sense from some part of the dream. And, if there is a felt sense, perhaps the asking of the question has interrupted the felt sense, so we must ask if it is there, or needs to come again freshly, so that the question can be addressed to the felt sense.

Some dream images are accompanied by an odd and indefinable feeling, a unique taste, an aura, a bodily quality, which, if focused on as such, is a felt sense. This can be a way for the client to discover what a felt sense is. Once the felt sense of that part of the dream has come, it will reveal itself as an intricately textured complexity, unique and new, yet with the person's own familiar quality.

In a bodily felt sense experiencing is whole: with its felt sense, anything from a dream is no longer an opaque dissociated image. From there it opens further. Every aspect of a dream can generate a unique felt sense. Once that unique sense has come, it has a life of its own. Even if we wanted to, we could not talk ourselves out of it, nor could we help it if it did not budge in reponse to some good idea. Then, when the sense finally opens, and a whole stream of detail emerges from it, the image is no longer a distant object about which we can only speculate. Only such an opening should count as a successful interpretation, rather than ideas that simply "fit," "click," or generate an intellectual "aha!"

Often the first procedure therapists undertake is asking for associations. Freud held that a dream consists of loose parts each of which is embedded in a series of associations. For Jung a dream is a single drama with a plot, characters, and a setting. In experiential therapy we often find that both are the case, and I will show how both can be used.

The client is left free if we first ask, open-endedly, "What comes, or already came to you in relation to the dream?"

Freud often looked for "day residues" (bits of events from the day before), and they often come up of course. We therefore ask, "What were you doing the day before the dream, and what went on inside you that day?" But when the client has a felt sense of some part of the dream, then we ask, "What in your life feels like that? What part of your life has the same quality?" In this way an association may lead to something that makes sense of the whole dream, or to nothing. After half a minute we move on when we see that nothing came. The client is soon comfortable as well that nothing came because nothing is urged on the client.

It is best to begin with open-ended questions, and leave hypotheses for later. We can take Jung's elements of a story and ask about the setting, characters, and plot. There is no fixed order but the setting is the safest one to ask about first: "The place, in the dream, was it inside or outside?" "In a room." "Can you sense the layout of the room. Where were the windows?" Then we do the focusing part: "Let your attention down into your body and get a felt sense of that room." And then, "Where in your life was there ever a room like that?"

Or perhaps the client might say: "It was inside but I didn't see the whole room, just a door." "Try to get the whole felt quality of that door. Where did you ever see a door like that?" "Oh, sure, that's my grandmother's closet, it was the spot where . . ." We would probably stay with that quality for a while and work with it.

After the setting come questions about the people. "Try to get the whole feeling that that figure gives you." Then, "What is an adjective or a phrase that would characterize the felt quality of that figure?" Then, "If that were a part of you, perhaps a part that you don't know very well, what part of you might it be? Can you feel it in your body?" If something comes we then say, "Does it do anything if we try out saying that you treat that part of you the way you treat this figure in the dream?" If this produces a breakthrough we have Jung to thank, but if the client only looks puzzled we go on after a minute.

Early questions of this nature are not based on the therapist's interpretations. They are simply open-ended questions about different parameters of the dream.

Many questions lead to nothing; some lead to important associations and emotions. They accumulate; we don't assume that they are diverse or that they belong together. Eventually one of the questions will open something deep. If there was only puzzlement before, now the client knows without doubt at least one aspect of real life that the dream is about. That part of the dream and that problem in the client's life have the same bodily felt sense. Other parts of the dream suddenly become meaningful as well.

Dreams seem to be about single situations, but really they are about the person, about what causes the person to be in such situations and act this way in them.

Asking open-ended questions of the felt sense is an elegant procedure. All the therapist does is ask questions, and the client soon knows what the dream is about.

However, although questioning such as was described above can sometimes lead to a concretely experienced therapeutic step forward, if the dream seems only to be a good metaphor for what the client already knew, it probably means no therapeutic step has come as yet.

The client may want to stop at this point and so we stop of course. It may be quite enough to identify what seemed so puzzling in the dream. Just to enjoy the dream work is a lot. The dream may also help the client to feel something more deeply, even if it was known before, and that can mean a great deal. But the dream has not yet made its essential contribution as long as we only have a metaphor for what we knew before the dream.

The dream's essential contribution lies in the striking fact that the dream has translated the client's problem into this particular set of images!

It is not enough to know what problem it is that is translated into the dream symbols. *The unique images themselves contain an implicit energy that can develop into a therapeutic step.* The following four procedures will show this, and illustrate ways in which we can let it happen.

THREE PROCEDURES TO FIND A NEW STEP

"Help" from the Dream: "Collecting One's Allies"

Before tackling a sensitive issue, it is well to look for what I call "help" from the dream. Some of the images do not represent the problem; rather they picture something that brings a positive energy with which to approach the problem.

Jung's ideas are grounded in mythological studies; when he says that the animal in fairy tales is always right and that its advice needs to be accepted, or when he says that something alive and green is positive, his "amplifications" can be very useful. If we use them experientially, we use them not as ideas about animals and green things, but as the bodily energy they bring, a bodily change for the better. We can let the theory guide us in asking about these things, but their successful interpretation will have a living quality, if it is found.

If this "help" reveals itself, it will make the body stronger and in a better state to cope with whatever problem the dream addresses. To seek such an experiential effect, we need not be sure in advance that it is there. We go directly to the client's body. We ask the dreamer to feel the quality of an animal in the dream, a green branch, a child, a beautiful stone, a loving person, or an enjoyable activity. For example, playful ice skating turned out to be "help" in an excerpt in Chapter 10.

We can look for help in any object in the dream. Associations made to those objects (or role playing them) may turn out to bring help. Help is anything that brings a new and freeing energy, a good or expansive quality, physically in the body. We want to have these good things with us, when we come to the difficult issue.

Jung says a boat takes one "across" a large challenge. But we would let the dreamer's body interpret the boat directly; for example, there was a boat in this client's dream. After other questions, the therapist asks,

T: What is a boat, to you? Where were you last on a boat?

C: (*Shakes his head*) I haven't seen a boat for years. When I was a kid we used to take the Staten Island Ferry.

T: What was that like?

C: The ferry — ah! — (*His face lights up and his whole body changes.*) The ferry was *glorious*. (*He tells more about it.*)

T: Let's take the feeling of being on the ferry with us, as we work on the rest of the dream. OK?

The client didn't have the feeling of the ferry experience until he was asked further about it. Then his body changed visibly. We will have better luck with the problem of the dream if the client's body first changes in this way.

Such "help" is one kind of energy some dream images contain.

Reversing Unnatural Negatives

There is often something in a dream that should be "help," but in the dream it looks or acts badly. For example, an animal acts in some unnatural way, perhaps the way the client does in life. The client may recognize the similarity or not.

For example, at a workshop, one participant told of a dream in which there was a sick turtle walking slowly down the road, with its entrails trailing behind it. The image gave the dreamer an awful but familiar feeling. She felt it physically and knew what it was, in her waking life, that gave her that feeling. It let her know without doubt what the dream was about. But the dream seemed to be saying only that the problem was indeed in bad shape. She was asked: "What would a healthy turtle be like?" At first she was thrown off by this question. "A healthy turtle? A *healthy* turtle? Well . . ." She inhaled and exhaled a long breath, and her posture and color changed. She seemed to expand like one of those Japanese compressed paper flowers when it is put into water. "A *healthy* turtle? Well . . ." "You don't need to describe it, just feel it in your body." Her response was, "That sure feels a lot better." "Can it mean anything to say that you could be this new way in that part of your life that your dream is about? The good way your body is *now*, could that be a way to handle that situation? Does it mean anything to say that?" "Yes, it has a lot of meaning. Yes." She was so content with this, that we went on to the next participant's dream. A little later she interrupted to tell us: "Now my turtle is up on its hind legs, dancing!"

We see that it isn't enough for the dream to be only an accurate metaphor for a dreamer's problem. We must also notice that the dream transcribes the situation *into turtles*. Although we don't know what to do about the waking problem in its own terms, a therapeutic change may emerge if the problem is put in terms of its images.

The turtle image has an incipient energy to engender certain changes. Sometimes such images can develop directly into change steps (for example, by letting the dream continue into waking imagery). But when something naturally positive is in the dream as sick or negative, we ask what a healthy, natural one would feel like. Here is another example of this sort of reversal:

C: There was a dead man lying stretched out on an altar. I know what that is. It's my creative part. It died.

T: Well, we can't leave your creative part to stay dead. Can that man on the altar stand up?

C: He stood up! When you said that, he just stood up.

T: In your body, can you feel him, standing up?

When this sort of thing happens we see that energy for further steps is present in dream images. We don't notice it if we keep them static and fail to ask them to move.

How do we determine whether to ask the client to role play a negative dream figure or to ask what the figure would be like if it were positive? We would suggest role playing a violent or opposite figure because aggressive energy can be good and freeing, but we would not have the client role play a sick turtle. That would not release a new and freeing energy. We ask her to play a *healthy* turtle, a *natural* turtle. In the next two chapters we will see more examples of negative elements that change into their natural positive version if we ask for it to come in the body.

But reversing something unnatural is needed only in special cases. The following are two examples of the more common way in which dream images implicitly contain a step.

Working with the Problem in Terms of the Dream Images

When the main problem in a dream is sensed in terms of the dream images, these can organically lead to steps of resolution.

C: I dreamed there was this motorcycle, biped, putt-putt something, and it wouldn't go. It had snow and ice on it. The repairman said it wouldn't fix it just to remove the snow and ice. I did anyway, and pushed it. It wouldn't go. Then the dream changed channels. There were all these women, one wore a blouse I designed. Another one was very important, and many other women came and lit cigarette lighters to warm the place.

"The place" must have been the vagina, the client hypothesized. She also found homoerotic implications in the dream. But nothing new happened as a result of these speculations. As before, she sensed the presence of a wish that her closed sexual dimension would open up, so that she could feel sexual. She tried "being" (role playing) the motorcycle, the ice, one of the women. Not much happened.

The breakthrough came with a regular question about the story, the plot. To ask about the story in a dream involves picking three main events in the dream, with an act of the dreamer in the middle: "First this happened, then you did this, and then that happened." The three-way summary is followed by: What in your life is like that?"

T: At first something cannot be fixed; *then there is something you design.* And then they warmed the place.

Her body changed and her face reddened. Of course! She designed the blouse. She loves to design clothes and other things.

C: Now I am the motorcycle and the ice is melting!

Her capacity to design things and her love of design dissolved the block to the whole issue. She designed doll clothes when she was 5. The feeling of design led her to her love of colors. Then many kinds of color came to her. She felt that her creative (and thus essential) self is frozen scared. This scared self does not open itself directly into the erotic dimension that she wishes she could feel. Rather it has another channel and that one is now open: It opens around color and design. The way to her erotic feelings turned out to open *from there.*

When the familiar sexual problem was worked with as the dream translated it into just these images of the dream, they turned out to have steps to resolution implicit in them.

In the next example, the client is involved in a battle with an unreasonable person who makes him very angry, too angry. Therefore this dream worried him.

C: A graph was shown next to the picture of a head, and it showed that if whatever was graphed went any higher, it would lead to a stroke. Then it [the dream] switched to the "control center." The repair crew was already there, but I couldn't go in, because the door was blocked by a saw horse — you know like the police use to block some place off.

T: Oh good. I'm glad the repair crew came. They know how to fix things under there. Can you be glad they're there?

C: (*Sighs*) Yes. I hope so.

Many questions following this produced no great result.

207

T: Can you *be* the saw horse?

C: (*Scrunches down, as if he were almost flat, looks very stubborn and strong, and grunts.*) I got put here. I don't know why and I don't care. I'm staying put. I'm staying put. And, hmm, if somebody jumps over me, that's none of my business. I'm staying put.

This seemed to be a specially designed way for him to keep his cool; it came to him from his own body, while embodying the saw horse from the dream.

When the Dream and the Dreamer Disagree

Now we come to conflicts, symptoms, Freudian "compromise formations," or the "opposites" Jung refers to. In my way of looking at it, there is a juncture in many dreams at which the dreamer rejects or denies what the dream says, or conversely, at which the dream refuses to do what the dreamer asks. For example, a dreamer finds a sheaf of papers in the toilet marked *Instructions for Spiderman.* He throws them away. I think that the dream puts those there for the dreamer to find, but the dreamer throws them out.

Or, the dreamer wants to go to a certain place, but the train takes him to a totally different place. Or, someone thought to be wise in the dream says, "We will now all jump off the top of the china closet," but the dreamer says it is a bad idea.

An interpretive idea need not be stated, but can lead us to formulate a question. As usual, we invite clients to address such a question to the felt sense, to see if anything budges. If there is no felt response, we let the question go.

Conflicts between dream and dreamer do need to be worked with in some way (if we have not stopped for other reasons), but neither side is simply right; this is evident from the fact that there is a split.

Looking at a conflict experientially, we cannot anticipate what the resolution will be (the examples below show why it is impossible in advance). We want to keep on asking questions with regard to the conflict, but there are no standard questions. This part of dream work is not elegant.

However, the experiential method has this advantage: Since the client already feels one side of the issue (the dreamer's side, naturally), when the other side is physically experienced, the change step that comes can take account of both sides.

For example, in the dream in which the wise person said to jump off the china closet and the dreamer refused, the dreamer's friend did jump and fell. The friend was not injured, but her heel broke the glass door of the china closet, and the fine glass figurines inside were damaged. In the dream the dreamer was very sad about this.

Dreams often present problems of coming to the ground: hanging at the end of a rope, falling. The dreamer's friend came to the ground, perhaps the friend's experience is the opposite side that should bring the good energy.

So, I had the dreamer role play the friend (who was described as a brave and solid person). We tried various questions such as "How might breaking the glass be a good thing?" A long series of other questions led nowhere. Then it turned out it was *her mother's* china closet. She was sad *for her mother's loss* of the figurines! The sadness was like her childhood experience of taking care of her mother. Now the energy moved; she said, "It makes me mad. I always had to take care of her, and be sad for her! I couldn't feel me. I'm done with that. I want to feel me."

It turned out to be worth the time spent asking questions of the spot where the dreamer refused the dream's instruction. Let me follow with another example of the dream and dreamer disagreeing. (This next dreamer is the same client who designed the blouse.)

C: A woman gave me a diamond necklace, lots of diamonds. I didn't want it, so she gave it to someone else. Later I was sorry. I could have sold it. I don't have any money.

T: Why don't you like diamonds?

C: I just don't.

Here the client's felt sense of not liking diamonds has to be invited and entered into. She doesn't like diamonds but the dream wants to give her a diamond necklace. With her usual attitude she sees only that she "could have sold it." We need to try for a step from the opposite side, the side that wants her to have diamonds.

Dreamers almost always bring their usual bias to a dream. They interpret the dream with the same attitude they had in the dream. They miss, in the dream and about the dream, exactly that which they tend to miss in waking life. Therefore we want to open the possibility (only the possibility) that a step might come from the side opposite to the dreamer's usual attitude. This is called "Bias Control" in my book on dream work (Gendlin, 1986a).

Which is right, the dreamer or the dream? Neither. In a process step the whole constellation will change. The step will be a new way of being. I would not try to combine the conflicting pieces because in a therapeutic step they *melt* and new pieces form.

The client's normal attitude is to reject diamonds, and she maintains it in interpreting her dream. If she had taken the diamonds she would have sold them. That is her side and she already lives from it. Therefore we can expect a step if we can add the other side.

She does not like diamonds but she does not know precisely why. There is no textured intricacy. Her dislike of diamonds is familiar but the felt sense of all that is involved in her dislike is still unknown. The therapist invites her to let a felt sense come:

T: Diamonds are valuable. There could be something valuable in them? What's your *whole sense* of diamonds?

C: (*Long pause*) Diamonds are for certain kinds of people . . . uh . . . hard, cold people. . . . Oh, yeah, sure! *Diamonds are ice! Like the ice on the motorcycle in the other dream!* . . . Yes, they make me feel *like that*, cold, frozen. My frozen sex. Hmm . . . yeah, I turn away from it, and I turn from design and art, too. . . . I feel it melting again.

The therapist was looking for a step from the opposite side in the dream. ("There could be something valuable in them?") The step did come from the diamonds, but more exactly from her felt sense of the diamonds.

Was the dream "right" to give her diamonds? No, because they were in their cold frozen form. Was she "right" to reject cold frozen things? No, because they were her sexuality, only frozen. Both sides are right, and wrong, until the constellation changes. The dream images have the change implicit in them, but the change actually comes only in the client's body.

In the client's next dream there is again a disagreement. The dream says she can have anything she wants; she disbelieves this (in the dream and afterwards).

C: I dreamed that there was this office supply company that sent me a catalogue and I could have anything I wanted out of it.

T: Wow! You could have anything you wanted?

C: Yes.

T: Anything you wanted!

C: You like that.

T: Well, is that the feeling quality of it, that you're offered anything you wanted out of it?

C: Yes it was! (*Breathes*) I can feel it, but I don't believe it.

T: You can sense both? There is something open so that you can have what you want, and also something that doesn't believe it.

C: It's . . . mmm . . . my family . . . uh . . . they're in the way.

The client's next dream continues on from this point. There is "help" in it.

C: We were right! I dreamed about Chuck [her "good" brother], loving him, and I knew when I woke up that it's not them all in my way. It's that Chuck left [when she was 5]. It's that pain-avoiding thing.

T: Chuck is back. *Let's keep him with us, be as you were with him.*

C: (*Silence, then a long breath*)

Chuck corroborates that progress was made, and he is surely a "help"; we want to keep him with us.

In the first phase of dream work we ask questions without any hypotheses. Then we look for "help" in the dream and take it with us if we found help. Finally we ask questions in the hope of a step from the negative or opposite part of the dream. When there is a step with positive bodily energy on the main issue, it is time to stop, even though much of the dream remains uninterpreted. A dream is inherently inexhausitble, and there will be many more dreams. If we continue on and on with this one, the client will lose hold of the new step. Instead of letting that happen, we make sure before stopping, that the bodily experience of the step can be found again, so that the client can "practice" being bodily alive in this new way.

Now I must refer the reader to my book on working with dreams (Gendlin, 1986a) because I cannot repeat all of it here.

We have seen that an energy in the direction of therapeutic change is implicit in dream images. This will stand us in good stead when we work with imagery generally, as we will see in the next chapter. It also raises the theoretical question: What are images that they should have this power?

CHAPTER 15

Imagery

IMAGES ARE POWERFUL, but we do not bring forth their full power if our work is only with images. Impressive strings of images can leave people unchanged. Therefore experts on imagery are now increasingly paying attention to the role of the body. With focusing, imagery becomes immediately connected to the body.

For example, while working on a problem a client pictures a heavy weight buried in the ground. Only the top of the weight shows. He attaches a chain to the weight and has a large crane pull it up. Long strings of extravagant and surprising images follow, a fascinating journey. One would think, from the nature of the images, that it must have been a deep process, and yet they created no real change in the client. Merely observing images is not usually a process that creates change. Some call it "watching the movies."

By attending to his body, this client finds the image of the buried weight again, as before. Now he notices that the buried weight is related to the heavy feeling in his stomach, created by the problem he had been discussing. Still attending to his body, he has the crane pull the weight up, as before, but as soon as the image is allowed to come spontaneously, the weight is back in the ground. He pulls it up deliberately many times, but the stubborn image always ends up with the weight in the ground again.

The reason the image resists is because the image is made from the weight in his stomach, from his body's sense of the problem, which is to say from how he lives in the situations in which he has the problem. The image is not merely a picture. The pictured weight remains in the ground because *the image is bodily connected*, and *there has not yet been a change in his body*. Pulling the weight up deliberately changes the image *only visually*. In the body's image the weight is still in the ground.

The bodily quality is a felt sense. By attending to it as such, new steps are possible. If the client asks the felt sense what it implicitly contains then it may open. Its opening is felt as a bodily shift, together with a new implicit knowing, and words will usually come to say what that is.

After a focusing step like this, if the image is allowed to come spontaneously, it will have changed (Olsen & Gendlin, 1970). It is an impressive effect. It shows that images are connected to the body.

The felt sense can be carried forward silently or by speaking, by interpersonal interaction, and in many other ways. With such focusing steps the physically felt weight in the example above will begin to move, or the earth in which it is buried will loosen, or another image will come as he finds why the problem is buried and what goes into making it so heavy.

It is natural to move from the felt sense of an image to words, feelings, and interactions. When one sits quietly in a safe and caring interaction, the interaction carries the body forward and can soon lead to a change in the image. Even though it seems that "nothing" has happened in between the images, it is the interaction that did the carrying forward. I will show this in some examples.

If an image that comes doesn't quite "match" the felt sense we can wait for others. We check each image, until there is a directly sensed effect on the felt sense, as if to say, "yes, that image captures the felt sense." The sense of this little "yes" is itself a small shift and will soon lead to a change in the felt sense.

Sometimes a client cannot get a felt sense at all. I can help such clients to learn focusing if they let an image of a problem come first, and only then ask what physical quality the image engenders in the body. "Suppose the whole problem were pictured on a large mural before you. . . . You might stand back to see it better. What image comes?"

Then I ask: "What sense does this image give you in your body. Wait, let it come in."

Let me show how focusing can be added to some standard therapeutic methods that deal with imagery.

In Simonton's healing method, cancer patients are shown pictures of cancer cells. They are then asked to form an image of a shark and visualize it killing the cancer cells. Simonton found this to be effective. He has also used focusing in various ways.

Continuing with this approach we would ask patients to sense their active shark energy and the shark's thrust in their bodies. Some patients might not be able to sense within their bodies and require some instructions and practice. The goal would be to show the client how to come to the middle of the body (most easily upward from the toes).

We would say: "Attend inside your body. Are you there? What quality do you find there?" (If the answer indicates a bodily quality such as one finds inside, we would continue. Otherwise we would work just to help the person find how to sense there. Next we would say: "Form an image of a shark. Let that image give you the bodily sense of being the shark." After a while we would ask: "What sort of body sense came?"

If some feeling seems to be blocking the way, we might work with *that* feeling for a while, trying to get its felt sense, and some steps from it. If the person still cannot feel a shark energy, perhaps getting the client to role play what the shark's energy might feel like could help.

Most of us have found that images flourish while we are deeply relaxed. Images come easily and seem to involve deeper aspects of the person. But during deep relaxation, unfortunately, there is no felt sense and no bodily feedback.

What are the criteria for relaxation that is too deep for the focusing process? Relaxation is too deep when the body no longer "talks back." In hypnosis, we may say, "my body is comfortable," and it will seem to be true. But if we say this during focusing, the sense of discomfort will come up even more sharply and clearly. The body talks back, gives feedback, a clear sense that, "No, not comfortable, rather *this*."

Even a light, barely noticed trance can be sufficient to prevent the body from talking back. Deep relaxation can be valuable in many ways, but a great deal will be missed if clients spend the whole therapy hour in relaxation. How can we obtain imagery without such deep relaxation? Unless they are in deep relaxation most people see no pictures when they close their eyes. But everyone easily sees images with their eyes *open*. I say, "Visualize where your bed is, where you sleep. Now walk to the bathroom." Almost everyone can do this even while they are looking right at me. Then I say, "Now there, in that image space, a picture can come to go with this felt sense you have now."

From Lazarus' (1971) Systematic Desensitization we learn that anxiety can be extinguished if a client maintains deep relaxation while gradually experiencing more and more images of something anxiety producing.

The procedure consists of a carefully structured series of images of something that makes the client anxious coming closer and closer. But Lazarus told me once that he often found more happening in the imagery than the method had planned. For example, for a woman having trouble relating sexually to her husband, the sequence was to bring him very gradually closer. Her first instruction was to visualize herself at the top of the stairs as her husband came in the front door. But when Lazarus asked her what she saw, she reported that he did indeed come in the door, but with his mother, whereupon the client found herself falling down the stairs and attacking her mother-in-law.

What actually transpires in the images is likely to go beyond a procedure. Therapy is the client's process, not the therapist's procedure. As Lazarus found, we need to relate to the client's actual process. We will then see that the other avenues are going on as well, and what the special powers of images are. No fixed procedure can reveal this.

Another method, Jung's Active Daydream, may sometimes involve a felt

214

sense. Jung spoke of a "fifth" sense, the moving center of a square of which sensation, feeling, thought, and intuition are the four sides. In some respects a felt sense is each and also none of these. Sometimes Jung tells a client to let images come "from the affect." He may not mean a *bodily* sensing. What he calls "affect" is more like an emotion than the *implicitly complex* felt sense. But one can easily use Jung's Active Daydream technique in a focusing manner, asking clients to attend in their bodies, to let a felt sense come there, and then let an image form from the felt sense.

Now let us see what we might learn and adopt from Jung's method. Once an image came, Jung would ask clients to be active in relation to the image, to respond to it as if it were real. For example, in one man's images his girlfriend dove into a lake and disappeared beneath the water. Jung would say something like: "Don't just sit there and watch this! What would you do in real life? In the image now, dive in actively and keep her from being lost!"

Jung would want the client, after acting in response to the image, to wait again, to give the image a chance to move on its own. We might at times adopt this alternation.

Once we have become proficient with several specific procedures they tend to break up into many small moves that we use flexibly at many junctures. Even just asking whether a client has an image can teach us a great deal. At many points in therapy we can ask, "Can an image come from that?" And when it comes, "What body sense does it give you?"

In Chapter 10 we saw some of the ways in which images can instruct us, often with new alternatives we could not have made up. The capacity of images to bring new alternatives is very sriking. We had only two alternatives: to stop or to go on. "Don't try to cross the fence here," the image says, "but further down, there is one place to cross." We do not instruct such images; we obey their instructions.

The turtle and the buried weight are images that contain an energy of their own, an energy that resists or generates new steps. We can sense their energy once a bodily felt sense comes from the images, and then the energy also moves to further steps.

What is unique about images?

In my philosophical works (Gendlin, 1962, 1992a, 1992b, 1996a, in press), I develop a system of terms with which I can carefully derive what I will say roughly here:

Every living body organizes, implies, and — if it can — enacts the next step of its own living process. If if cannot enact the next step, the implying of it continues. This may be painfully experienced over and over again in a way similar to pangs of hunger, in the sense that it implies feeding without its happening.

Images are projections (virtual objects) that the body creates in order to carry what it is implying forward in ways not possible in actual situations. An image is an intervening solution, a home-made object that carries forward what cannot (or cannot yet) be carried forward in reality. That is why a focusing step to solve a problem can come first in an image.

The sense we try to convey when we speak is a result of crossing. A great many factors go into "what we want to say," and words come to us to say *that*. An image comes similarly from the crossing of many factors. The image might come just from thinking about some situation. Then, if we get a felt sense and focus on it, we may find some of the myriad factors that crossed to generate the image.

If the image were of a plastic shield, we might think: "I could be there and the hostility wouldn't get to me, yet I could still see everything that goes on. And the shield is invisible, so no one would know I had it. And it would be just like in that movie, where . . . Yes, that would handle the situation exactly. It would give me the confidence I'm always looking for; it makes people who have it much safer. Yes, it fits all those factors!" (If we went on, we would think of others.)

Thus, images bring new and more intricate possibilities. Ordinary objects and alternatives are poor and few compared to the vast number of strands that cross in an image. But why is it that alternatives that come in images move toward solutions? It is similar to the reason a wound heals, or why when we are hungry we seem luckily to hit upon the idea of food.

Of course, there is no such thing as an invisible plastic shield that would let a person get around normally and confidently in threatening situations. But there *is* a bodily implied step or series of steps to bring this kind of invulnerability and confidence. Before the image came, the person was feeling threatened, only wishing for an invulnerability born of confidence. It is exactly the point that in reality there is no such thing. What is needed next is impossible, yet it comes, an organic carrying forward. It lets an impossible invulnerability and confidence actually happen!

Because the client cannot really obtain a plastic shield it could be said that we are stuck. If we had only the image as such, we would be stuck. But if the image has come from the felt sense, if it fits and carries that felt sense forward, if the client lets the felt sense come *from the image*, that felt sense will lead further. The new felt sense comes in this (usually threatened) person's body, and it implicitly contains the threatening facets of that person's experience, but now the felt sense includes the body feeling that is invulnerable and confident. The whole experiential mesh has changed.

If the person enters this felt sense and articulates various strands, each new bit of finding carries the felt sense further so that it changes in the body. This new and more forward way of being now exists in the body as a possible, already experienced, way of being that is ready when the person meets the actual situation.

On all avenues the next of the body's implied steps can instruct us. In order to do this we try to reflect the felt sense, for example, "I wish I had the confidence of people who feel invulnerable." The therapist might say, "You have a sense right there that you would be confident if you assumed you were invul-

216

nerable." But with the power of the image's plastic shield, the client actually begins to live invulnerably and confidently.

I will now continue with the imagery process I began to tell about in Chapter 11. (The following excerpts were reconstructed from notes. They involved more steps than are represented here.)

Sometimes clients have an image but don't mention it. At other times an image is invited by a question like "Can you see her?" A simple question like this can lead to a long sequence of healing steps. I may also ask, "What is she doing?" or "Is she sitting or standing?"

In this example, we need only to insure that the client feels herself as a safe adult, and that she attends to her bodily felt sense of herself as a child. With two safe adults to protect her (her adult self and the therapist), the child part can begin to live and heal.

Images have not been mentioned with this client before. As this excerpt begins, the client is sensing the whole of how she feels hurt. She has a felt sense. This is then carried forward at many points in the following sequence.

C: That [child] part of me is *so* hurt.

T: You can feel the hurt in this child part.

C: Yes. (*Silence*)

T: Can you see her?

C: Yes.

T: What is she doing?

C: I see her. (*Cries softly*) She's all rolled up in fetal position with her arms over her head.

T: You and I will just sit by her, quietly. We won't say or push anything. We'll just be here. You and I will keep her quiet company.

(*Silence*)

T: We will protect her. We won't let anyone in here. Other than that, we'll just sit here.

C: She's never had anybody protect her (*cries*).

T: In that time she didn't have anyone to protect her. That felt very bad. Now we are here, you the big lady sitting here, and me.

(*Silence*)

C: Oh, she's looking around!

Suddenly the child in the image begins to heal! But notice that the therapist did not attempt to arrange this as an imagery procedure by saying something like "Watch her; she will move and change."

217

"Keeping someone company" is a highly therapeutic interaction. It is naturally part of the therapy, and imagery is not an abruptly different therapeutic procedure. Keeping the client company fits into what was already happening, but it radically changes the context of the *child*, from her being alone and helpless to being kept company and protected.

It came as a surprise to the client that the child soon looked up. I believe the movement from inside would not have happened if the therapist had tried to anticipate what the child would do, or even that she would do something.

This example contains a process I have now experienced with 20 or so clients. It happens often when clients feel themselves as very young children when I say, "Can you see her (or him)?" and then ask, "What is she doing?"

Before I ask this, I want to make sure that the client has a warm feeling toward the child. This is easy for some clients but requires work with others. A warmly receptive attitude is vital in processing *any* part of oneself (not because we should view everything positively, but because the felt sense won't open otherwise). A warm feeling is especially important in relation to one's child part.

Many people are firmly turned away from the child part. When they encounter it inside, they want to ignore it. It is "too much trouble," or they think it is not legitimate or realistic. They are impatient with it, and hostile. They respond to it the way others did in their past. Sometimes they consider its very existence a weakness. They identify with the superego's attitude and are angry at and contemptuous of the child. But when they reject the child inside, they are unconsciously being *only* the child. Because, when the child is rejected it is left lonely, that is to say it is *only* the child, without a supportive adult.

"You are not *just* the child," I say. "You are the big lady who is sitting on my couch, and you *have* the child with you." Or I say, "Be both. When you are the big person caring for the child, then you are being both."

Many people are warm and caring toward other children, just not toward their inner child. If this is so it helps to imagine first another child, so that the warmth can be felt. Then we can work to realize that "The child you were is simply a child like any other."

I ask, "How would you feel toward *another* child to whom all this happened. Suppose one like that were sitting on the steps outside?" The client will usually say, "Oh . . . I would hug her." The impulse to do that is the warm feeling we need.

"What if she is too scared to let you hug her?" I might then ask. "We could just quietly sit down next to her."

It is not enough to urge clients to feel warmly toward the child. If I tell them to do it, they feel they must do it *alone*. That is the way it was for the client in the past. The child had to take care of the child. Therefore I say, "*We* will keep her company. *You and I* will protect her." Together we can do it.

We are keeping the child company *but without doing anything*. We refrain from anything that could be frightening. I say, "We won't do anything. We won't say anything smart. We know we don't know much. We'll just sit here and keep her company."

I might also say any of this without any intention of having the client generate images. When there is a child part, or anything tender or sore, it can help to suggest that the client and I are two protective adults. I will refer back to this in some examples in other chapters.

This approach brings together many principles. This way of being with something painful is akin to "making a space," neither avoiding nor pushing in. It is also similar to pure listening in that it refrains from imposing anything. Although it might seem that we are unable to do anything, what happens is that the lonely and unprotected experience is carried forward into an interaction of contact and unconditional regard.

Sometimes this keeping company lasts for only a few minutes. At other times the therapist and client might stay and watch for most of a therapy hour.

One client, without my having mentioned images, saw a little girl in the woods where there was a bed of pine needles that felt soft and safe. Later she was with a large bear who protected her. She had a felt sense of each of these images. She felt strong emotions and often cried softly. At times the client would wave her hand rapidly in front of her chest — indicating almost too much affect.

In the next session she did not mention any of this, but toward the end of the hour I asked her about the little girl and there were more events of this sort.

T: Can you still see that little girl?

C: Yes . . . oh . . . she's stuck up a ladder!

T: Well, let's keep her company.

C: Oh — I know what it is!

Her felt sense connected the image to something that had happened during the week. We waited until a way came for her to come down from the ladder, and the client's whole body eased.

Here is another example. A client had had a physical breathing problem for many years, and she wanted to work on it in this hour. After a while, sensing back into her childhood, she felt herself as she had been then.

T: Can you see her?

C: Yes.

T: What is she doing?

C: She's all curled up in a ball. She's like a ball.

T: Let's you and me big people keep her company and make it safe. We'll make it safe now, because it wasn't safe then.

C: She's rolled under the bed now.

T: Is it safe there?

C: No. It's *safer* but they can find her there too.

T: There is terror?

C: She's not breathing because she thinks that makes her invisible. It doesn't make sense.

T: Sure it does. Making no sound feels like they won't know she's there. She feels invisible.

C: Yes.

(*Silence*)

C: Now she wants her toys and books.

T: Let's bring them.

(*Silence*)

C: She says she doesn't know me (*crying*), but she appreciates the toys and books.

(*Silence*)

(*At this point a good figure from a dream she had had came, and a part of her jumped into his lap! But another part stayed under the bed.*)

C: One jumped into his lap! But the other one stayed.

(*Silence*)

C: The one still under the bed is very sick.

T: That one is very sick.

C: She's despaired, despaired (*exhales loudly*).

(*Silence*)

Now other people come and stand all around her, protectively.

Does such a sequence indicate that real change has taken place in the person? The changes in the images cause changes in the felt sense, and these are often changes that the client has not experienced before. Indeed, for some clients it is highly unlikely that the bodily feelings that accompanied these images would ever have arisen. We can use images to engender small changes that make large contributions to therapy.

Used with the body and in interaction, we discover that dreams and images have an incipient energy for movement. I find that this movement is always positive, always a gradual turning toward life, interest, connection, and healing.

CHAPTER 16

Emotional Catharsis, Reliving

THIS CHAPTER IS DEVOTED to the spontaneous coming of emotions and the "catharsis" (also called "discharge") of those emotions. A group of methods utilizes catharsis and I will unpack their procedures so that we can use small-scale moves.

WHEN CATHARSIS COMES OF ITS OWN ACCORD

Catharsis may involve screaming, intense sobbing, a runny nose, coughing. Clients may pound the wall with their fists. (See Chapter 10, Excerpts C and L.) In the last chapter we saw that the presence of the therapist and the client as two quietly protective adults can provide childhood experiences the client needs. Instead of simply reliving an early experience just as it was in the past this new approach allows new steps to come. In contrast, one relives the past in catharsis just as it actually happened, but with the great difference that one expresses and fully feels emotions that were blocked at the time. To some extent this happens in all therapy. We call it "catharsis" or "discharge" when there is a great deal of physical expression that has a certain unstoppable quality. If the discharge of such emotions is new for the client and comes of its own accord it can be very valuable.

Therapists who are unfamiliar with catharsis are often frightened by it because it seems "out of control." But we should not be frightened of the discharge because it comes to a natural completion within a few minutes. Interrupting it because we are afraid can have long-lasting bad effects. Clients who are stopped are likely to feel that there is some terrible force inside them, which is always close to going out of control. Fearing this unknown force can make everything inside them seem threatening. The client becomes afraid of becoming crazy, and all inner work is blocked. Clients can carry a fear like this for years. And all because a therapist was unfamiliar with the quite natural process of emotional discharge.

If the therapist had not stopped the discharge, the client would have yelled, cried, or pounded the desk for a little while longer and the energy would have been spent. If the client happens to be pounding on something hard, the therapist should simply slip a pillow in between.

Catharsis feels very different to the person experiencing it than to the person observing it. The inexperienced observer feels it as being bad. This is because the waves of emotional intensity are coming at the observer. Anger and pain coming toward oneself do not feel good. But for the client, when those same waves of energy roll outward from inside, they feel very good.

In traumatic childhood events there is usually a double oppression, not only from the events themselves, but also from the fact that one is not allowed to cry, tremble, or "throw a tantrum." Tantrums are a very natural process for living organisms. When the long-blocked child is at last allowed to cry, it thereby also experiences itself being whole again. Such times are precious and catharsis can have a deep personal value.

A common problem with catharsis is that people find themselves discharging the same emotion in the same way over and over again. I usually interrupt discharges that a client has had a great many times before. Something beyond this is required, but if it is not repetitious and wells up of its own accord, it should be welcomed and made safe.

Because catharsis is natural, it is always being rediscovered. But it is insufficient as therapy and therefore tends to be discarded soon by therapists. Freud found it and then discarded it. Dianetics found it again in the 1950s and overstated the case for it. Primal Therapy has found it again more recently, but has also overstated its value, regarding it as all one needs for therapy. Catharsis can be induced in nearly everyone, but whether it should be induced is an open question. What is certain is that when catharsis comes of its own accord it ought to be received and respected as a natural part of that particular client's therapy.

Early in therapy, or when the therapist senses that catharsis might be of value, it can be presented as a possibility. I tell clients to feel free to do something like scream, pound on the couch, or punch a pillow. I say, "You might want to do *this* at some time or other," and then demonstrate by kneeling and pounding the couch myself. I want clients to feel that they could do this if such an expression ever feels right to them. Some clients follow my suggestion immediately, others at a later time, but most of them never do.

Catharsis fits in well with other avenues if we make it an option, but without inducing it, and if we welcome it if it happens.

222

WHAT CATHARSIS LACKS:
THE PRESENT SENSE OF THE PAST

The exclusive use of catharsis loses the *fresh sense of the present*, including the *present* sense of the situation in the past and the way the sense of the present can allow us to take new steps that would have been impossible in the past. We have seen new steps of this type throughout this book, particularly in the last chapter.

Clients in Primal therapy do work on a problem by feeling it in their bodies, but they do it *only* for the purpose of letting a *past* experience come up. A vivid experience from the past quickly arises, but usually it is one the client has gone through before. They intensely relive that familiar experience again. They physically feel its pain and fury; they cry and scream, presumably as they needed to, and could not, do at the time. Their attention is wholly on the past experience; they have no felt sense of the present life situation on which they wanted to work. Clients in Primal therapy are often quite disoriented about their present lives and personalities because they work so consistently on every problem as if it existed *only* in the past.

The pitfall of working *only* on the past may also take place in focusing if clients are first deeply relaxed and then asked to attend to whatever comes up without the requisite reference to a specific problem. Reliving and catharsis of early childhood events are likely to happen in this relaxed state without reference to one's present life.

Catharsis involves a certain regression that is akin to hypnosis. For example, even though no relaxation is induced in Reevaluation Counseling (Jaekins, 1962), a method that features emotional discharge, at the end of each session clients are asked to "return to present time." To insure that they have indeed returned, the client is asked to describe an object in the room. But that is the end of the session! One's present life and the present sense of the past are not worked with as such.

Intense emotionality causes a narrowing of experience even without relaxation and regression. From the common advice that we should count to 10 when we are angry we can see that intense emotion narrows our experiencing in such a way that we lose track of much that is usually implicit in it. Both regression and intensity have this narrowing effect on experiencing. (See my "A Theory of Personality Change," Gendlin, 1964, and my theory of emotions in "On Emotions in Therapy," Gendlin, 1991b. See also McGuire, 1991, on catharsis.)

By contrast, the felt sense is *wider* than ordinary experiencing. The felt sense of "all that" is much *more* than we would sense in ordinary experience. It has many more implicit strands and edges. It is from these that new further steps develop.

There is an optimal degree of relaxation: just enough to let things come, but not so much that it is difficult to react fully in the present. With very little ordinary relaxation one reaches an optimal point where bits of material can come, but the client is fully present and can immediately respond to what comes. That is what happens in focusing (Gendlin, 1996b).

FOR CATHARSIS SOME EXPERIENTIAL STEPS MIGHT FIRST BE NEEDED

The client in the excerpts in Chapter 10 probably would not have been able to tolerate the past experiences that came up early in her therapy if she had not pounded the mattress when her rage became too intense to bear. And yet we saw how carefully, a little later in therapy, she sensed for the proper time to do more of it. Then she refrained from emotional discharge for a long time. It was important to extend an equal welcome to both alternatives.

The client sensed that a certain kind of work needed to take place before it would be advisable for her to confront directly what was left of her affect.

If clients are afraid of a lot of anger from the past, there may need to be a long series of little steps that gradually bring them closer to the anger. Bit by bit such clients become able to stand their ground "next to" the anger. As they become stronger, they are able to touch the anger more directly. All the while the therapist may have known how to make the anger come out, but it was better to refrain. Clients develop staying power in relation to their anger.

Over time, a client's whole person develops. New aspects begin to stir. These may be important in their own right, but they may need to be present before the anger can be processed.

Here is an example: "I have this . . . very hurt . . . feeling. I can hardly talk about it . . . uh." At *this* stage the therapist would not want to increase the intensity of this hurt. It is quite enough for the client to touch it slightly, for now. The therapist's ongoing company is helping the client spend time standing this much as it is.

Or, for example, a client says, "That's where I got stopped. . . . That was too much for me. . . . I fought so hard. . . . Oh, I'm *not* a bad person!" (Neither client nor therapist had been aware that something in her thought she was a bad person.)

The client may suddenly reconnect to healthy times before the traumatic events. "Oh . . . that's how I was. . . . (*Sighs*) That's the last time I was hopeful . . . way back there, that's where I got stopped." The client may look visibly more alive in bringing that long-lost way of being forward. What is going on is not only a product of the past, since the client in the present now lives some moments in this way. Such steps make the client much more whole, and stronger. We can well understand why a client might need to live in a new way before reliving traumatic events, so that explosive anger can have a different outcome than in the past (Grove, 1995).

As therapists we are not in a position to decide that one client needs such steps or that another is ready for catharsis. The precision with which the next small steps come, one after the other, shows that the decision is best left to those steps themselves.

On the other hand, if an emotion is right there, we welcome it. When I hear anger, I say, "I hear anger, is that right?" When a client first cries, I might say, "The tears are welcome. I hope you can welcome the tears." If I see a client suppressing tears, I ask about it. If the client says, "I can feel tears, but I can't cry," I usually say, "Please send a message down there to let the tears through whenever they do come." Children are taught that they must not cry. The therapeutic ethos now says that we must cry. Both are artificial. Far down in us there is a little guardhouse that stops tears. If we leave a message with the guard there, "Let the tears through whenever they come," then when they come up naturally, they are let by.

FELT SENSE COMPARED TO EMOTIONS

The felt sense can often be very slight, whereas anger is very intense. The felt sense of all that went into becoming angry is wider and much less intense than the anger itself.

People accustomed to catharsis may have difficulty recognizing a felt sense, even when it comes. They are used to the extreme intensity and drama of long pent-up emotion. Compared to a situation in which the client is screaming and sobbing, one in which a client is quietly sensing an unclear whole may seem as if not much is happening. But intensity is not a criterion of effectiveness. Very intense emotions sometimes do come out of a felt sense, but having a felt sense is usually quiet.

Sometimes the past needs to be relived and completed at the point where its emotions were blocked. Hypnosis can also help at certain junctures. (One client reported being greatly helped by hypnosis without any suggestions being given during it. The "multiple" parts could be all on one plane for the first time. Later that was possible without hypnosis.) Meditation is a kind of deep relaxation that is valuable in many ways. We do not know everything that deep relaxation might provide. I am not speaking against these states. But why insist on regression during most of every therapy hour?

Sometimes a client consistently sits in a meditation position and I can tell that the client has practiced meditation. I might then say, "If your body is accustomed to meditation, it will go there as soon as you sit like that. Then the body doesn't talk back the way we might need it to do here. Please sit a little differently, and more loosely."

Clients can choose whether to sit up on the couch, or stretch out on it, or do either at times. I would not prevent them from dipping down deeply into a relaxed state. At times I might ask a client to sit forward and come out of too relaxed a posture. At other times I might ask a client to relax, lean back, and let go of being so mobilized.

We can best acknowledge the importance of the therapeutic avenue of cathartic discharge by letting clients know it will be welcome if it comes, or if they feel the need for it, and then leave them free to employ it or not.

CHAPTER 17

Action Steps

ARISTOTLE SAID that people are able to change only by *practicing* the right actions. Habits are powerful forces that cannot be overcome all at once; rather, they are changed by practice over time. So far in Part 2 of this book we have considered avenues of *inner* change that result in outer change. But one can also change from the outside in.

In this chapter I incorporate the essence of another group of therapies, those that employ the avenue of actions.

Operant Behavior therapists (Skinner and his students) have discovered an effective way for people to change their habitual behavior; it is to make *very tiny* steps toward the new behavior. We can incorporate this and some of Operant Behavior therapy's other innovations. Part of an hour of therapy can be spent devising a small new step in the direction of change in action to be undertaken between sessions. It can be the primary emphasis of therapy or it can require only a few minutes.

Inner and outer change go together and require each other. We may be convinced that inner change will lead to outer change, but it may not always be sufficient.

Inner change may precede outer change, as in the case of a lonely client who suddenly finds a life partner soon after overcoming certain unconscious fears and developing an inner readiness to attract someone. But it is also true that something like this can only happen if there has been a change in the client's behavior out among people. The client may be inwardly ready, but the desired person will not come to the door and ring the bell. The purpose of therapy is for the client to have a better life, and most of life takes place with other people.

Some clients are inclined to wait until their feelings have changed *entirely* before beginning a small new action. But inner change is hard to complete

227

without at least some concrete outward action, and this is not only because of the change in events and opportunities a change in action brings. Performing a new action is also a physical change process. A new action changes the body because it requires a new manner of bodily experiencing. Inner difficulties will be experienced in a new and different way. A small act, therefore, insignificant in itself, has the potential to shift the whole inner complexity of a problem. A small change in action can also let one encounter one's inner obstacles more directly.

I will now discuss several kinds of action steps that can be easily used in the context of psychotherapy.

HARMLESS ACTIONS

Therapists can help clients make changes in their actions in such a way that the actions seldom have negative consequences, for example, getting information, calling someone, looking in the newspaper, or bringing resources to a problem. Clients often discuss something like changing their jobs or careers as if they had no options at all. They very likely do know agencies and people who might have information but they avoid them because of their inner fears. Nevertheless, a call to renew an aquaintance or to obtain information might be manageable. A series of harmless moves can change everything. It can open a whole new range of possibilities.

ACTIONS TO PRACTICE HAVING
A NEW BODILY ENERGY

When a client experiences a new bodily energy during therapy, it is sometimes a good idea to ask what change in action the client could make to ensure that the new bodily energy does not fade, and to manifest this change. It need not be a major action. Even a small action can embody the new manner of being in such a way that the client can practice it during the week.

One client, a recently divorced woman, planned to go to a dance at her church. She knew that her ex-husband would come and bring his new lady. He didn't usually go to her church and she saw this as a deliberate attempt on his part to upset her. She said, "I will call him and tell him this is my space and he shouldn't come. I'm scared to call him. It's hard to do. And I know he will come, anyway. But it's still right for me to do it. It's a step forward."

To identify and perform such actions it is often necessary to leave aside a concern for immediate results. We call this "doing it for practice." In doing something just as practice by definition we cannot fail. We have already succeeded simply by performing the action. It does not matter if it is done well or poorly. In fact, we expect to do something awkwardly at first.

A client one time made this comment about such an action: "It would have made a lot of difference years ago. It's too late now, but you have to do those things anyway. If you actually do them, the body *gets* that you mean to be different now."

A small action can embody the new manner of being and let one live in it. For example, after finding a new level of assertiveness in a therapy session, the client searched for an action that would be an instance of his new manner. He decided, "From now on I will go to the bathroom as soon as I need to, rather than waiting until someone is through talking."

Let us examine this as an action step. First of all what he has resolved to do is totally within his power. He might find it difficult to do, but the only impediment to its being done is in himself. Notice also that the action is private. Only he knows that it is a large step for him to interrupt others for his own needs. Yet, the step is *an instance of* the new assertiveness that he has found. If he succeeds in only this action he will have the chance to live in this new way of being many times a day, and in doing so regains the new quality of energy he found during therapy.

In experientializing behavioral methods, we examine the effects of actions on experiencing. Actions can do more than *keep* a new energy; they *continue it into interaction*. Bodily "energy" implies and moves into interaction with the environment. If an energy is new, it has not had its continuation into interaction. Its primitve pattern is not ready for real situations. But small actions enable its patterning to change in major ways, as it becomes connected.

In the example above, the man's new assertiveness may at first be simplistic and primitive and linked to desperate, hostile motivation, because blocked energy creates circular, noninteractional patterns. If he tries to manifest this energy in this form in important situations, he will be obliged to abandon it and fall back on his old, overly considerate ways. But in a small action the energy can be lived even in its primitive form, and it will be able to connect so that it can gradually develop its differentiated continuations. This represents a major *intra*psychic change.

Clients do not usually think of practicing desired transformations in safe situations first. They want to rectify major problematic situations immediately. To try this will be too big a step and nothing will change.

For example, a client had gradually developed greater strength and confidence. He had come to feel that his perceptions of his work situation were accurate. It created a new sense of fearlessness in his body, a new energy that might let him assert himself and take more latitude and initiative for himself. Now he said,

C: I want to go in there [his boss's office] and tell him off. But I can't do it. *Right now I feel almost like I could,* but I know when it comes to it, I can't.

T: *Is there some other person or situation where it would be safe, and easier to practice acting like that?* Is there something somewhere that you feel like calling a halt to, where you're sure it would be right and OK to do it?

C: I think I'll participate more. Connie [his wife] is always saying I don't participate, but then she doesn't like how I do things if I do participate.

T: You're thinking of doing more and . . . I wasn't sure . . . caring less about whether she likes it?

C: No, I wasn't thinking of that, only that I should participate more. She's right.

In this example the client knows that the action step of telling off his boss is too large, and he takes up the therapist's idea of finding an easier first step. The therapist may well have been correct since the client seemed to have already lost his new energy ("She's right"). Of course we have no final way of knowing. Perhaps he knows that she is right. Perhaps he knows that he only pretends to participate. If the therapist had pushed the suggestion (of "caring less about whether she likes it"), and the client had accepted it, the therapist would be functioning like the client's boss and his wife, knowing better than he and telling him what to do.

So far what I have discussed are "harmless" actions that are instances of a new way of bodily being. Let me discuss another kind:

A PROGRAM OF TINY STEPS: OPERANT THERAPY

Using Skinner's theory of operant behavior, Goldiamond developed an effective system of progressive steps for changing behavior. Here is what we can learn from Goldiamond's approach:

First of all he has a general formula, a "program," an outline of typical steps. For example, in a *dating program* the first three steps might be: Buy a newspaper that advertises events for singles, make phone calls to get announcements of social events, and make a list of places to which you might conceivably go to meet people. Note how small these steps are.

A further step might be to get dressed up once a week on a certain day — and then stay home. When this has become easy, the next step might be actually to go to one of the places — but not to go in. Just succeed in actually getting there. Then go home. Give yourself a big reward.

Later might come the step of going into the establishment and looking around. The next step might be to relate to one person, then go home. Still later the goal is to stay a specified amount of time or talk to a number of people. Be sure to reward yourself at each step — just for doing the step, whatever else happens. A further step might be to look around and notice when someone happens to be looking at you. Along this rough trajectory, the actual steps can vary with each person.

Such a program differs very greatly from mere willpower. Exercise of willpower consists in forcing oneself and can build up huge counterforces that eventually wear down the strongest resolution. Small steps avoid this.

In another contrast with small steps: A regimen driven by willpower can be lost in just one failure. This happens when one is under pressure. A program of small steps can be adjusted: One client says, "When my parents come to visit I put my smoking program back to one every 15 minutes [from one every 45]." He loses a little ground but he does not lose his program.

In the following example, note how almost absurdly small the steps are. This client profited also from other aspects of therapy, which always took up more than half of his session. But he did especially well with this program of small steps. A lonely man, now 55 years old, he had had only one brief sexual experience, in his youth. Now he wanted to become able to relate to women. We had already worked on many of the usual topics, especially his relationship with his mother. After a month or two I suggested an action step, which revealed that he had difficulty even with the act of getting dressed up. Where he worked the dress code was casual, but he said that even there he was known to dress poorly. Our first steps involved his buying clothes.

An early step of our program consisted of his getting dressed up every Wednesday evening, then celebrating that he had done so, hanging up his clothes again and staying home. Keeping up the practice of getting dressed up Wednesday nights, he went on to making a list of places he might go to meet women. He knew a street where there were such places. The next step was going there, and then going home. Then came looking inside one place, and then going home.

The client always knew that he could and would do the next week's step, both because we had devised it to suit him, and because the step was always so small. We did not settle for a step unless I heard his energy almost laughing, saying, "That one I know I can do."

The next step was the crucial one: Going inside, saying hello to one woman, perhaps exchanging a few words as long as the conversation is easy, then going home. Soon he went on to saying hello to two women. "What if I do even more than the two we said?" "Fine," I answered, "but take a minute to celebrate when you have spoken to the two." After a while he was saying hello to five women a night. From being so hesitant that he could hardly bring himself to do anything, he became active and optimistic.

By the time this stage had become easy, it was possible for him to spend the evening talking with one woman. Then came asking a woman to go have coffee down the street.

We continued to work on all dimensions of therapy, spending only perhaps 15 minutes on the program. He worked on his relationship with his mother who had died recently. But all along he had assured me that if he ever actually succeeded in getting into bed with a woman, everything would go very well from there. I accepted that, although I thought it unlikely. I was prepared to work on the "underlying" problem that I thought would appear when that opportunity came.

The next step was to provide for the possibility of his being with a woman. If a woman sugested going to her house, that would be fine. But, he asked, "What if she suggests going to *my* house?" This led us to a series of steps to do something about his ugly bare mattress, the only sleeping accommodation in his apartment. This involved various steps of calling stores and arranging deliveries. Meanwhile the time came, but it was her house the woman suggested. And what happened? No trouble at all.

He stayed in one relationship for a while. Then he met many other women. He reported that women his age look very attractive and much younger during intercourse. It had something to do with blood circulation.

HOW TO EXPERIENTIALIZE THE OPERANT METHOD

The usual Operant Behavior therapy takes up the whole therapy hour. In the first hour the client chooses a "target behavior" to be created and increased (or decreased and eliminated). The first step is to *keep a record*, writing down each time the behavior happens and recording just what preceded and followed it. In following sessions client and therapist examine the record together. This reveals that the behavior in question occurs much more frequently before or after certain events. Clients reward (or "reinforce") themselves with something they buy or enjoy doing. The reward is selected in advance. There is a reward for the labor of keeping a record and for each subsequent small step. In addition the therapist rewards the client with praise and interest. Some behavior therapists use candy.

Let me point out how some of this was done better in an experiential way. From being interested only in behavior, we shift to an interest in how the method is experienced. We achieve behavioral results more effectively if we also look for the experiential sources and effects of each step.

Selecting the Target Behavior

Some behavior therapists commit an error psychotherapists would not make. They ask the client to choose a "target behavior" in the first hour. Many months may then be spent on that behavior. In the context of psychotherapy behavioral goals will emerge as part of a longer and deeper process. At the beginning people tend to pick targets along the lines of their present attitudes, which are likely to change as therapy progresses.

All psychological change poses this paradox: The person must choose the direction of change, but the choice is likely to be an instance of (rather than a way to change) the aspect of the person that is most in need of change. Therefore, although clients must pick their own targets, it should be done within a deeper, more self-interactive therapy process. Especially in focusing, genuine targets gradually emerge from a fresh sense of what one really needs in one's life.

232

Rewarding (Reinforcing) Each Small Step

Rewards are important. Operant therapists suggest candy, a small purchase, or a pleasant activity. These things are effective rewards. But a vital *experiential* kind of reward is for the client to spend a few moments celebrating having done the step.

People are accustomed to punishing themselves, quite routinely, for every effort they make to improve their situation. It sounds odd, but whenever most people try something new, something brave, a little step forward to change their situation, they punish themselves immediately afterward.

For example, a lonely person will exert a great deal of effort in going somewhere to meet someone of the opposite sex. But if a likely partner does not turn up that evening, the person will go home more depressed than ever about being alone, and self-critical about having lived just to end up alone. With this as the consequence it will naturally be harder to go out and try again. Just spending the evening at home watching television does not bring this punishment.

With small steps, a depressed reaction like this can also take place. One has indeed gotten dressed up, or whatever the small step may be, but this does not produce a positive result. Instead one has a vivid sense of being far from a result.

The operant principle of working with *immediate* consequences is very sound indeed. The usual rewards are good and should be used. But the best way to avoid the self-punishment is to develop a specific positive self-response as the reward. A bit of private celebration does just that. Like other rewards it must be planned in advance and done as soon as the step is completed.

The therapist should prepare the client by saying something like, "But will you actually celebrate when you make the list of places to go? If you do the step, will you take a minute then, just to say, 'Wow, I did my step, I'm on my way! I've got a program going'? Will you take time to be pleased?" The client will probably say, "sure, I'll be pleased," perhaps in a flat tone of voice. The therapist then may need to ask a focusing question: "Well, imagine you've just done it. How does it feel?" Then the client may say, "I wish I didn't have to do this — it's because I avoided this problem for so many years." There is the self-punishing again. It takes some work to overcome the tendency to punish a step rather than rewarding it.

A feeling like the one above needs to be reflected ("It's painful, and some part of you blames you about it.") and followed with steps of focusing and listening. We can try later to structure the self-reward, explaining it again from the beginning. "Now, when you actually made that list, will you then really celebrate?" And the focusing question: "Check and see. Will you be able to celebrate?"

Emphasizing the Tinyness of Steps

It is essential that the steps be *very* small, so small that one cannot find oneself unable to do them. To buy the paper and make a list of places to go? No, that is several steps. Just buy the paper. Or perhaps just notice where they carry the paper that lists events. Even that is a lot. Perhaps just check the papers on one newsstand. "Sure I can do that." Even so, lets ask: "Where do you pass a newsstand and is there time to do it?"

A good step is not likely to be the first one proposed. We need to experientialize the way in which we devise small steps in order to find a good one. We say, "Check, and sense, would you actually do it?" "I will, I will." "Well imagine going to do it now. What's your sense of it?" If the situation is prepared for in this way, the reasons the person might get held up appear in advance. These impediments can then be dealt with in a more usual therapeutic way. Meanwhile the client can find a different action step, one that can surely be done.

The right step, when found and checked in this way, is energy-giving. "Yeah, now *that*, I *know* I could do *that!*" A bit of happy energy and relief comes when the step is right.

INCORPORATING THE USE OF ACTION STEPS IN THE USUAL THERAPY

Action steps require only a small part of most therapy hours. If the rest of therapy is moving well, I may bring up but do not insist on action steps (nor any other of the avenues outlined in this book). If the therapy is stuck, I am more ready to bring up an avenue on which we have not yet worked.

I ask a client who is lonely, "Where do you ever go, where you might meet *new* people?" This can mean people of the opposite sex or just friends. "Oh, I meet new people, I do, I do," the client says. "Well, where?" I press. "Oh, next August I am going to a convention." "But now it's December," I say. Most lonely people never go where new people to fit them could be found.

I might say, "Could you make a list of places to go? Don't go there, just make the list." Of course I instantly listen again to whatever the client says in response. We then work on whatever came. I bring up action again at some other time.

Or I ask, "What sort of person would you like to meet? What sort of activity would that kind of person enjoy doing? Let's see if you could go, not just to a place for singles, but to an activity that would be natural for you and for such a person to attend. Then you can stand being there better, and it's much more likely that someone you could like would be there."

I also say, "It probably takes checking out 50 possible people to find one you could really like. But that is possible because it takes just 5 minutes to check most people out."

I've seen a good success rate with this method. The most dramatic example of this was a divorced woman who had five children, old enough to give her time to return to school for her Ph.D. When asked what sort of person she was looking for she said she would like to meet a divorced man. So I said, "Why don't you do your thesis research on divorced men?" A typical study requires about 25 research subjects, but in her research she interviewed 150 divorced men, found three real prospects, and married one of them.

More recently a wealthy female client responded to a similar question by saying that she would like to meet a rich and successful man. I asked about activities such men were likely to engage in. After a while she hit on it: "I'll do a lot of flying *first class.*" Within weeks she had found a very compatible man whom she eventually married.

To suggest a change in action takes only a moment. Then one can listen to the response. The interaction always has priority. For example, if the client says, "Yes, doctor," warmly with a laugh, it's all right. But if the response means, "Stop pushing stuff on me," I will say, "You don't want me to push stuff on you, it makes you feel . . . how?" Anger is welcome, too, of course.

Reactions like this happen most often when I first introduce action steps. One such reaction might be, "I'll get to that stage." I say, "OK," and reflect that. ("You're telling me to stop pushing this, there will be a time when you naturally get to it in your own process. OK.") A month later, perhaps, I bring it up again, although with some clients I might not suggest it again.

It doesn't hurt a good therapeutic relationship to spend some time searching for small action steps to do. For example:

C: I saw a girl I could be interested in, and I thought of asking her for a date. But then I thought I couldn't handle it.

T: Have you often asked girls for a date?

C: Never.

T: Well, *some* action can be very important. You don't need to get into a situation you feel you can't handle. Could you take her out for coffee in the afternoon, or some other smaller action? It has to be small enough so it just bites into where you're afraid a little bit. Even deciding to think about an action is a kind of action.

In the next session the situation developed like this:

C: I am getting clearer and clearer dreams, but my life hasn't changed one iota as yet. Is it supposed to be that way for a while?

T: Yes, it can be that way. But some action might help connect your inner process with your ongoing life.

C: It turned out I wasn't interested in that girl.

T: Can we find some action?

C: The way it is here, if I hit on a girl, I'll hear about it for a year.

T: Must be things people do that don't commit themselves, like talking while standing in line, or on the way home. Or, people make remarks or just look at each other. Could you observe what people do there, that doesn't commit them?

C: I can do that.

This was a lot of talk from me, but the client seemed to welcome it, so I added:

T: To observe that way would be an action. Also, that way you can relate to whatever you run into, inside you.

C: Yes, in [another type of situation] I am trying things, and I run into fear.

T: Don't push into the fear but don't run away either, just back up a couple steps. Then see, "What was that?"

Typically action steps work by freeing the present from the felt blockage of the past. When a client can feel exactly how a maladaptive pattern in the present is linked to early experience, a necessary change can come about through a change in action in present. Here is an example:

C: When I got home I realized I hadn't bought the one I really wanted. I spent all weekend on it. I know what that was, of course.

She has worked for a long time on a deep block against wanting anything or trying to get something she wants that stems from an early experience of abuse that happened when she tried to get a toy that she wanted.

C: How long am I going to miss out on life because I'm trying to prevent what already happened? It keeps being the same.

One week later she said,

C: I brought that one back to the store and I got them to give me the one I wanted. It was hard to do, it was so deep. But when I got home I knew: *I got that toy!!*

Still later, she said,

236

C: From now on I want to change the past by living in the present, instead of missing the present by living in the past.

THE CONNECTION BETWEEN PSYCHE AND ACTION

There is no true opposition between *psycho*therapy and *behavior* therapy. In a human being the inner and the outer are two sides of the same life process. Action-oriented people sometimes ask me whether focusing might merely make them feel better without changing their life — as if anyone *could* really feel better without their life having changed. We "live" our situations with our bodies. When the felt sense changes, what we are then able to perceive and do also changes. Conversely it may happen that in spite of our best efforts nothing changes. But our bodily feelings cannot change when our life and actions do not.

From the other side, very introspective people resist trying action steps directly. They think it is artificial. They believe that it must be ineffective to act in a way that does not come directly from how they feel. In a difficult situation, instead of attempting an action, they eagerly find some familiar inner conflict. It is as if they said, "What a relief; there is still an inward problem that can be worked on, so it's not yet time for action." But a change in action can alter the whole body, and may bring just the feeling that is most lacking.

For example, it is true that dreams are never *only* about a difficulty in a specific situation, but are also about the whole personality. A person cannot have a difficulty in a situation without also having the kind of personality that is generally instanced by that difficulty. Precisely because it is instanced in the particular situation the deeper difficulty is implicitly changed by a new action in that situation. Whether intrapsychic or in outward action, a change produces and requires new bodily living in the present.

In this chapter I have tried to familiarize the reader with a variety of action steps; harmless actions, actions that instance a new bodily energy, and the tiny action steps of an operant program. A therapist can suggest any of them. We have also seen how to employ them in such a way that they carry forward a new energy that can come from focusing and listening, from working with the bodily dimension, and from role playing a dream.

CHAPTER 18

Cognitive Therapy

SOME CHANGES IN CLIENTS' cognitive categories take place in all forms of therapy, but it is well known that cognitive change *alone* produces little real change in people. It can therefore seem that cognitive change as such has no role in therapy. This is a wrong conclusion.

A similar mistake is often made when focusing is described as if cognition plays no role in it. Focusing is a conversation between the felt sense and the cognitive side.

Let me first discuss standard cognitive therapy and how we can employ it as cognitive therapists would, but as brief moves, only at certain times. Then I will show how focusing changes the cognitive dimension altogether.

METHODS OF STANDARD COGNITIVE THERAPY

Combatting Negative Thoughts

In its usual form, cognitive therapy counters the tendency of clients to make negative interpretations of events and themselves. It has been found especially useful with depression. Depressed people tend to have negative thoughts of a certain type. "It's no use," they say to themselves, and the very act of saying it makes them feel worse. To recognize and combat such thoughts can be of crucial importance.

Remembering last week, depressed clients say, "Oh, then I could still laugh. Today that's impossible." Instead of letting those thoughts go unchallenged cognitive therapy encourages clients to examine and question such a thought process, for example, by recalling times when they got over previous depressions, times when they felt good.

Cognitive therapy works on what clients say to themselves. It is a major therapeutic step if clients can come to recognize this type of thought. They can then stop and change it before its effect goes very far. They can substitute a thought they know will have a positive effect. For example, in the morning clients may think, "I'll feel better if I just stay in bed." But perhaps they have learned that staying in bed during the day makes their depression worse. Therefore, they can think, "Yesterday it helped me to get up and stay up."

Any therapist can employ these discoveries of cognitive therapy with clients who may need them. A therapist need not take up cognitive therapy as an exclusive method, nor should it involve lecturing clients, putting them into a passive role. Briefly offering these ways of helping themselves now and then can be sufficient.

Alternative Ways of Seeing a Problem

In addition to combatting negative thoughts certain concepts also have the potential to change the quality of experience. For example, the whole sense of a situation may change if one considers it as a challenge. Similarly, if new behavior is hard to do, thinking of it as "practice" makes it much easier. We saw this in the previous chapter. Rather than desperately try to succeed at a new way of acting that one cannot yet do well one is certain of success if the immediate goal is to do one's practice.

Cognitive therapists say that such concepts as challenging and practicing counter unconscious assumptions, for example the assumption that one *has to* succeed, that one *must be* ashamed if one fails. Recognizing the inevitability that one is merely human and full of faults may lift the discouragement that "perfectionism" brings.

THE EXPERIENTIAL USE OF COGNITIVE METHODS DURING THERAPY

Although a certain concept has made a big difference to one client, we should not assume the same notion will help a different client. It might even mean dullness or defeat to that client. We have to work not just with notions, but with their experiential effects in each person.

When a cognitive method succeeds, it changes deeper layers implicitly. When it fails, it suggests that the deeper layers need other kinds of work. It can then seem foolish to have tried a seemingly "superficial" way of dealing with a problem. Nevertheless, cognitive work can be worth the brief time it requires. For example:

C: I give a lot. But there is the ultimate hypocrisy: I want something for myself.

(Her face is distorted with an expression of disgust.)

T: Are you assuming that's bad? I'm glad you want something for yourself too. That shows you're alive. It seems sound to me.

It is often useful for a therapist to offer an alternative way of thinking. It is best done as an expression of the therapist's own convictions. It lets the therapist be real and present, without *imposing* something on the client.

Now I turn to the discussion of some theoretical issues. Even if I succeed in clarifying them, the thoughtful reader will see that I am doing more than that. I am using what I have worked out and presented in my philosophical works. See Gendlin, 1962, 1992a, 1992b, 1996a, and in press.

IS COGNITION THE BASIC ORGANIZATION OF EXPERIENCE?

There is a basic theoretical difference between cognitive therapy and other therapies. We do not need to settle it, but we should understand it. Cognitive therapy assumes that all human experience is determined by cognitions, by conscious or unconscious "assumptions." The opposite view is that cognitive assumptions are superficial, and merely hide deeper factors of biological, interpersonal and psychic life. Both theories are simplistic.

Our bodies and our interactions are organized by many more basic factors, and cognition is only a *further* organizing of human experience. We see that animals act in accordance with certain relationships in their environment, but we do not assume that the animals think of abstract relationships *separately* as pure cognitions. Neither is most human experience organized by separate cognitions.

When we first state cognitive relationships, were they actually there in the form in which we now state them? The answer is no. If they "fit," then the activity of saying them *overtly* is a *new* and *further* experiencing.

WHAT IS EXPERIENTIALLY CONNECTED THINKING?

Thinking is an important human ability; it builds and rebuilds our world. It cannot very well be considered useless in human development. It has gotten a bad name as an avenue of therapy because it is so easily misused. When thinking is cut off from the other kinds of experience, it is called "intellectualizing" and brings little psychological change.

Most people do not know that an experientially connected kind of thinking is even possible. We have been taught to think at a great distance from experience. Even when we want to think about a specific experience, we often leave our direct sense of it behind, in order to think about it. As soon as we have one thought about it, we think from that thought to another and another, without ever returning to the experience to see if our thoughts do justice to it. People say, "I think what I'm feeling is such and such," and then they think on from that thought. They draw conclusions from that thought, without turning back to check whether they are doing violence to the experience, or whether the experience has opened and expanded.

Such effects can be noticed, for example, when we discuss a powerful film with someone. Analyzing the film may cause us to lose its impact. The thoughts may fail to express the impact of the film, shriveling it down until it dies away. Then we are sorry we tried to analyze the film. But it may also happen that analyzing the impact lets us feel it more and more, discover what it is and its import, so that it is developed and maximized. What determines the difference?

We can know the difference — and guide ourselves — if we check back from each little step of thought, rather than waiting until the end of the sequence. At each step we can sense how that thought affects the experience we are talking about. If the experience shrivels as a result of the thought, we can quickly shelve that thought, and seek another that will maximize it.

Sometimes we may wish to pursue a series of consecutive logical steps for a purely logical result, but then we can turn back to check what that result does to our experiential sense of the topic.

Usually we can drop a thought swiftly if it makes us lose hold of the experience. We can wait for a thought that connects with it and maximizes it. After a while there is a thought to which the experience responds. Then we pursue not only what the thought itself implies, but also what has opened in the experience.

This is the kind of thinking we welcome in and about therapy. It is not "intellectualizing" because the concepts and words are not allowed to function alone. They must carry the experience forward. We cannot decide just from the concepts alone whether they do that or not. We can know it only if the client attends to directly sensed experience.

But there is more: The experience has to be able to maximize and develop. Therefore it needs to be *the felt sense of* the event, emotion, or problem. However intractable something seems to be right now, the felt sense of it can open and move forward.

Some cognitive therapies recognize that cognitions alone are not very effective. Ellis changed the name of his "Rational Therapy" to "Rational-Emotive Therapy" (Ellis, 1962). But emotion is not the crucial kind of experience either. When one moves to a felt sense one discovers that emotions also are embedded in a whole mesh. A shift in the felt sense brings new emotions and new cognitions that move life forward.

THE COGNITIVE AND THE NONCOGNITIVE
ARE ONLY TEMPORARILY DISTINCT

For example, in focusing it is a cognitive move to say to oneself, "Let me get a felt sense of all that." On the other hand, the bodily attention and the coming of a felt sense are not cognitive moves. But again it is a cognitive move to ask: "What is the quality of all that?"

When a felt sense opens and something comes the thing that comes needs to be welcomed, and the welcoming is a deliberate cognitive response that must usually be learned. One shelves (one does not discard) one's disagreements with and reservations about what comes so that what comes can develop and lead to further steps. Then, if the cognitive side still differs, one asks questions of the felt sense until the two sides both change so that they are no longer distinct.

Beliefs are embedded in experience and may take many steps before they can be thought separately. For example, one of my clients felt that if a man wanted to have sexual intercourse with her, she had no choice but to agree. Therefore she avoided sexual situations. This did not change in therapy for a long time. Yet cognitively we both affirmed her right to refuse intercourse if she did not want it. We also affirmed her right to have it if she did want it. Both of these rights seemed cognitively valid to her, but they failed to connect with her feeling that she had no choice. The bodily felt sense of this "no choice" led her to many therapeutic steps. But only after much else changed, did the lack of choice open. Then she found, "Oh, I have the right to refuse it when I don't want it, but if I *do* want it, do I have the right to refuse?"

This example illustrates (1) how cognitions alone may be ineffective, and (2) what cognitive therapists call an "unconscious belief" (that if she was sexually aroused, she had no right to refuse).

Could the right cognitive statement have helped this client at an earlier time? Perhaps. A cognitive therapist who was familiar with beliefs like hers might have brought out such a statement and saved time. But the example also shows that a cognitive therapist who was not familiar with beliefs like hers would have needed to know how to work at the felt edge, until the relevant, specific belief emerged, because neither therapist nor client in this situation knew all that was involved in her inability to refuse. Therefore simply changing the cognitive side did nothing.

If a cognitive effort fails, we listen to the felt sense, give it space, let it open, and let it tell us what is in it. Then, depending on what emerges, the felt sense might dissolve or we might need further steps from both sides.

HOW IS COGNITIVE REFRAMING EVEN POSSIBLE?

Cognitive therapy spends the whole therapy hour "reframing" how clients interpret their situations and experiences. The client is urged to impose a new interpretive "frame." Sometimes it makes for genuine changes that enable the client to live better. How is this possible? If the interpretation changes the experience, it seems that the events we have experienced have no intrinsic interpretation of their own.

Of course, if only one interpretation is correct, and if it is already contained in the experience, then other interpretations must be delusional. Postmodernists correctly reject this assumption. They know that how we think about an experience can change the experience. But they can easily fall into the opposite simplistic assumption that experience has no order of its own at all. If it were organized *only* by cognitive categories, it could take any interpretation we impose. If that were so, we would all be healthy, happy, and rich, if that is what we wanted. So it is obvious that experience accepts some reinterpretations but not others. This is obvious, but it is hard to explain.

Experiences and situations always do have some character, but experiencing is a living process that can go on, *further*. Saying how experience "was" or "is," is always a going on further.

But we cannot just pick any way to go on from an experience; experience always implies its own going further, but the implied way to go further is not a cognitive form.

WHEN IS REFRAMING EFFECTIVE?

Only the directly sensed experience can let us know whether a reinterpretation has carried the experience forward. It is easy to invent reframings that are merely intellectualizations. At best they have no effect; sometimes they block experiencing. It is not only therapists who propose such blocking interpretations. Clients also do it. They relate a situation to other events which have no immediate connection to their directly sensed experiencing. A lot of time can be spent on reframings that obscure experience or make no difference in the client's life. But if reframings are kept closely connected to bodily sensed experience, the useless ones are swiftly dropped so that there is room for an effective one to arise.

An effective reframing has a directly sensed effect. A weight is lifted; there is a physical freeing and new bodily energy. The client feels able to do what seemed impossible before. Such a reframing is obviously not simply intellectualization. Other noticeable effects might be newly recovered memories or a clarified sense of an issue that had been unclear. Effective cognitions do not always have such results immediately. Their first effect can be slight. If there is a slight effect one needs to stay with it, to let it come through fully. As we have seen in other instances, this requires attention to the body. When what concerns a life issue has long been dull and silent, *sensing that it stirs* can bring hope and energy. But most people will miss such a stirring because it may not be intense. Say, for example, in response to a particular statement, the client senses something stirring. Instead of the old familiar feeling, there is a slight eagerness to hear the

243

statement. What can a therapist do in such a circumstance? Surely the meaningful statement could be repeated. The client might then need the therapist to repeat it many more times until eventually the feeling can be kept and entered and further steps finally ensue.

Such openings will not be missed, if the therapist and client are on the lookout for an unfamiliar energy, a new quality, a loosening, some seepage that slowly suffuses the body. It may be very slight.

Conversely, an attempted reframing can cause a sense of dullness. Although valid, its usefulness may have long been exhausted for this client. Or, perhaps the statement makes the problem feel more oppressive than before. There may be a sense of closing, boredom, the loss of what had seemed alive moments before. Such cognitions need to be discarded quickly, so that the experiential sense one had before can be regained.

A statement may have a soggy, unsound quality indicating that there is some error, something inappropriate in the statement. For example,

C: I told him I had decided to see him. He said, "Are you sure?" I said, "No." He said, "*If one isn't sure that something is OK, one shouldn't do it!* But I think *life couldn't ever get different if we only did what we're sure of.*"

Please examine the two principles in italics. They are two cognitions. There are many ways in which either could be seen as true, but the question is, How does each affect this client's experience? What role does each play *here*? What difference does each statement make to this person? Of course only the client can sense this.

This client had often discussed a pattern of being pulled into the wrong situations with men. If that was the sense of "not being sure," she ought not to see him again. On the other hand, she also has a pattern of not living, of just waiting.

The difference turns on the role the statement plays in the client's experiencing. Its role is accessible if she attends to the physical quality: Does "not sure" reek of her old pattern of getting herself in a destructive situation? Or does it let her feel something fresh and untried? To answer these questions requires attending for the felt sense that might come from their assertion. As general statements such cognitions are neither true nor false, nor helpful or unhelpful.

The role played by a cognition cannot be evaluated on the basis of the cognition alone. The client must know to sense at the experiential edge. That is where we can find the difference the cognition makes.

WHEN A COGNITION IS EFFECTIVE, WHAT IS TO BE PURSUED NEXT?

Many people assume that when a cognition is effective, we should proceed by examining its implications. But the value of a cognition lies in its experiential effect. In therapy we pursue the difference in experience a thought produces. Otherwise we might miss the change and be left with just the thought. When a thought opens something experiential, we enter it and see what further comes there. Then we can react to it from the cognitive side again.

WHAT THOUGHT IS, AND WHAT IT IS NOT

In genuinely fresh thinking one pursues a new edge that is only vaguely sensed. At the edge of a scientific discovery, at the furthest end of a logical progression, there is something troubling, new and exciting, not yet articulate or organized. To think freshly involves *sensing*, after every step of thought: Does that get at it? Does that open something up? Does that enter into the unclear lead that I am pursuing? Or does it cover up my sense of that lead?

Fresh thinking is like psychotherapy in this respect. In both cases all categories are open in principle. If it could be thought of entirely in the old categories, it would not be an unclear edge.

At a new edge in therapy, as in philosophy or mathematics, the person is both helped and blocked by already formed notions. The edge is unclear. It will easily be lost if one forces it to be clear before it has generated new categories according to which it can be articulated. Most of us can easily fashion several interesting, clear assertions at any stage in a thought process. To stay with the unclear, never-before-formed edge is harder, both in theoretical thinking and in therapy.

AGAIN THE BASIC QUESTION: IS THE ORDER OF EXPERIENCE DERIVED FROM COGNITIONS?

When people freshly articulate something from their implicit experiencing, they often find that beliefs and notions they thought were natural were actually "trained into them," so to speak. Our experience is partly shaped by such introjected beliefs, and we are not aware of them as such. From this it is only a small, but erroneous, jump to the conclusion that human experience *derives from* learned beliefs.

People often reject a portion of these ingrained beliefs once they discover them. Their rejection is therefore experiential. But it can be misunderstood and seem as if the rejection is itself simply a cognitive operation that substitutes one cognition for another. But we can reject a cognition as we become aware of it, because of a dissatisfaction with it is implicit in the more intricate order of our experience. This intricate order can be made known in turn, but this is a carrying forward. It might then seem that the rejection was due to the cognitive expression of that intricate order. But this is not so.

For example, let us say a client has found that she has been living largely in accordance with a self-evaluation she learned early in her life, that said: "You exist only to serve others." The moment she finds this, she rejects it. It can seem that her rejection is based on the cognitive belief that her life is worth more than that. But this is not so. The belief is rejected by the whole of her organic, animal life process as elaborated by all the situations, experiences, and cognitions of her life. Physical and biological processes are more intricate and more capable of novel configurations than cognitive systems. Elaborations of them increase their intricacy. Certainly this client's organic process included the cognitive teachings of Western individualism. But those cognitions were comparatively thin and poor; even the habits and situational patterns that go with them were only a small segment of her organic life. The client may well state one of those old principles as an expression of her revulsion at living only for others. But that cognition will be nothing like the thick organic living process that immediately rejected the belief.

When there is a problem a whole aspect of life may come to a halt and remain blocked; that aspect of life can no longer be carried forward in a way that has worked before. If the person pursues the blockage as it is felt by the body its intricacy may require more cognitive distinctions than the person has ever articulated before.

WHY COGNITIVE INTERVENTIONS CAN (AND MUST) BE OCCASIONAL AND BRIEF

We are not making a compromise if we decide to use cognitive methods only occasionally and briefly. In terms of their effectiveness in the experiential process, cognitive interventions are brief by nature: Suppose a client tries out a new thought, and this produces an immediate felt shift. Now we listen and respond in such a way that helps the client pursue the experiential effect. Cognitive interventions are therefore brief when they are successful in producing an experiential effect.

But what if a proposed cognition had no effect, what is needed then? An experiential change, some forward movement may need to happen first. Lacking this, if the therapist argues for the cognition, the client might agree with the wisdom of the suggestion, but nothing will really change. Even so, the new cognition may still have been worthwhile. The client has heard it; it has therefore become part of the client's general repertoire. Later it may have some effect. The therapist can also mention it again at a later time. However, continued attention to the new cognition would only build up counterproductive pressure. From this we see that cognitive interventions that fail will also be brief.

CHAPTER 19

A Process View
of the Superego

EVEN WHEN THE THERAPIST is respectful of every one of the client's feelings, a very critical negative "therapist" is at work *inside* most clients. Freud called it the "superego." It is an inner voice that criticizes and interrupts a person's every hopeful move. Even the most neutral therapist would surely intercede to defend the client's process if this negative voice were an interruption by some other person who is visibly present.

Superego attacks are one of the main concerns of cognitive and interpretive therapies. In this chapter I discuss how to prevent the superego from constantly stopping the therapeutic process, how to enable clients to recognize superego attacks, and how to work on what the superego implicitly contains.

MOVING THE SUPEREGO ASIDE

Although therapists should generally listen neutrally, this does not apply to superego attacks. We can intervene and identify such attacks. Then we can try to get back to what the client was feeling just before the attack. Here is an example:

C: I feel . . . [a few words about the feeling]. . . . But that's just stupid [or lazy, selfish, etc.] because . . .

T: Something attacks you there and says it's stupid, but *you* were feeling . . . [I reflect what was said about the feeling.]

Without such a response, the client would continue with why the superego thinks it's stupid and leave behind the feeling that precipitated the attack. My

247

main procedure here is to move the superego aside, to help the client reestablish contact with what was trying to come. It is often sufficient just to recall and reflect what was inwardly sensed when the attack interrupted it. Then the client can continue from what came before the attack.

But even so, the client may continue from the superego side:

C: It's just stupid to think that I could know about this. I must just be trying to be superior.

T: Something attacks and says you can't know about this, but *you* were trying to feel into your own sense of this thing. You were saying, . . .

C: It's not something. That's me attacking me. That's what's wrong with me, I'm always attacking myself.

T: (*Gives a short description of the superego.*)

C: I still think it's me. I do it a lot.

T: OK. To you it feels like that is *you* attacking you, and you find yourself doing it often. Before that, you started to say that you feel . . . (*I again reflect what was said before the superego attack.*)

Usually my response is designed only to have us return to what was trying to come, but sometimes I point out superego attacks so that they become recognizable. Gradually the client becomes able to recognize an attack, to notice that something has interrupted what was trying to come up from inside. If the superego attack is not recognized, the client will be diverted without even noticing.

THE SUPEREGO IS UNIVERSAL

Everyone is familiar with the experience of being attacked from within. Something — some people call it a "voice" — says, "You're no good" or "You do everything wrong. Just look at this and this . . ." (It keeps a long record of your mistakes.) Or, if you are trying to do something brave and new, it says, "It won't work. It's stupid." If you are pursuing a new idea of your own, it says, "If it's your own idea, it must be wrong."

This "voice" has little understanding and no compassion. If you feel bad, it is not likely to ask why. Rather, it will say something like, "It's all your own fault. You should have done. . . . You could have done. . . . How often have I told you . . . ?"

Sometimes the superego is not like a voice but rather more like a sudden thud. One feels a sudden constriction. Sometimes after describing the superego to an audience, I say, "If anyone here doesn't have one of these, let me know. I'd like to study you." The audience laughs.

Everyone who has studied people has found this part of a person. We recognize it under various names: "the superego," "the inner critic," "the bad parent."

Although the superego has a lot to do with one's parents, it is more unreasonable and destructive than one's parents ever were. It contains a residue of parental preaching and criticism, but it is much more than that.

Freud (1923/1960) said quite rightly, "The superego dips deeply into the id." He meant that it is crazy. It is primitive. The superego absorbs the aggression and violence that the conscious person rejects. The less aggression a person lives out, the more destructive the person's superego probably is. Many lovely, sensitive people are inwardly brutalized and oppressed by their superegos. They would never treat others as their superego treats them.

What the superego says is usually quite wrong. It reacts to some single facet of a situation (for example one's attempt to reach out to someone). It does not involve a judgment of the whole of the situation.

Cognitive therapy works largely with superego messages (although it does not call them by that name). The cognitive therapist tries to show the client that this type of message is wrong and unreasonable. For example, when clients think or say, "should" or "should have," they are urged to replace it with, "It would have been nice if . . ." Cognitive therapy combats the assumptions implied in the superego's messages, such as that one ought to be able to control events, that one's value consists in how one compares to others, that one "should" not be angry, that one "should" be able to obtain all the good things one knows about, that one "should" please other people, or that one can be perfect.

The experiential method adds ways to process the superego that go far beyond combating the mere messages.

What makes superego messages destructive is not so much their *content*, but rather *the characteristic manner* in which the messages are delivered and experienced.

Some people may have succeeded in discarding the old parental precepts they learned as children, and in replacing them with their own better values and convictions. But this does not help much if their own values come back at them in the *manner* of superego attacks.

Let me describe the hallmarks of the superego as a *manner* of experiencing.

RECOGNIZABLE MARKS OF THE SUPEREGO'S MANNER

The therapist can recognize the following signs and sometimes point them out as well.

The Difference between "At Me" and "From Me"

The superego is experienced as coming "at me." It is like an authority standing above the person, lecturing, pointing a finger, "How many times have I told you . . . ?" It comes as if from the top down, or from the outside in, at the person.

We discussed a similar difference in regard to role play, when the direction of the energy is reversed. The dream figure is scary when it *comes at* the dreamer, but the energy feels good when it *moves out from* the dreamer. We also saw that catharsis of negative affect feels good when it rolls out *from* the person, but painful when it *comes at* an observer who is not familiar with it.

The direction of the energy is crucial also in the client–therapist relationship. We are glad when a shy client gets angry at us, or is otherwise more assertive with us. We do not want to attempt therapy primarily by teaching or arguing, since that makes the client the passive object of our energy.

People usually think that their superego attacks are part of themselves. And of course, in some sense it is they who are attacking themselves, because it is certainly no one else. But in another respect, when thought of as the *manner* of experiencing it is, the superego is inherently "not me." *What we call "me" pulls back, defends itself, hides, and becomes constricted under the attack.*

For example, say I sit down to write something. Now I feel (my superego says) that I should have written it years ago. The act of writing derives no benefit from "should have written it." I can write only if what I want to say comes to me, from inside. "Should have written it" cannot help me bring that forward. I have to move that voice aside, so that I can hear what I want to say. Without being didactic about it, we need clients to recognize the fact that superego attacks are not something reaching up and trying to live, to expand into the world. They come *at*, rather than *from* the client.

The Superego's Negative Tone and Destructive Attitude

If we attend only to the words we may be fooled. But if we sense the tone, we can recognize the superego by its unreasonable, negative, destructive attitude. It is the voice of a prosecuting attorney. People think that these inner attacks may help to keep them hardworking. But on closer examination we see that the superego's negativity only gets in the way. When we constrict, we are less able to do well. It does not strengthen us for the task. We do our best work when it is not attacking us. When it attacks we become heavy, sodden, constricted, and much less able to do well — even if we wish to do just what the voice tells us. The superego's attitude toward us is not one of helpfulness.

The Superego Does Not Know the Facts

The superego automatically says that you did something wrong, regardless of the situation. For example, you come away from a situation feeling self-critical about having talked too much. As you go back over the situation you decide that you actually did not say enough. Instantly you feel attacked again, and in the same way, but this time for not having stood up for your beliefs. As you think more about it, perhaps you cannot really decide whether you should have spoken more or less. Superego attacks are not based on the facts.

The superego is not in possession of the facts at all. The information about a situation is not in the superego. To find it, you have to enter the implicitly complex felt sense of the situation. The superego blocks that; it has no channel into it.

The Superego's Criticisms Are Simplistic

Clients often say that they are "just lazy" or "just scared" or "just" something. Superego attacks tend to be simplistic. The superego completely misses the intricacy of any situation. Of course a person may be lazy, but never *"just"* lazy. The felt sense of any circumstance will reveal more intricacy than that.

The Superego Is Extremely Repetitious

The superego's messages tend always to be the same. They have been compared to tape recordings. The message will be one of a familiar group, heard many times before. Superego messages are boringly familiar.

The Superego Is Not Moral

Freud said that the superego is the "conscience," but this cannot be so. The Bible says the conscience is "a still small voice." The superego is anything but a still small voice; it is the loudest voice inside us. However, it does mix itself into most people's morality. It needs to be differentiated from morality.

For example, suppose you have hurt someone. The superego attacks you and grinds you down; it makes you feel guilty. It is all about you and only you. This shows that it is *not* concerned with morality.

Only when the superego attack has subsided, do you become concerned about the other person whom you have hurt. *From you* arises your care for that person; you can now think about what to do for that person. Rather than constricting you as the superego does, your care and concern causes you to expand. You come forth more; you reach outward. You judge that something should be done. You wonder how you might fix the situation. Should you write? Should you call? Now you want to find out where the event left the other person, and how you might still help. *That* is morality.

The Superego Has a Familiar Quality

These characteristics of superego messages make them easy to recognize. But superego attacks can occur without overt messages like these. Then the super-ego is harder to recognize.

For example, a client had a sharp pain in her side whenever she brought up certain feelings. It took both of us a while before we understood that her pains came from a prohibition against the way of feeling she was trying to explore.

When clients are used to focusing, they come to recognize the effects of superego attacks whether or not there is an identifiable verbal message. It is felt as a thud, a constriction, a collapse of energy in the body. It is recognizable by its familiar manner and repetitious quality, whereas focusing moves are new and unique.

When we teach focusing, we alert people to this difference. A felt sense may at first be slight. A person may wonder if anything is happening at all. It only begins to come, very shyly. Before it can come in fully, there may be a super-ego attack — a distinct strong thud in the stomach, or a constriction in the chest. The person new to focusing may think, "That must be the felt sense!" Not at all! The felt sense is the intricate and unique sense of the problem at issue. The thud is instead a typical, familiar effect that accompanies the commonplace super-ego attack.

Poorly conducted psychoanalytic therapy leads to a similar need to recognize the effects of superego attacks. The therapist listens silently for a long while, then "shoots" an interpretation at the client. The client freezes. Neither person knows how to make use of the interpretation. The interpretation *itself* is supposed to be the therapy.

Ex-patients from such "therapy" often use this approach on themselves. They have learned some concepts from which any number of interpretations can easily be generated. The moment they have a feeling, they think some interpretive thought — usually a negative one. Then they feel the emotional impact *of the negative thought* (actually a superego attack). They would like to go on from this to work on the problem, but cannot. The felt "thud" in reaction to the thought is not the sense of the problem. But they cannot find or even look for how the problem makes them feel, because they think that they *are* feeling it. So they do not discover where and how something can be found, that can lead on, and lead to the resolution of a problem. One needs to recognize the "thud," and distinguish it from what one is working on. This distinction is important for everyone, because everyone has such "interpretive" thoughts at times.

IMMEDIATE HELP WITH THE SUPEREGO

Here are some strategies for counteracting the superego that can be immediately helpful. Later I will consider more long-range work with the superego.

It is sometimes possible to respond to a client's superego attack by referring directly to the feelings implicit in the superego. For example,

C: I probably don't have a real talent for drawing.

T: You're *scared* to think you might have?

C: (*Silence*) Then they would make me do it all the time.

Here is another example.

C: And so I did that kind of thing again. I do everything wrong. When will I ever not do that sort of thing?

T: You're so tired of that. I also hear anger and I think fear. Is that right?

Notice that the feelings of anger and fear are implicit *in the superego*. They are *not* the feelings of the person considered as a victim of the attack.

Disrespecting the Superego

An attitude of disrespect is helpful. Disrespect means one has discovered that the superego is not informed, not moral, not a helpful authority, but rather is silly and destructive. To acquire this disrespect, one need only notice how unreasonable, negative, stupid, and repetitious it is.

At Least Do Not Believe It

Most people believe the superego messages. But since they are not based on information, knowing not to believe them is a step forward. One knows this best if one knows how and where to find an accurate account of what happened; this comes from the felt sense of what happened, the wider sense of oneself and the situation in question.

But really finding this out takes a few minutes of peace and quiet. It may be hard to do while one still feels the effects of the superego attack. Perhaps one can do it better a little later.

Humor Helps

Because the superego is so repetitious, one can say to it, "Come back when you have something new to say." Since it has no information, one can say, "You might be right — but if so it would be by accident." About its attitude one can say, "Anyone who talks to me in *that* tone of voice is not trying to help me." Or, just roll your eyes.

What Was Happening Just before It Hit?

Superego attacks disrupt a person's inward attention. From focusing we learn one of the best ways to recover from an attack. We are able to ask what was being attended to just before the attack so that our attention moves back down to what was felt or being worked on. Even just trying to find it moves us out of the superego's ambience.

Waving the Superego Off

One should not spend much time arguing with, defending against, or verbally countering the superego. One should say, "Yes, yes. I've heard all that. I don't need to listen to it again." It is even better to say nothing, just waving the hand to move the superego away.

This is like living with a nagging old relative who refuses to keep quiet. The nagging goes on and on, and it's no use arguing with the person. So one says, "Yes yes, but move aside so I can hear myself think."

Sometimes it helps first to grant the urgency the superego seems to feel the issue warrants; then we set the superego aside so we can work on what is so urgent.

"Let us put it over there," I will say to a client, pointing to the corner of the room. Or I say, "It needs to wait outside." Then we check. If it actually went there, the client will feel physically lighter and more energetic, more able to be active.

Rapid progress can be made with these simple procedures. I told one client about them in her first interview. She had said, "Every morning something tells me to kill myself. I shouldn't be alive. It's horrible. . . ." Two weeks later she reported, "I used to be near killing myself every morning. Now when it tells me I shouldn't be alive, I tell it to fuck off. I just laugh at it. It always says the same stuff. It's really remarkable."

Her achievement stayed firm, but we made very little progress on her other issues for the rest of the year she was in therapy with me. People do not usually change so quickly. But a client may feel a great immediate effect from being alerted to the fact that these are superego messages and that they are not true.

LONG-RANGE WAYS TO PROCESS THE SUPEREGO

Role Reversal

Since there is only one organism, the superego's energy is really one's own energy — turned against oneself. One aspect of working on the superego therefore is to get one's energy back from it. Here is an example.

C: It used to give me a thump in the middle. It was a signal to feel terrible. Now it's a signal to get mad. It's like somebody kicked me. "You stop that!" is my reaction.

As the person becomes stronger, the superego becomes smaller. The superego can be role played much like an aggressive dream figure, with a similar shift in the direction of bodily energy.

The superego is not *just* a "voice" — it has attitudes. It is usually negative, angry, hostile, attacking, mean, petty; it enjoys oppressing a person. These attitudes can be felt from inside it, when clients "play" the superego.

Sensing Fear and Hysteria in the Superego

The superego has a quality similar to the "macho," in that a lot of fear and insecurity lies beneath its aggressiveness.

Rose Katz (1981) describes this side of the superego: In group therapy, she says, there is often a member who avoids opening up. As the first few weeks go by, the other members share things about themselves, but the one member only comments on what the others say, criticizes them, and puts them down. After five or six sessions, there comes a time when the others turn to this one: "What is with *you*?" they ask. "We notice *you* never say anything about yourself. You only criticize. Today it's your turn. We wonder what *your* feelings are." Then that member breaks down and cries.

It is as if the superego were such a person. When focusing becomes familiar, the client can sense the superego as a subpersonality. Something like fear, hysteria, or insecurity can be expected behind its attacking front.

I sometimes describe the superego as being like the Wizard of Oz. From the front it has a big bullhorn, but let us walk around and go up the steps behind the curtain. There is a *small* person in there. How does that person feel? From that felt sense we can work on the superego as we would on anything else.

Sensing Why the Superego Hit When It Did

Having returned to the point at which the superego interrupted, one can ask, "Why would my superego attack just when I was doing or feeling this?" Then one can sense what the superego was trying to do. "I was feeling shaky and vulnerable. Oh, it won't let me have *those* feelings." Or, "I felt like being close to you. Oh, it wants to protect me from that. As a child I tried so many times. It says: 'Don't you know enough not to try that again?'"

For example, one client felt that she should be able to speak, and that I was critical of her for not speaking. I told her to wave the superego off and allow herself some quiet time. But she said,

C: Don't tell me to wave it away — I have to take it in and ask what makes it come on *now*. It says, "Go home if you can't say anything. You can't just sit here silent." I know I don't have to talk here. I know you don't care if I'm quiet, and I don't either. And, sure it always says that to me. But I took it in to see why it said that *now* . . . and . . . that led me to my hurt place. It's what I have to work on next, but I'm not ready to do it today.

This client can do all this because she has learned not to fall for what her superego says. Only in this spirit can she sense behind it, or "take it in" with good results. Otherwise "taking it in" would be unwise. This client has become strong enough to be the active one in relation to her superego. *She* takes it in; she exmaines it; she makes it answer her. Done in this manner her efforts have good prospects.

Psychosexual Concepts

Superego attacks can be conceptualized as castrating in their manner and effects (for both men and women). Freud's concept can help us to recognize a pattern of which superego attacks are a part. The pattern is characterized by guilt, shame, humiliation, blame, fear, the inability to act freely, the avoidance of competition, the wish to give up one's power, the conviction that one can never get what one needs, the habit of stopping oneself from acting to get what one wants, and many other variants. These avoidances of life and living are related to superego attacks. When these larger patterns are left behind, the superego attacks might stop. A therapist can mention various versions of such patterns, which may help clients to find theirs.

Owning One's Evil

Freud and Jung (in different vocabularies) have found that people need to come into active ownership of their evil or negative desires and actions (whether really evil or evil only by someone's definition). In superego attacks by contrast, people are passive. They do feel responsible, but condemn the relevant part of themselves as if they knew it only through observing it from the outside. How they feel it *from inside* is split off. The motto "A murder a day keeps the psychoanalyst away" expresses the difference: On hearing it, people laugh because the motto frees them *to side with* the evil desires from inside, while knowing that actions are a different question. Actions have consequences for others and ourselves. But "owning one's evil" from inside lets one be whole, rather than the passive victim of an active part of oneself that is split off.

Finding the Person under Covert Superego Attacks

Chronic outward expression of anger is not a reliable sign that the direction of their energy is necessarily forward. Clients may be trying to defend themselves in response to superego attacks which we cannot see. They perseverate about trivial events, and self-righteously blame everyone but themselves; all the while they are only trying to ward off being inwardly decimated. Such self-defense is not at all the freeing energy of good whole-bodied anger. But even this kind needs to be respected.

It helped one client to hear me state my conviction, each time she expressed anger, that her anger was at least *some* way for her to stay alive and come through. When she could begin to sense herself more directly, then she could sense the *inner* attack to which she was really reacting, and from which she was defending herself by fighting against other people.

By endorsing the anger, we could find her sense of herself and move her out from under the superego attack. She had felt the superego attack only dimly while she was blaming everyone else. As she grew to sense it better, she found that her superego was attacking her child part, calling it ugly, worthless, saying it failed at everything, and that it should be dead.

IT COMES DOWN TO SIMPLY BYPASSING
THE SUPEREGO'S ATTACK

Just before the exchange recorded in the following excerpt, the client had wondered if her father had hit her. She did not remember that he ever had. Her father had scared her, and she felt this in the bones of her chest and in her hands. She has been exploring a deep-felt fear, of her father, of hellfire. She is, and has often been, angry at her family for "fucking with her head." She is exploring the direct fear of her father, which has sexual overtones, and the more general (also very real) fear of hellfire she experienced as a child. But now this exploration is interrupted.

C1: That's what formed my personality, being scared of everything, everybody, my whole body stiff with fear. That's my personality, formed then. Nothing I can do about it.

T1: That's not your personality.

C2: What is it then?

T2: That's what's in the way of your personality.

C3: (*Long silence*) I can feel the green on the other side of this! Free for seeing and hearing and sunlight. It feels like ice melting.

T3: Yeah.

C4: It must have been masturbation but I don't have a hold of that. . . . My hands . . . I can feel my body relax when I say that.

As strong as T1 and T2 sound, the therapist would immediately go back to listening if the client had disagreed. But she more than corroborated T2. From being all sunken she moved in those moments to the other side of the fear, to green vegetation, sunlight, and ice melting. She had had some hint that there was this other side before.

Notice that there is a difference in C4 between the sensation which is in her hands, and the one that involves a whole-body response. It was not the sensation in her hands that opened; rather, the first change came in her body. It was a change in her felt sense, her present body's fresh sense of herself. But this did not avoid, rather, it opened the problem about her hands. Her superego attack had interrupted her in the process of dealing with the sexual issue. The therapist interrupted the interruption.

The *main* procedure is to move the superego out of the way of the process. The simplest way is to restore and respond to what the client was feeling just before the superego attack.

CHAPTER 20

The Life-Forward
Direction

THIS CHAPTER CONCERNS therapist responses to early bits of
movement in the direction I call "life forward." A life-forward direction has
already been an aspect of a number of the examples in other chapters. Let me
now present the life-forward direction in its own right.

Therapists need to recognize and respond to life-forward movement when
it happens. At first it may be shy, or only implicit. We also need to sense where
it *might* come, so that we can look for it there. So we need to know what it looks
like.

A client may feel something stirring inside, where before everything was
long numb and dead. We want to notice such a stirring, if it is new and leads to
more life. What might it be that points "toward more life"? It might be to let
oneself have feelings (if they have been blocked), or to assert one's own perceptions (if one has long discounted them). It might be to say something one has
long felt but not said. It might be to permit oneself to feel a little bit of hope.

We need to look for and respond to new health, a belly laugh, shy bits of
trying something new, a feeling of interest (in anything); or the desire to give
oneself space, more self-respect, a gift, the room to learn something, a new
personal project, a bit of playfulness; or to discover something more of what is
characteristic of one's essence, perhaps finding oneself being more creative or
stronger.

When a therapist senses a life-forward process beginning, the first shy bits
need response and confirmation. The therapist does not need to be sure it is
happening in order to respond. Nothing is lost if it was not life-forward movement after all. The therapist's response will have been brief and the client can
correct it. Then the therapist can reflect the correction: "Oh, I see, it's . . ." Only

the client's sense of life-forward movement can corroborate whether a given move was life forward for the client. If it is corroborated, the therapist can repeat it to make sure the client does not just run past it.

Therapists are often deeply trained to respond only to negative matters. We work with negatives because from them something better may arrive. Surely we don't want to push that aside when it comes. We don't want to greet something new by saying, "This must be another instance of your old pattern."

Here is an example of welcoming new forward steps:

C: I'm just angry at myself for always letting everybody talk me out of things. I knew *I wanted to go and try that*, and now I didn't again.

T: You're really *angry* that you got conned out of it, but there was, or is . . . *Is it still there*, . . . *a real appetite for trying that*?

From having worked with action steps we can see that people tend to punish their forward attempts because the attempts don't go all the way. In the excerpt above there is something new ("I wanted to go and try that"), but it would have been easy to miss because as it was expressed it was already defeated and lost. The therapist hears it as a new step of hers. Of course the defeat needs to be responded to as well, but we would not want to miss the new step! A bit of *appetite* for trying something new is revealed here in midst of the superego attack.

Here is another example:

T: Give that feeling space there for a minute. Just sense it.

C: No, I won't!

T: OK.

In this example a shy client's tone is suddenly very assertive. She rejects the familiar focusing suggestion with a new and energetic assertiveness that has never been there before. The therapist at first is taken aback, then is happy to have heard a healthy from-the-belly energy, then feels a desire to praise the client, then realizes that praise can be patronizing, and decides the best response is just to say OK.

If the client had then criticized herself for it ("I'm so negative"), the therapist would have said something like, "It sounded like you were taking room for yourself, when you pushed my suggestion off. Wasn't there some good strength in it? Did it feel like that?" Later one could ask, "I think your saying, '*No, I won't*,' felt really good. Did it?"

We should not be so ecstatic that a client would hate to disappoint us. But it is well if clients learn that the therapist will welcome their getting stronger. Clients are not always welcomed for becoming stronger in most other situations.

Here is a similar example. The therapist needed the client to narrate her dream in a certain way and became grumpy and irritated when she wanted to tell it her way.

C: I want to tell you my dream. There was this person at work and it turned out they wanted me to take them on, and I already have too many people.

T: Is this your dream?

C: No, it happened at work. They're always asking me to . . .

T: Please, when you tell your dream, tell just your dream.

C: I can't do it that way.

T: Well, I need to know what's your dream and what actually happened, if you could separate which is which.

C: (*Not hearing the distinction*) I can't just tell my dream, it goes on into stuff and I need to say it.

T: Just so I know which is which, OK?

C: My dream, there was this person at work . . .

T: (*Half-shouting*) I can't stand it when I don't know if you dreamed that or it happened!

C: (*Shouting*) You're not going to tell me how to do my dream! (*Really yelling now*) I'm not going to split myself anymore, not for you, not for God, not for anybody! Not anybody!

T: (*Silence*)

C: Are you upset?

T: I just need a minute to recover. . . . I *loved* what you screamed.

C: I know I get scattered.

T: No, no, I'm used to how you do that sometimes. This is me, I do something funny with a dream, I get all open for it in a certain way. It's me, we'll look at it later. I loved your screaming! You're not gonna split yourself, *not for anybody*, not me, not God, not anybody!

C: That's right!

T: It's great!

C: I know what you need, I don't have to mix it up so you don't know if it's the dream.

T: Well, something in me gets funny, I can tell it's me. I feel it real clearly. I'm OK now.

C: I know. But I *can* keep them separate. I thought you wanted me to tell just the dream, only, all the way through.

T: What matters is, you "won't split yourself, not for anybody!"

C: I can't *do* it anymore! I can't!

T: Feels good.

C: Sure does.

A client once wrote me: "Sometimes I find you relating to my growth even when I'm trying to ignore it. Then I'm forced (if I want to be honest) to try to look at it, or let it be. I thought, 'Gene expected me to have my center, no matter how many people raped me.' It put me in my center. The rape is true, but your relationship is less with the ugly pathology than with my center. You had such a big response about my Dad giving me money for piano lessons when he had to charge our groceries . . . that [it helped me understand that] my Dad would want me to have my center. Letting me lose my center when I just partly found it—your attitude was silently that it's my choice. I lost it when I denied it—then you reflected my not liking to lose it.

"I asked you if what's left of the pathology doesn't need to be worked with more, first, before I try to 'get there.' You said, 'Well, why don't you get there first and then we'll do something if we need to.' "

Her letter confirms that the life-forward movement is the essence of a person (she calls it her center). It needed to be responded to before we could be sure that it was there. When we suspect that it is behind fear and shyness, the person's desire to live needs our response.

To define or identify pathology is never itself the point or the purpose of therapy. Pathology is only what is in the way. But in the way . . . of what? That (whatever you call it) must have priority. It is what leads out of the swamp. I call what is blocked by pathology the life-forward process.

The concept that there is a life-forward direction does not mean that a certain thing is good for everyone. It does not mean for instance that self-assertion is the right direction for everyone at every point in life. Right now a self-assertive step might be *you* coming forward, coming alive where before you had been silenced and numb. But self-assertion may be your middle name, and you always take up more than your share of space. Therefore, it might be life forward for you to notice how fascinating others are, or to wonder and wait to sense what they might feel before asserting something to them.

After a few steps, a life-forward direction might require something that looks like the opposite of what transpired in the earlier steps. For example, for one client it is a great step for her to fight and not retreat and hide. To overcome her earlier pattern of hiding she fights openly, visibly, flamboyantly. But later on it turns out that she fights more effectively by no longer doing it so visibly. Therefore it is a step for her to fight more covertly. Someone might think this is the opposite, that now she is hiding again. But *this* hiding is not the same pattern of retreating and hiding from before. The definition of what leads in the same direction may change many times.

From the verbal content alone we cannot decide what is a life-forward direction for a given person. But when something life forward comes inside the person, it is very clear. Yet it can be easily postponed, ignored, or denied. Therapists should respond tentatively when they cannot be certain that a given thing is experienced in a life-forward way. But when it becomes clear that it is life forward, and the client still ignores it, then the therapist must take a stand in favor of giving it priority.

CHAPTER 21

Values

SOME THERAPISTS BELIEVE that they must decide the goal of therapy for a client. They think of therapy as a way to help people reorient their values. The assumption is that goals and values are inculcated into people *from outside*, by society. Freud (1940/1949) held that the infant is only a bundle of chaotic drives "which has no relations with the outside world" (p. 108) so that all organized behavior must be learned. The ego is entirely a product of each society. Freud wrote that it is as if the ego had "Made in Germany" stamped on it, just like an industrial product. He assumed that nothing inside organizes or directs life. Although most therapists since Freud have rejected this assumption, it still inheres in many concepts and attitudes about therapy.

Something quite basic in the human being is lost sight of, when people think that "entering treatment" involves giving themselves over to a therapist. People are inherently at the driver's wheel of their lives. An attempt to give up this control silences or weakens just that in the person which we hope to strengthen in therapy. There may be deeply important therapy hours when the client lives as a child and the therapist is the good parent whom the client did not have, but this must occur within the wider understanding that clients remain inherently in charge of their own human life process.

It follows that therapists must be value neutral according to the very nature of their attempt to help *another* person lead a human life. Ultimately this value-neutrality should indeed be maintained, but, as I tried to show in the last chapter, the therapist can take a stand in favor of a client's life-forward direction, and may need to do so long before it has emerged for the client. Of course the ultimate criterion is the client's own further experiencing and differentiating.

A client's *inwardly arising* life-forward direction is more precise and more finely organized than any generalized values. The steps that come in focusing and experiential therapy are much more finely differentiated than generalizations. Observing these steps leads to a new understanding of values. Let me show the difference:

Values are often thought of as *general* principles or preferences, for example that sex is good, or that it is bad, that death is a natural part of life not to be feared, or that death is a calamity one must avoid at all costs, that children deserve everything we can give them, or that adults must try to save something for themselves in life. In our society people differ greatly in regard to such values, so there is no basis for therapists' trying to impose their preferences on clients.

We need to recognize a valuing process that is much deeper than such generalizations. I will present several examples of seemingly opposite "values" that helped different clients. We will see that they are not actual opposites. Experiential values do not have opposites. In context their meanings are more precise and more differentiated than statements of them. Their experiential meaning moves a whole mass of intricate experiencing forward.

As an example, one woman berates herself for being irritable and impatient with her children when she comes home after work. I ask her to put her attention in her body and sense her impatience, to give it room so that we can listen to it.

She finds a longing to have time for herself. But she says,

C: I arrange things so as never to take time for myself.

T: *People have a right to at least some time for themselves. Everyone has a right to that. What is the feeling that goes with never arranging it?*

I believe that individuals must direct their own lives. It might seem that I am stating a universal value (people have a right to at least some time for themselves), but I am not concerned with the universals. I sense that the client is reporting a stoppage of her living. I ask her to focus specifically on *why* she doesn't take any time for herself. I am hearing that *her* forward-moving direction is being suppressed.

I invite her to sense and listen to what in her body opposes giving herself time for herself. She focuses briefly.

C: I don't believe in needing anything for myself.

T: Please let your body give you the sense of all that goes with that belief.

After some moments, her own needs as a child emerge. But she says she doesn't want to have those needs.

T: What is the sense you have there, that makes you not want them?

She focuses and finds it.

C: My needs were not cared for when I was a child, and they never will be. They never can be.

T: *Every child should be cared about.* Let us, you and me, care now for that child you were.

A long silence ensues. We spend the time quietly together, she and I and the child still in her. She cries quietly during the silence. Then she says,

C: I wanted so badly not to need anything. But it was because I knew I could never get care.

And after another long silence she says,

C: Oh . . . I have been teaching my children the same thing! When they need something, *I tell them to be strong.* I have been setting them up never to get anything in life. I am so glad I found this.

The issue here is not really a matter of having time for herself, nor of having her needs met, nor even of feeling that her needs could sometimes be met. People can stand not getting what they need. The worst effect happens when people cannot permit themselves to feel their needs. Because of the conviction that her needs cannot be met, she pushes them away. Therefore having time for herself expresses a life-forward direction.

Of course this client's care for her children is real and comes from inside. Notice that she has *not changed* her value, that the children matter most. She wanted to work on her impatience because she was concerned about mistreating her children. And now what is it that means the most to her about what just came to her in focusing? It is that it helps her not to teach something detrimental to her children. Her set of values has not changed to another set of values. Rather, it is a special kind of "change": an experiential differentiation, as I will now explain.

In this example we can see what it means to "differentiate" one's experience. It is not like making a *conceptual* distinction. One might mistakenly say that she has made a distinction: Before *only* the children mattered; now she will give some care to herself, and some to her children. But this is not so. What matters most is still the children. If they need all her time after she comes home from her job, she will still give it all to them.

The *experiential* differentiation happens between two kinds of "being strong." She has not thought about it verbally, but of course she did not conclude that one should be weak. She has discovered *directly in her experiencing* that her old "being strong" meant pushing needs away so that they would not even be there, making it impossible for her to get anything in life. As soon as she finds this, she rejects it. The rejection is inherent, internal to the further step of the experience of this kind of "strong."

Experiencing generates more differentiated values from itself. Such values are not imposed from outside. But then what about the therapist's statements, such as, "Every child should be cared about"? Another person's statement can have a carrying-forward effect, or it can engender blockage and difficulties. Therefore, if my statement gets in the way, I drop it. I might quietly reaffirm it once, but if there is no carrying-forward step, I go back to reflecting the client's side. For example, this man says,

C: I could never give my mother what she needed emotionally.

T: You felt her need, but you could never give her enough of what she needed.

C: And that always made me feel insufficient, inadequate; I ought to be able to do better and I can't.

T: This shouldn't have been that way—you shouldn't have had to try to give her what she needed. *She* should have tried to give *you* what *you* needed. A little child should be mothered. The mother shouldn't mostly need to be mothered.

C: Oh well. It sure wasn't like that.

T: But you *do* know you should not have had to meet her needs and feel insufficient?

C: Well, not really I don't know it. It sounds good. But I still feel the same way. I have to try, and I'm always insufficient.

T: Can we touch where that boy you were *still* feels he should have been able to do it? Can we tell him he shouldn't have had to?

C: (*Silence*) Sort of. (*Silence*) There's a hopeless feeling. I can never do it right.

My assertion has moved nothing at all. Therefore I now pursue the feeling he finds there, the one he tried to express at the outset:

T It feels hopeless to you. It's a feeling of "You can never do it right."

In the next example my statement did help.

C: It's so hard to reconcile that she [his wife] might die [of cancer].

T: (*Listens for a long while.*) This shouldn't be happening. A person in their forties with a small child—that's not the right time to die. That shouldn't be happening. It's not right. (*He stares at me, and then a huge amount of relief shows in his face and body. Tears come. He sits a long while, just exhaling long breaths. I did not know why, until he explained:*)

C: I was trying to feel that it is a *right* thing to happen.

What I said so briefly had connected to and carried forward something inside him that had been pushed down and silenced.

In the case of a calamity, some people do more than just *face* reality, which of course they should do. They also try to convince themselves that since it is happening, it must be right. They have a relationship with God which they never mention. They think that whatever happens is what God wills. But calamities are not what the inner organismic rightness wants. It wants to heal, to move in a life-forward direction.

In this instance I did not sense in advance that this man's life-forward direction was being turned back and defeated. I simply stated my own conviction and would have been willing to drop it at once if it had gotten in the way.

With another person at another time the conceptual content might seem to be the opposite:

C: He [a close friend] was my age, and he died. I've been scared and tense ever since, as if I am holding myself together. (*He focuses. Then he exhales a great sigh of relief.*) Oh . . . it is permissible to die. It is permissible to die. This sentence is important to me. It is permissible to die.

T: The tension eases if you say, "It is permissible to die." It is not something that is not allowed.

Looked at as a generalized value, this seems to be the opposite of the previous example. But here I understood that this man's whole body had been holding itself tense against the possibility of death. In focusing he found that his tension was not the fear of death which it had seemed to be. It was rather the sense that dying is inherently wrong and utterly prohibited. As soon as he found this distinction, it differentiated itself from the fear of death and loosened.

The *experiential* meaning here is not the opposite of that in the previous example. It did not mean that the dying was "right," as the man in the previous example had tried to think. Without the experiential mesh that a statement carries forward, we do not know what it means: Without entering into the felt sense and carrying it forward into further experiencing, the person saying it may not know what it means. Although the statement may be affirmed and kept as such, how it carries experiencing forward is what it means just then. Experiencing is always more intricate than concepts. (See Gendlin, 1967, 1982, 1986b.)

A therapist cannot know in advance which general statement will be life-forward for a client. I might easily have told the second man what I told the first.

If I had said that his friend's death wasn't right he probably would have confirmed such a statement, but it would not have had any experiential effect because his implicit prohibition against death needed to be found through focusing.

Is this to suggest that the meaning of all statements is purely individual. No, not at all. Most people can appreciate another's experiential differentiations, once they understand them. There is something interhuman about experiential differentiation.

Is the sense of organismic rightness based on nature? For example, that "every child should be protected" seems true of animal infants in nature. But my next pair of examples shows that the bodily sense of rightness is not *simply* based on the facts of nature. Consider the following example: A client seemed to remember himself vividly as a newborn. His two older brothers looked down on him and shook their heads. "No good," they said. "No good at all."

C: I felt such contempt. I was just no good, not worth anything. And I couldn't defend myself against them. I didn't have language. I couldn't talk back!

T: They dumped contempt on you and you had no language to defend yourself. That wasn't fair. *It shouldn't have been like that. You should have had some way to defend yourself.*

It was a turning point. He visibly expanded, his shoulders straightened, as if he was throwing a weight off. He breathed better.

C: Yes. I should have had a way to talk back. I've lived under that contempt all my life, and I don't have to anymore.

Nature gives us no way to talk back when we first arrive here. So my assertions do not come just from the way things are in nature. I value the example because it shows this so clearly.

My counterexample comes from a recent Russian emigré who said to me about his good life here:

C: How we live here is not reality. Only a few people live this way. The human reality in the world is how my mother and my brothers and I lived in one room and spent all our time just surviving. I need to find a way to tell my children that this is not the human reality.

My value statements about what should be, what would be more right than nature and society provide for, can seem to obscure just that knowledge which this man values and needs his children to have. The fact that we can appreciate both shows that there is something universal about both (and about any experiential differentiation).

269

In the first of my next pair of examples, the client had been sexually abused in her childhood. She had been finding a great deal of painful experience. At one point I said,

T: That should not have happened. I know it did, but it shouldn't have happened. It wasn't right.

C: No. That's not how the world is. Anybody can do anything to anybody.

Still, something glistened in her eyes. I could see that something inside was moved. Something came to life, stirred, uncramped. There is something inside a person that knows, *and always knew*, that abuse should not have happened. It is not necessary that this be agreed to in words.

Following her response I shook my head and reaffirmed what I know. "No. That should have happened. I know it did but it shouldn't have. I'm sure. Every child should be protected. But I know you're saying no, anything can be done to anybody." She simply went on with something different.

When the child is mistreated an inner sense that something wrong has happened may be silenced, but it never wholly disappears. It is discouraged, confused, defeated, weighed down by actual events, but it remains and can be carried forward.

The next, seemingly opposite example (with someone who is not a client) shows that the general sort of concept I adhere to, that an organism has an innate sense of rightness, can be made irrelevant by the way someone else makes an experiential differentiation. And, as with all experiential differentiations, we can of course appreciate this one.

I often suggest that something should not have happened. Her reaction was strong:

"I hate what you say. I have finally lived past all those things that happened to me. Now you are telling me to go back to some time before them, as if they hadn't happened. I'm bigger now because I got through them. You're telling me to be smaller again!"

Because this woman was not a client and I was interested in the general issue, I did not move my statement out of the way quickly enough. By the time I stopped explaining my view, it had done some damage. When I saw her the next day she said

"It took me most of a sleepless night to get back to the good way I had been feeling."

We see how senseless and even damaging it can be to push a generalized value statement on someone without knowing the experiential effect it has in them. We cannot know what a statement means inside another person or in ourselves, unless its experiential effect is entered into, through focusing.

We can feel how great is the capacity of human life to be carried forward in many ways. Its intricacy enables so many differentiations that are valuable, even indispensable once we have them. We also see how poor and few our statements are.

ORGANISMIC RIGHTNESS WITHOUT KNOWING WHAT IS RIGHT

We can also affirm organismic rightness without any statement and without thinking that we know in which direction something right would move. In focusing, when we ask, "What would be a right next step?" the "rightness" is left cognitively open. We become accustomed to employing a sense of "right," without defining what "right" means in advance.

Sometimes I might say to a client in a conflict: "Would it help not to have to decide between them. Try just deciding that you want everything that is right, and nothing that isn't."

This soon becomes a valuable move because it melts the conflicted block and brings physical relief and openness. "Oh . . . I want whatever would be right."

One client had done some Gestalt therapy to integrate two of her "multiple personality" clusters. Then she felt a great loss. Integration turned out to be wrong in this case.

C: Something went wrong there. I integrated and I lost something.

When I understood her I responded:

T: Oh yes, that kind of integration can be wrong. I know a kid who plays both the violin and the piano. He practices each for half an hour every day. Those integration people would ask him to practice them mixed at the same time.

C: But I don't know what to do. Something seems to push me to integrate, to mush them together. (*She looks nauseous and in pain about it.*) I don't know what to do.

T: Don't decide. Just ask for what would be right, and leave it open what that would be.

C: I don't want to integrate; I just want whatever is right.

It brought relief. At certain times now, when she feels inwardly caught, she says, "I just want whatever is right," and it frees her.

One can decide to want "whatever should happen" or "whatever would be right," leaving open what that is. This has a large effect in the body. If one says

271

this and the body responds to it, one is no longer conflicted. One no longer plays one thing against another. Instead, one is *all in one piece* in one's wanting. It gives one a breath, one's whole body straightens. Experiencing moves on past the stoppage. Then, *from the further experiencing*, a new way can later be formulated.

Sometimes this also brings false or unsound commitments to the surface. "Oh," a client might suddenly feel, "I *want* it to be bad for me, because I'm so mad." Then that can be entered into.

Unsound or twisted things are not always recognizable, of course, but sometimes they have a certain soggy, swampy, reeking quality to them. Or, they are frozen shut, so that one cannot enter and sense them. These qualities become familiar.

Affirming an unknown but physically felt rightness is a useful procedure.

No formulated standard determines when experiencing is carried forward. No goal or value brought to the therapy process determines its direction and its steps.

Now it might seem that generalized value statements are useless since we may do better with a content-free sense of rightness, and since (as we saw earlier) we cannot know what statements mean without knowing their experiential effects. But general value statements matter a great deal, and precisely because they *can* have great experiential effects.

A bodily shift similar to a bodily shift during focusing may happen as we discover or recall a value. The moment we reaffirm it, the whole way we feel can change right in front of our attention. If one works on a problem, this large change alters the whole context around the problem. Value affirmation lets the problem be felt in the context of a life-forward direction. This does not solve the problem, but now the problem brings a new felt sense, so that steps toward solving it can come. Therefore values constitute an avenue of therapy.

People state such values in many different ways, for example, in terms of self-development, or in ethical, aesthetic, political, or spiritual terms. Let me give some examples.

For the purpose of our discussion I define *political* as opposition to oppression of any sort. If a person is conversant with opposing political oppression, some of these attitudes can be transferred to combatting psychological oppression.

If a client happens to be certain that political or social oppression is wrong, this certainty can help us if it is applied, for example, to the way the superego oppresses a person. Without this analogy clients might believe that the superego is right. But once recognizing the inner oppression they are convinced it is wrong.

This *political* attitude can also generate a truthful self-respect. For example, instead of being ashamed of bad grammar a poorly educated person can say: "See, they didn't even teach me to talk right." We want to oppose oppression; we would be joining it if we were to look down on the wounds and the marks it has left, instead of having respect for them.

A client of mine was hit as a child whenever she said she wanted anything. Now she finds her stomach violently wrenching whenever she is about to say certain things like that she wants to own herself. When her body now still shrinks together to avoid the beating, she berates herself as a coward. I tell her about a guy I knew who—6 months after coming home from war—still jumped under a table whenever he heard the noise of an airplane overhead. "The rest of us all respected him," I tell her. "We knew how he got that way."

I am inviting her to have respect for her body's response as being that of a veteran warrior. It should be respected in this way, should it not?

This type of change in attitude can alter the context of a trouble and affect the way the whole thing exists in the person's body.

The certainty that oppression is wrong and equality is right can also transfer to personal relationships in which it highlights the client's implicit rights, and also those of others that the client might be violating.

Political, spiritual, and psychological vocabularies seem to cover very different topics, but if taken experientially they are all one implicitly. Each is opposed to oppression, but the different vocabularies give one different leverage with it.

Spiritual literature, as rich as it is, mostly fails to discuss the implicit. Once one has gained access to the implicit, one might find that it is written all over the spiritual literature. (Similarly, you can say that every method of therapy does concern itself with the implicit.) But it does not show it to people who do not already have it.

Teachers of Eastern religions say people must find their own internal guru; then some of them proceed to impose an external guru in grossly authoritarian ways. Psychiatric and spiritual authorities seem quite similar to me in this way. The change we need can happen politically and spiritually only if individuals discover their own inner source of direction. But the spiritual language makes this source sound so rarified that ordinary people think they cannot expect to find it.

Spiritual values can produce a global change in a person. Spiritual literature contains many powerful ways of changing the whole context around a problem. Modern people may have to work to understand the language of this change experientially. New words and phrases can help one to carry forward a sense of experienced vastness and significance that exceeds mundane conceptions.

For example, a great change comes from imagining the end of one's life and then returning from there. It can let one recognize the few things that feel important in one's life. Here is an example of such a shift: During meditation merely personal troubles may seem small. It can seem to us that we will never again be upset by such small matters. (And yet soon after, they may weigh us down just as before. I will discuss this question below.)

Much like the political context, the spiritual context can reverse the positive and negative value of an aspect of our lives. Again what most of society devalues now appears valuable, and vice versa. Recalling the reversal can bring a shift in how any particular problem is felt.

Now let us consider how such a shift relates to working on our personal life problems. For example, a spiritual value may seem to say that personal problems are not real. How can they be? They are only small "ego concerns"—a Zen master would not be bothered by them. One may feel a great relief in one's body in response to this. But that is not the end of the personal problems.

Some of the relief provided by such an approach is appropriate. As with any felt shift in focusing, one needs to let it complete itself. After the shift has gone as far as it can, one needs to sense for what is left of the difficulty.

A spiritual value can make one feel so good, it can release so much tension and heaviness that one can easily make the mistake of ignoring what is left of the problem.

For example, while feeling bad in the midst of some problem, a person reflects: "There are so many human stories—mine is only one more. I need not 'identify' with what weighs on me so heavily. I am not the story! I am the human aliveness that looks out from behind my eyes." This is true.

Logically it follows from such a concept that nothing need remain of one's personal difficulty. But what is left of a problem still exists although it does not appear in terms of such universals. If the person senses for what is left of the problem, it will still be there, much lighter though it may be.

If the person will focus on what is left of the problem while it feels lighter, steps to solve it come more easily. But people must still work on their unique personal mesh, even after a value generates a bodily shift. One cannot skip over the felt texture of a situation, as if one could get rid of all its demands and opportunities for development.

Specific situations are opportunities to develop specific strengths. Sometimes these give us trouble just where we most need to develop, the spot where newly specific meanings and actions can originate. In between the high spiritual truths and the murky situation is the debris, the anger, fear, and sadness, interwoven with the relevant events. To skip this whole personal mesh and try to live only in universals would avoid personal development in just these areas of our lives that now call for it. No universal principles can replace real interactive learning in the intricacy of life.

A monk appears to escape from life situations, to live entirely in contemplation. But soon he is envious because Brother Edward is closer to the Abbot. Being human involves being challenged to develop in specific ways every day. The universals are not in conflict with the need to meet specific personal challenges. Rather, the specific challenges can be more easily met within the universal context.

When a whole problem seems spiritually solved, we can know that this only gives us a good context in which to process the problem. We may already feel fine or nearly so and go about our business, noticing that we still have a slightly restless feeling. If that is happening we should say, "Grab that! Stay with it a moment, don't let it creep into you further." We would not want to ignore it, but we also would not want to see it as if we were only backsliding from the earlier relief the spiritual solution gave us. Rather, this is the bodily version of the problem, this small nervous feeling, which could easily be ignored. This is the sign that our body knows what we have not yet coped with in the problem. "OK, what's still 'nervous' about it?" we ask the nervous feeling ("nervous" is only the handle word for the overall quality).

Values need to have a life-enhancing, energy-giving, forward-moving effect. If they push the person's energy back, they are not being used in an experientially sound way. Spiritual terminology can be a form of oppression. It needs to bring a sense of widening, not narrowing and resignation. One must *sense* whether widening or narrowing is actually happening, so that one can avoid constricting oneself. If a given value statement constricts, one can focus and expect a truer, more differentiated version to come.

As I have tried to show in many examples, the experiential effect of a statement cannot be known from the statement alone. The statement may have many unintended effects in the person's intricate experiential mesh.

How can we reconcile the universality of values with the uniqueness, intricacy, and variety of people? Our human capacities are constantly increasing and becoming more various. No concept of a universal human nature can limit the wild and ever-increasing gamut of human possibilities. There is no universal human content. We can see the universal only in the fact that we can always understand any person's steps of experiential differentiation, if we are permitted to accompany the person. In that respect we are all the same, just like tulip bulbs from which only tulips will emerge. But in the human case the body develops ever new forms to carry forward the very same process that is prefigured in the bulb.

CHAPTER 22

It Fills Itself In

THE ORGANISM CAN fill in what should have happened in its infancy and early childhood. It can even do it relatively quickly. People wrongly assume that this cannot happen anymore because the person is now an adult. Of course the present interaction is not one of nursing or child care. But the present interaction can implicitly and concretely provide the actual continuation of processes that were stopped in childhood. The body has implied the next steps ever since, and will enact them if the interaction makes it possible.

In Chapter 15, on imagery, I showed that such a continuation can happen with images if they arise from a *bodily* process in a safe, protective, company-keeping *interaction*. In the example of the woman who arranged no time for herself I showed that it can happen also without images.

I pointed out that we can articulate this safe protective attitude as if we felt it about a child. I often ask clients how they would feel toward a child. Then I say "*we*" will keep the child company because I know the client cannot usually do this alone. I explain that "we" adults do not know anything and should be wise enough not to push anything on the child. We only protect the child and keep it company.

For example, the neglected care of the child happens as the woman who arranges no time for herself sits silently with me, both adults caring for the child she was.

Here is another example: The client laments the total absence of good female "models" in her childhood. As she talks and also attends to the bodily sense of what she is saying, it becomes clear just how badly those models were lacking. As she goes on, she makes what was missing more detailed and vivid. These models are so vivid, they could almost *be* here. Their presence *would* be felt concretely, if it were not for the fact that the client is filled with sadness, anger, and regret about the fact that she never had them. The old sadness and anger have been felt and reflected before. Since they occupy her body, she cannot feel herself as she would have felt with such models. A therapist who knows how to work with bodily energy knows that the client might physically feel how it is to be with these female models, if her body were not occupied with her familiar anger and regret.

Now she mentions a woman who would have made a good female model. "If only someone like her could have been there when I was little." I say something like, "Let this woman be right here now," and I ask her to feel *how her body feels* with the woman here now. She feels this quite palpably; her whole body changes.

I work to help her keep this feeling for some minutes, and to get it back when it seems to have gone.

Then I ask her for one or two more women, actual women she knows, who are like that.

C: X and yes, also in a way Y. How I wish I could have [the first woman] and X and Y right here, with me, and all the time.

As she goes on to say more, the felt effect disappears. She falls to lamenting again. I ask her again how her body physically feels with all three women here. Again the whole sense of her body shifts.

C: Yes, now I have them *all around me*. I'm fine. I would love to have one in front, one on the side, and one in back of me. I want them all the way around me, like a circle.

It is happening now. In her body, deep in there, some tissues are changing and growing.

Over the period of some months she lets her body shift like this, again and again. A more permanent physical change gradually seeps in. After a while other problems become central, and I notice that *this* lack has (what I call) *"filled itself in."*

I don't know if this client had images. Whether she did nor not, the change-steps came from letting herself bodily experience being with these female models. Our concrete interaction provides the reality in which these processes occur. A quiet, contactful kind of being together over a long period *implicitly* provides the continuation of all sorts of stopped processes. The organism can fill the gaps in, even when the client only reports the week's events. It is more likely to happen when the client discusses what was lacking and is deeply heard and understood. I observe that the organism is most likely to fill in the gaps when there is attention to the bodily quality of being with what needed to happen.

Here is another example: The client has had a lot of previous therapy, and can say some deep things very easily. She says that her husband is something like her father in not being very expressive:

C: I'd like to get them both out from behind their newspaper. I always had to work to attract his attention. I couldn't ever get it.

As I hear this I hope that the present interaction with me is one of getting attention, not one of having to work for it and never getting it.

In a subsequent therapy hour she said something like:

C: It made me feel only like a half. I mean half girl, half boy. I always have to do everything myself. It's my boy part that always has to do something. I can never just be, and let something come to me. If I were all girl then I could just rely on his being there, without having to *do* something. I could just let go. Just be.

I could feel the longing in this description. The longed-for father is there so solidly and reliably that she can rest on him without strain or tension, instead of having to work to pull him. At some point she is very close to feeling with him as he is needed. She says,

C: I wish I could sit on his lap.

Then I could say,

T: You could try this: Feel yourself physically sitting on his lap, actually sitting on his lap, just being there.

She sat "on his lap" for a long time, silently, perhaps 20 minutes. Many steps must have happened in the process. Afterward, she said,

C: At one point just now, I was sitting on the floor in front of him, and his sexual organs were hanging down over my head, like a bunch of grapes.

It certainly seemed to be a deep physical tissue-process, and I assumed that it was good. But I had to ask:

T: Was that good?
C: Oh, yes (*sighs*).

These short examples written down some time after the hour do not convey the process well. They don't show the long-term, concretely ongoing interaction that implicitly provides the reality in which the bodily experience occurs. My instructions seem abrupt, as if the therapist directs the whole process. But when clients are already very close to this process, when they vividly feel what is needed, I can provide the suggestion that they can let *their bodies* feel the longed-for thing as *actually happening*. Then what is needed fills itself in, if our present interaction is already the kind in which it implicitly happens.

Nothing has happened, at times, when I have suggested this too early. I have also found that I cannot explain it to a client. It sounds fictional, like wishful thinking, a substitute for a real solution, and is therefore discouraging. Of course the process is anything but a substitute. It is the concrete happening, not merely symbolic. But a description of it sounds like fantasy, because there is no way to say that the concrete interaction is the implicit occurrence of these things.

I do not think we should direct clients to vividly experience what was missing early on, for the purpose of then being able to suggest this process. It would be artificial and therefore thin. But when it happens of its own accord, I need only say at some point, "Let yourself feel *in your body* how it is to *be* there."

As we have seen throughout, bringing the body into the therapy process can be quite vital. One client tells me that he does focusing during his daily 20 minutes of exercise on his treadmill. I am not certain of course, but I think it means he disconnects from his body and lets it go on treading automatically, while he does what he thinks of as focusing. Similarly, many clients disconnect from their bodies during their therapy hours. The body is left sitting there, immobile, whether slumped or upright. It just waits till the end of the hour. Much more therapeutic change can happen if the body participates.

In the examples here my asking clients to feel the being cared for in their bodies gets around the sad conviction that the need can never be met. The client's body is filled with anger, sadness, and various ways of autistic coping. All this is in the way, even if the present interaction could implicitly meet the need. As one client said, slumping into a hopeless posture: "Inside me I already gave up on getting loved. I won't beg. I go away, poor but proud." (She laughs and points her nose high.) "Or I make the other person feel good." Of course we work on the old patterns that have formed around the long-unmet need, as well as the anger and sadness. And of course we work on them within an interaction in which the need is concretely being met. But the brief suggestion to let her body feel it actually *happening* can cut through the accumulated patterns and feelings of its not happening, so that it really does.

Another main lack which can fill itself in, is being "grounded." Everywhere in the world infants sleep on their mothers' bodies. In Western society infants sleep alone. That probably explains why so many people in our culture lack the sense of groundedness. This is a bodily sense of continuity with the earth. It is a sense of solidity under us, which carries us, somewhat like lying in the grass, feeling the big earth under us. Many people are never able to let all their weight down.

I may tell a client about the comedian who says he is scared of flying. He doesn't trust the airplane, so he holds himself up by his elbows. He never lets his weight down into the chair. After we laugh, I ask clients to feel the support of the couch, the floor, and the earth, so that they can rest and let their weight down.

Dreams often show the problem. Common themes in dreams are, for example, hanging from a rope, being in an attic without stairs, on a rickety ladder, or in an elevator that won't go down. Falling out a window *to the ground* is a sign that one is reaching the ground, but not yet in a regular way.

A mother is a bridge between the infant and the ground. She holds the infant securely. Some clients had especially unnurturing mothers whose lack of care continues in them as adults. When such a client's body becomes genuinely grounded, I may say, "A mother is a bridge to the ground. Now that you have your own ground, you don't need her for that anymore."

Grounding happens implicitly in most good therapy hours, but especially when the two people sit quietly in a deep contact which they both feel. In such times the total restfulness and security of early grounding can fill itself in.

HOW CAN WE THINK THEORETICALLY ABOUT THIS FILLING IN?

Now let us ask how it is that the organism can fill in the gaps, the needed and implied events that never happened. If we can understand this theoretically, our work with images, dreams, bodily energy, and concrete implicit interaction will become more understandable.

Most current theories assume—quite wrongly—that one knows only what one has in fact experienced. Not so. An infant's organism *knows* before birth how it should be received by a mother. That includes being received by arms that pick the infant up and cuddle it, and by nipples that bring first a certain fluid and then later milk. Infant and mother are one system together, and the whole system is prepared.

Jung said that every organism has not only the experience of its actual mother and father; it also has an internal (he called it "archetypal") mother and father. He made it sound mysterious and in a way it is. But we can think about it with my theory:

The infant and the mother are one system together, both when the child is in the womb and later. The child emerges ready for the breast, and the breast is prepared for the child. If there is no breast, the child cries and starves. But, if there is no child, the breast too is in bad shape. If the child dies or is taken away, the breast hurts, impacts, and has to be pumped.

If a kitten disappears, the mother cat searches for it all over. When aborted at a late stage she also searches, and will pick up and carry little toy figures, or the closest things she finds to what might have been her young.

280

Some people say, "I never experienced being loved, so I wouldn't know what that is." Not so. Every organism is carried forward by being loved or cared for. The conscious person might misconstrue, might perceive old patterns instead, but the body will take a carrying-forward step if it can happen in the interaction.

In one respect what should have happened is only an idea; what actually happened is real. But in another sense what should have happened is *more real*. After all, what happened was due to the foibles and disturbed lives of the limited people who were a person's parents. How they behaved was an accident. On the other hand, what is planned for in the organism is as real as the organs of the body. How each is meant to operate is given along with it. We are born not only with lungs but also with knowing how they breathe.[1]

I ask my class, "How do children learn to walk?" They answer, "They copy the adults." I ask, "How do they learn to crawl?" Then the students laugh. But of course they are young; they have not observed how a child pulls itself to standing, lets itself fall down and then stands up again, until it has systematically mastered every position between sitting and standing. Then it insists on trying to walk till it walks. The body comes not only with legs, but also with the human walk.

The body has not only a stomach but also the complex process of digesting. It implies its processes, and its processes are all interactions. It can digest food—*if* there is food. The body implies how things and people will interact with it. Since breathing is implied, the air is also implied. By implying walking, the body implies how the ground pushes back. Digestion and sucking imply milk, nipples, and a nursing mother.

The infant organism knows (feels, is, implies . . .) its next bit of life process, which means how it will be *with* a mother and father. It implies how its life process will be carried forward by them. Just as it "knows" how to inhale the air into its lungs, so it "knows" how it will be held, nursed, welcomed, and protected.

The bodily implying is always still there. If it can generate the missing interactional events, it will.

THERE IS INTRICATE NOVELTY

Since these early universal patterns seem fixed and always the same, how do they generate the novel and intricate experiential steps which I have emphasized up to now?

When a cardboard partition is put into a beehive, some bees are soon born with scissorlike appendages that cut through it. When an amoeba is put into a fluid that contains a chemical new to it, the amoeba develops certain complicated reactions that keep the chemical out. This bodily novelty also can happen in relation to language and culture.

We saw a duality like this in dreams. They manifest the universal patterns that Freud and Jung described. The dream knows about primitive culture, myths, turtles, and sexuality. But each dream is also new. Each dream brings more intricacy than interpretations can exhaust. The images allude to *this* person's life. They bring uniquely designed steps for just this person in this situation. It is important to know that such steps come of their own accord. If we don't know it, we work tensely; we try to design something to fix a trouble. We cannot and need not do this. The organism can fill *itself* in. The steps come from the body just as, when there is a wound or a cut, our part is only to clean it. *It* knows how to heal, how to match up all the capillaries.

NOTE

1. David Grove (1995) has developed a carefully formulated series of questions for working with early abuse. Among these, are: "Where do you feel this?" (some location on or in the body.) Later in the series, he asks: "What would you like to have happened?" Something deeply needed (for example something felt as protective) may then appear. In this different way he also finds that what should have happened, can fill itself in.

CHAPTER 23

The Client-Therapist Relationship

INTERPERSONAL INTERACTION IS the most important therapeutic avenue. Its quality affects all the other avenues, because they all happen *within* the interaction. This has been evident throughout this book. Now let us take up the therapeutic interaction in its own right.

Interaction is a therapeutic avenue in two different senses: In the primary sense it is always concretely going on. In a narrower sense it is an avenue when we work on the interaction as such. Some clients criticize the therapist, become angry, doubt that they are cared about, complain that the therapist is not genuine, miss sessions, resent paying, react to the therapist with hurt feelings, impute certain feelings to the therapist, make difficult requests; or they have overly positive feelings for the therapist, want to meet outside of therapy, raise sexual issues, and so on. With such clients therapy may consist largely of such interactive events.

Other clients hardly ever do these things, and rarely speak about the relationship. They speak about themselves. Only occasionally do they relate overtly to the therapist.

Simply because an aspect of therapy is essential for some clients, this does not mean that it should be imposed on all clients all the time. As with the other avenues, it is an error to try to turn every hour of therapy into a discussion of relational events. We need only respond overtly to issues of the interaction when they arise.

Later in this chapter I will discuss specific ways of working overtly with relational events. First I will consider the interaction that is always going on, whether it is spoken of or not.

THE ONGOING INTERACTION:
WHETHER AN ISSUE OR NOT

Everything we do in therapy is interaction. Therefore we must ask about anything we do: *What kind of interaction is happening?*

The therapeutic effect of each procedure discussed in this book has relied not only on the procedure as such, but also on the implicit interaction that it is.

For example, if the therapist pushes the client into doing role play, the client may be passive in the implicitly ongoing interaction. This is not always the case, but it certainly can be. Perhaps the therapist says, "Put yourself into it, exaggerate it, be active," and in saying this makes the client passive. Then the ongoing interaction negates the one being talked about. Sometimes this cannot be helped, but the therapist should be conscious of the kind of concrete interaction at work.

Here is an example of a positive implicit interaction: During reflective listening the implicit interaction is one in which the client determines what the therapist takes in; the client corrects the therapist, and the client's autistic, long-stopped feelings flow into the concrete interaction. Many pathologies and negative patterns can be thought of as stopped interactions between the client and other people. If the concrete living process that is halted in such a pattern can be made to continue in therapy beyond the point it has always been stopped and turned in, therapeutic change happens. The therapist reflects back, "You feel so lonely and isolated," but the implicit interaction is one in which the client has reached another person and is being kept company. Or the therapist reflects back, "Talking feels useless." But the implicit interaction experienced by the client's body is that the client has just affected someone (the exact opposite of the verbal statement). The therapist reflects, "You're saying that no one would like you if you really showed yourself," but the concrete implicit interaction is one of being liked while really showing oneself. In reflective listening the concrete interaction is positive even though the verbal content is still negative.

But it can be the reverse: If I were to tell the client, "Look here, just now when I said this back to you, you were not isolated. Your feeling reached me, and when I responded you felt my company"—what kind of concrete interaction would that be? Of course it would depend on the client, and on the context of the moment and the tone, but probably it would be an interaction of catching the client in a contradiction, winning a point, being the one who saw it first, putting the client in the position of having to take my point in, having to admit something, having to learn from me, having to make room for what I say, perhaps pushing back the lonely part that had just been speaking. The concrete interaction might be the opposite of the things I would be saying.

The experienced relationship is bodily and concrete; it is not what is said about the relationship. Neither is it how the two people perceive or think of each other. The relationship is each time the concretely ongoing interaction.

THE MOST COMMON UNTHERAPEUTIC INTERACTION

If the therapist interprets the relationship for the client, the actual relationship may be that the therapist tells and the client is told. Or, if the therapist asks about the relationship, the actual relating may be one of interrogation, with the patient having to answer.

Whether this happens or not depends chiefly on whether therapist and client share an old-fashioned set of ideas about authority. If they both understand that authority resides in the client's process, then it may not matter so much just what is done at some moments. Or it may.

Even when I only tell the client, "We can be silent for a while," it may be an interaction of client-being-told-how-to-feel. The anxious client may think: "He wants me to feel a way I don't feel" or "We can be silent is easy for *you* to say." The interaction consists of client-being-told (what we can and cannot do here).

But since I am the therapist, can I avoid saying what we can and cannot do here? Of course I do it at times. But it does repeat the being-told interaction, which everyone has experienced throughout childhood, and since. This cannot be the new kind of interaction we need, the kind in which the client changes.

Of course we sometimes ask questions. But then we can notice whether the client moves into active self-expressive steps, or is forced into self-defense. If we are aware of the concrete interaction, we can judge what to do, and how often.

In therapy the interaction should not too often duplicate the common childhood type in which someone defines reality for the client, and the client is supposed to listen. Everyone has had that kind of interaction with parents, teachers, experts, overweening friends, perhaps also with unskilled therapists.

In such an interaction *the other person* is active, animated, perceiving clearly, explaining clearly, taking up space, defining the world, moving ahead— just the interactional modes that the client needs to discover. Meanwhile the client is passive, is impinged upon, is expected to listen and put away the thoughts and feelings that are already there, pushing them back, crowding everything in further so as to make room for what is being expressed, then to wait till the other comes to the point, follow the other's reasoning, and see the other's good sense.

This is the most common type of concrete interaction that should be avoided most of the time in therapy. Little new will happen in it, however valuable what we say may be. Such times should be brief and rare, and they should stop if arguing ensues.

But what if we are already expounding or arguing by the time we notice it? We can shift instantly by changing over to reflective listening. We can say: "Now I want to grasp what *you* really mean. Let me see now, you were saying . . ."

Then it is well to listen *purely* for a while. It does not help to mix listening and arguing.

Problems do not get resolved in interactions that duplicate the kind in which the problem was generated. On the concrete level they generate the problem all over again. We need a new kind of interaction, one in which the client actually lives in a new way beyond the old stoppage. The more forward and more intricate experiencing will have new implicit edges that will bring change.

CONCEPTS PERTAINING TO THE OVERALL INTERACTION

"Putting Nothing Between"

The first constant relational "procedure" I want to discuss is what I call "putting nothing between."

When I expect a client, I put my own feelings and concerns to one side. I don't put them far, because I need to sense when something registers there. I also put aside theories and procedures, all that I have discussed so far in this book. All that is on the side. In front of me the space is free, ready for the other person.

Let me explain the difference this makes. For example, right now I am in a certain mood from my private struggles. I am also preoccupied with rewriting this chapter. If you suddenly walked into my office, there would be a third cluster: social guidelines for greeting someone properly. I would respond to you drawing on those. Or if you were an old friend, I would respond from something that draws on our familiarity. If you then wanted to relate more personally, it would take me a minute to put our usual ways of relating aside, to put my concerns about this chapter away, and to roll my mood over so that I am no longer inside it. Then I would be there with nothing between. But it would be much easier for me to remain behind all that.

To be with a client, I keep nothing in front of me. Of course I know I can defend myself. I can also work according to guidelines for responding. For example, I can always reflect a client's feelings, however I might feel. But I do not want the attitude of being ready to respond *between* me and the client. Because I keep nothing between, the client can look into my eyes and find me. Many clients do not look, of course. For a long time some of them cannot. But if they do, I won't hide. Then the client may see a very insufficient person. I could not allow this, if it took a special kind of human being to be a therapist, a wise or good one with pure motivations, one who lives life really well, or who is an untroubled person. But fortunately no particular kind of person is required, just *a* person. This fact makes a thick peacefulness. I need only be here so that I can be found.

Putting nothing between is the first constantly applicable relational "procedure" I want to specify.

"The Person in There"

Now I want to describe my sense of the client. I relate to what I call "the person in there."

In my student days, one of the most useful things anyone told me was: "There is always a person in there." In infants and senile people, seemingly worthless people and seemingly stupid children, there is someone in there. Usually it is an embattled person struggling to live somehow with (or in spite of) all the inner and the outer content.

A few years later I worked with hospitalized patients who sat bent over, staring at the floor between their knees. I thought: There is somebody in there! I would sit next to such a patient, and explain what I was doing. I would say: "I am keeping you company." Every few minutes I would say something. The patient might never move or speak. But I found another thing to say, and another. The nurses gave me funny looks. They found it amusing that I kept on talking. Saying all those things put me far out on a limb. Yet months later the patient would become verbal. Then one patient asked me: "Why did you say so little? Don't you know it helps people when you talk?" (See Gendlin, 1972.)

I have frequently discussed with other therapists Rogers' three "necessary conditions" for therapy. *Empathy* is understood, but many people wonder: How can one be *genuine* and feel *unconditional positive regard* at the same time? There is often so much unlovely stuff in a client, which cannot genuinely be regarded positively. But I see no contradiction because, as I formulate it, unconditional positive regard is for the embattled person in there, not for the stuff. The person in there is up against that same stuff, struggling to live with or in spite of it, all the time. I do not mean that it is always easy to feel for every person struggling inside, only that there is no contradiction here.

Many people look at a person and see someone smart, or a jerk, a neurotic, a shy person, a Ukrainian, a psychologist, or a salesman. People are these things, of course, but much more importantly, people are the one that is in there.

There are various ways to think about this. We can elevate the person as a spiritual essence, or reduce the person to an absurd bit of temporary flotsam. But either way the person is in there, struggling, trying to live. When we meet someone's glance, someone is there, looking back. That might feel good or make us nervous, but someone is there.

Who looks back is not the person's traits or experiences, not the felt sense either. A person is not a felt sense; a person *has* a felt sense. The person looking at you is none of the content. Content does not look at you.

Whether the client looks or not, someone is in there. The basic interactional framework in which I practice therapy consists of putting nothing between, and sitting down with the person in there.

A Deeper Continuity

I know that every person has a deeper continuity even if at present it seems to be missing. The client who looks out at me may feel thin and helpless. The deeper continuity may be lost or covered over, silenced, shut away since early childhood. But I know it is still there.

Instead of living from themselves, many people can only select what seems the best way one *might* feel. Then they try to believe that they feel that. In spite of this, there may still be a lot of anger, bitterness, and fear, a shakiness and no continuity, deep down.

Clients sometimes report a loss of self: "I feel empty inside" or "I don't think I have any real self." The person looking at me reports the loss or lack of a deeper self.

Such clients value the moments during therapy when they come inwardly alive. In an earlier chapter I mentioned a client who suddenly felt that *she* was present at a moment when she spontaneously disagreed with me.

When a client reports having no self, being dead or absent inside, I say: "I know there is a *you* way under there, and we won't stop till we find it.

I say it briefly and I never argue about it. I affirm it quietly once or twice, without any expectation of agreement. Something inside may hear. The client need not believe it at all. Although seemingly lost or dead, the deeper one *is* there somewhere, always still.

It is like a person lost beneath the ruins of a gutted building. As we walk through we might hear a tapping from far down. Surely we would not walk by just because it is slight.

Sometimes the client *says*, "I died." Or, from the felt sense something may say, "I died." There it is, speaking! But we also need to know that it is true that this part died. It is always still there, but it *did* die, if it says it did. A child who was abused may very well have been unable to breathe and was actually near death. The child experienced dying. The child part that "died" may have been lost or closed off.

In focusing, one client came in contact with a long-lost childhood part. She spoke as an "I" from it, reporting feelings and events step by step, for half an hour. Then suddenly at the next step, she told me:

C: And then I went out.

T: (*Silence*) What did you mean? Did you go outside?

C: No, I went *out*, like a candle. After that I wasn't there anymore.

When vital parts of a person stop, the client feels thin and ungrounded. But the part-selves are not the deeper self. The deeper one is a kind of continuity from far down, and it is often found only after the part-selves are found. Without the deeper one, the person's directly felt *wanting* is also missing. The person wants what others want, or what seems appropriate, but has no inner energy to reach for something.

One man I know got so weary with never really wanting anything that he borrowed some money and stopped doing anything. He sat in his room every day for more than a month, stubbornly and desperately waiting for some impulse to do something that would feel real. At last he wanted to go outside, but by then it was snowing. He had no overcoat and found to his great relief, that he *wanted* one. It was a great step. He went out and bought an overcoat.

In the example of the woman who would not arrange any time for herself, suppose we ask her what she would do in such a situation? She would probably say that she does not know. But if she arranged some weekly hours just for herself, she would be relating to that deeper person in her, which has always been pushed aside. Eventually a wanting would come.

A therapist I know had an acquaintance (not her client) who always spoke of himself in a kind of jest. She asked him: "When you say things like that, are you joking or serious?" He thought for a while and then said, "I don't know," and smiled. "There," she said, "you're doing it again." Later he came back and said, "Thank you." She said, "You mean because I went looking for you?" He said, "Yes."

One client often said: "If I didn't hold on to this [old painful stuff], I would be nothing." But after a while there was a feeling that "I *could* be different." Still there was the problem: "But if I am free to be different, then who am I?" This disconcerting gap may be where one's deeper sense of self can come. Late in therapy it is often as if the client's old ways of being are lying about, fallen away, but by then there is no scary emptiness. Instead, the client feels much more alive. Everything looks vivid, as when the windows were just washed. One client says: "Most of the time, now, whatever I'm doing, *I'm* doing it."

Providing Safety

It will be evident from the above that I consider therapy a plain real relationship between the two people. This reality is not diminished by the fact that psychotherapy has a distinct well-known "frame," which provides a certain safety. Every relationship has its frame, and the frame is always part of its reality.

The client needs to be free and safe to express all feelings. The safety requires that the therapist will not *act* in response to a client's feelings of sexual attraction, or a client's report of unlawful behavior. These things will not lead therapists to act as they usually would. To keep this safety unshakable is part of the reality of a therapy relationship. The world offers many sexual opportunities, and there are also a great many police; the therapy relationship is rare and has another purpose. This makes it narrower in acceptable conduct, but deeper than most other relationships.

The safety of the person in there supersedes all procedures, theories, diagnoses, interpretations, all thoughts and contents. The one who says "I" is the one with whom we are dealing, and the one who should be safe with us.

The safety can be lost when we put the fascinating activity of psychotherapy ahead of the person. We try to push the person to do what the activity requires. This is understandable but when we catch ourselves, we can recall that the person in there matters more than our wish to make something happen right at this moment.

I may forget this when some process I wish the client to try seems very promising to me. Or, some insight or content may seem terribly important. I may be attending *only* to what my client *said*. But suddenly I see her there again, perhaps oddly small and tense, pushed back into her chair, nevertheless *someone there*, looking at me. How could I have lost track? What else matters? Just my recalling her is enough to let us meet for a moment. Our contact is restored. She is more important than what she said, and what I will say.

Whether our eyes meet or not, there is contact without my doing anything to bring it about. Perhaps my voice and posture convey my sense of the presence of the person, but I do not need to think about that. I only need to recall that the person is in there.

Now I want to mention some examples of specific therapist responses:

Often, when we are stuck or the client is in pain, or when our relationship is off and I don't know what to do, I simply say, *"Hello!"* (as if the client had just arrived). This is not an interruption; it gives the process a better chance with whatever is to be worked on.

I have already said that therapists should not usually interrupt silences. But does the client feel my presence in a silence? If I have the impression that the client feels alone, I might cough or shift in my chair. I want my presence to be part of the client's inner process.

One client, who had an abusive experience as a child, could imagine no way she could ever heal, except to make it "unhappen." Eventually she said she would have been all right in those years if there had been someone to talk to about it. Nothing could have made it unhappen, of course, but she and the person could have "sat on a log together." I am here in such a way that a client can sit on a log with me.

This means that we do not need to have an answer to the client's stuck places. Sometimes there are real answers. However, usually we have answers because we have not yet understood the problem. When we reach the stage where we have no answer either, then we have really understood.

Sometimes I offer answers to help the process go further, where the client is stopped. I know so many procedures. I am never without something further that we can try. But we can try it later. We must not miss the real and thick process that happens in those moments when the client and I sit *on a log*.

In our society people find it hard to sit together in silence. If I think the silence makes the client uncomfortable, I might say, "Here we are, you and I, and for the moment we don't have a way with this." Or, "You are feeling the pain of this, and for the moment there is nothing to say." Or I might just say, "pain."

Such statements indicate that we need not hunt desperately for something to say. I might add: "We can just be here for a while." In words or, more usually, in silence I indicate that our being together *is* something real that we are doing, even if there is nothing to say.

In the Interaction We Are Still Separate People

Contact is not merger; quite the contrary: It is the keen sense of the reality of the other person's presence as another being. In merger we feel as if the other person consisted of our sense of that person. When we discover that the person is just now feeling something utterly different than we had thought, merger breaks, but contact is heightened.

With one client whose trouble with separateness gradually made her an expert on the subject, I had this exchange:

C: You have to hear this: I am so glad you are the way you are!

T: I will try to take that in.

C: You just have to hear it. Whether you take it in is your business.

Contact involves the fresh impact of the other's otherness and separateness. We can welcome and enjoy the moments of surprise. Such moments dispel projections and show that one is in touch with the actual other person.

OVERTLY INTERACTIONAL RESPONSES

Let me now turn to the narrower meaning of "interaction," the occasional difficulties that are also opportunities for therapy.

How Interactional Trouble Can Become a Therapeutic Interaction

Therapists who do not work consciously on the interactional avenue may think of interactional conflicts merely as difficulties. But these are opportunities for therapy. The approach to such difficulties in classical psychoanalysis would have been to interpret them. This was done in terms of the client's resistance, interpersonal dynamics, projection, and transference, a repetition of the client's past.

More recently many therapists have learned how to turn the interaction into a therapeutic opportunity. The general principle is this: clients are not stopped, nor are they just tolerated, but are responded to so as to continue the present interaction in a way that goes beyond their old pattern. This enables clients to discover themselves living in new ways. As therapists we need to be on the lookout for such opportunities.

Here are some examples:

When Something Covert Is a Trouble between Us

If something is out of kilter in the relationship it must be straightened out before any other therapeutic means can be expected to have good effects.

The troubled aspect of the interaction *needs* to be verbalized, and it has immediate priority over other avenues. We may already be in a conflicted interaction and are pretending not to be. When we are darkly struggling while pretending nothing has happened, then it is necessary and freeing for the therapist to allude to the difficulty. We may both even feel a distinct zest when the therapist brings things like the following into the open.

I may say:

"I know we don't agree about this."

Here are other examples:

"Thank you for agreeing to my having changed your appointment, but I know you might still have some feelings about it."
"Maybe you're still mad about that stupid thing I said last time?"
"I think you're trying to say that you feel we aren't getting anywhere."

The client may be afraid to express a reaction to the therapist directly and so may hint at it. For example:

C: I'm mad at everybody.

T: You're mad at everybody, probably me included.

THE THERAPIST'S INTERNAL REACTIONS AS A WAY OF REGISTERING INTERACTIONAL PROBLEMS

Personal feelings about a client should not be allowed to build up in us to the point where they explode and we dump them on the client. (The same is true of interpretations that seem to come to mind over and over again.)

The client is not here for our needs or to understand and satisfy us. Therefore most of a therapist's personal reactions fall away, or these issues need to be worked on in our own terms, away from the client. However, we must say or do something if our feelings indicate that the therapeutic interaction is going wrong.

I have said that I welcome it when a shy client tells me to keep quiet, or directs me in some other way. But don't some clients need exactly the opposite, to run into limits, to cope with the reality of another person? What about clients who are overbearing and impose on everyone until they are justly rejected? In ordinary social situations I might find it easy to ignore a behavior, but in therapy it is my responsibility to speak up, to meet the attempt to impose on me, and do it in a manner that will help the client.

When I reflect a client's anger at me, I firmly stand my ground very solidly, so that the client's anger can come out more. I don't want the client to pull back in guilt for fear of hurting me. I am vividly undamaged when I reflect: "I think I did all right, but *you* feel I did . . ." In the implicit concrete interaction we are *both* solid and undefeated.

As a therapist I may be glad the anger came out more. But before I *say*, "I am glad your anger can come out more," I have to consider what interaction this would be. Some clients might experience such a statement as patronizing, that somehow I am out of reach of their anger. I could say this to other clients who share a reflective level with me. I might say it also to a client who feels that by getting angry she will lose me.

"You and I are now like this," I sometimes say, bumping my fists together. "I don't think you're right, but I know *you* feel . . ." I want the implicit interaction to be one in which there is equality and room for conflict.

The Negative Can Be Considered a Stopped but Positive Process

Another way to respond to negative and self-defeating ways of relating is to think of them as positive ways that are as yet incomplete, stopped, or twisted back on themselves. Therapists might ask themselves: What life-forward direction might conceivably be implicit here? The client may *already* be going in that direction but it is inhibited, partial, or turned in. The therapist can respond to that right intention, as if it were obviously there. Whatever the actual life-forward direction is, it may then emerge.

For example, the client may tell of real or imagined mistreatment (by others or the therapist), resent it, but always end up going along. A stronger person would firmly call a halt. Now we can imagine that the client *is doing that*, only not far enough. We can try responding: "You are *calling a halt* to that. And I can see why, if that is what you felt he (or I) was doing." This could help the client move forward more strongly: "Yes, and you (he) shouldn't be doing that."

Even if such a response from the therapist is wrong, it invites the client to come out with whatever the positive direction is. Perhaps the client says, "No, I'm not calling a halt to anything. But I feel you don't care about me." Then we can welcome that. "You feel you should be cared about and that I should care.

Yes, you should be cared about. I think I care a lot, but you want to feel it and you don't."

The troubles clients talk about may manifest themselves in their relation to their therapists. Sometimes I make this overt and say, "Good. Now *we* have the problem you spoke about, so it's alive and we can work on it. I'm glad it's here." That can change it from a discouraging hiatus to an exciting agenda. "Well, what are we going to do with it?" the client may ask. "We don't know yet," I answer, "but we've got it here, now."

ISSUES OF TRANSFERENCE

Clients sometimes know that something we would characterize as transference is involved in the interaction. For example, a client may say: "I'm mad at you! Well, not really you, uh, only partly you . . . uh, it's confused . . ." I respond so as to keep both the present and the past open: "You are saying (both at me and at someone else here), that you are really mad at me."

Sometimes the client feels a quick alternation or merger between past and present, which can be painful. A therapist's easy understanding of this phenomenon helps. I say, "I know I am both myself and this other person, just now."

I represent simultaneously myself and someone from the client's past. This client is aware of the duality. Clients who are not aware of the duality also need to be responded to in both ways. Insofar as the anger is directed at me I am ready to meet it as I said above. Insofar as it is directed at the person in the past, I am ready to let it come out at me but I will not respond to it as myself. If I nod and reflect, I am implicitly and concretely responding so that both levels can be here.

In classical psychoanalysis all relational moves and feelings about the analyst were interpreted as really being directed at people in the past. Currently some analysts reverse this. They insist on interpreting patients' feelings about their parents as really being directed at the analyst. Of course there is an aspect of the present relationship in every moment of therapy. And the past is involved in every present moment. Why decide which of the two it "really" is? Both are generally involved, and both can be dealt with.

It is now well understood that there is never a pure transference; it is never *only* issues from the past. The issue is usually raised by something that has just happened. Sometimes it is easier for the client to sense and work on the past if what the client expresses about the present is first acknowledged. In Chapter 10 we often saw that the therapist responded to *both* past and present, usually first reflecting what the client said about the present, then inviting the client to sense whether something from the past is involved *as well*.

Similarly, when clients speak of the past, it should first be reflected, even when a verbal response to the present relationship is needed *as well*.

When a Therapist's Self-Expression Is Needed

In interactional difficulties with a client I assume that I am often part of the problem. It does not surprise me when this is the case.

When there is a relational problem, there are four directions that can be pursued: the present and the past from both the client's and the therapist's sides. All four are always involved, but rarely must all four be worked with.

Sometimes expressing something from the therapist's experience may be utterly necessary for some clients. Others badly need the therapist *not* to do that. A tentative amount of expression of the therapist's side can reveal this about a client. Some lose track of their own process and are prevented from working their projection through. Such clients may say: "I need to ask you a question, but—please don't answer it."

Other clients are stopped if what happened for the therapist cannot be opened, so that they can experience it. For example, one of my clients says: "I saw your reaction just then. What was it?" I become aware that a painful reaction crossed my inner space and must have shown on my face.

If something showed on my face I am not going to insist that nothing was there. It never helps to deny something real. But because the client needs room to express and explore what happened to her, and my answer might stop her, I reflect and let her go first. Or I say: "I *can* go into that if you need me to, but *you* felt interrupted, criticized, something like that?" The client might say, "I felt I did something bad to you" and move on into her side. Then she may not need my side.

But if she asks again, I will probably go into it. A whole texture will be implicit in my own felt sense. I will say only what matters now. At rare times clients have needed me to explore further.

Perhaps if she insists, I will go into my side before she explores hers. Afterwards I will surely invite her to enter into her felt sense, perhaps both in respect to the present interaction and her own past.

Suppose what showed was something private that occurred to me. If she asks again, I can say that it was unrelated to her. If that isn't enough, I might share a bit of it, and how I came into it.

If my reaction belongs in our interaction, I express it if requested to do so, or I might decide to volunteer it.

Without truth and acknowledgment of reality, the interaction can be stopped and blocked, and can reinstance earlier stoppages and projections. In the past the client's perceptions were often denied. The client sensed something in the other person, but was not allowed to reach it. The interaction stopped; the client was left alone in autistic space. We do not want to duplicate this kind of stoppage.

But it may be enough simply to acknowledge, "Yes, I did that. I know what you are referring to. I *can* go inside myself and see what it came from. What did it mean to you? What is your felt sense of it?"

Inside myself I will enter into my own reactions regardless. If I feel something troubling, I need to ask what it is: Annoyance? Impatience? Anger? It need not have a label. More importantly: "What is *in* this feeling?" "What does it say to me about what is happening between myself and my client?"

My reactions contain information about the ongoing therapy. I am an instrument on which the client registers. Since my personal complications are familiar to me, I can usually recognize what I sense in the client. Then I can find a therapeutic way to respond *to the client*. This may or may not be a verbal statement about the relationship. Whatever it is verbally, it will be something that might enable the concrete *implicit* interaction to become unblocked where it had been stopped, turned, and autistic.

Therapy cannot happen meaningfully when the past is explored in an interaction in such a way that it only reinstances that past. We may find the causes of the client's troubles but be at a loss as to how to change anything. We need the finding out to happen in the context of a wider process in which the client is changed and moved beyond what is being found out. We need the very process of exploring the past to be simultaneously a further development.

Two Ways to Move beyond Mere Repetition in Transference

(1) What comes from a felt sense has uniqueness and specificity. If I express something from my own felt sense it will be unique and specific. It lets my client *experience* that what I say has my particular quality. This is likely to dissolve transferences and projections. The therapist's being present and sometimes expressing unique experience is one way of doing this.

(2) Exactly reflecting the client's feelings is a second way to move beyond (and thereby resolve) transferences. Even if verbal content is only about the past, reflecting provides a new interactional context. An exception is clients whose parents were indecisive and made them long for structure and models and to encounter limits and the reality of others. Then reflecting can seem to reinstance how their past was for them. Reflecting is *concretely* the opposite of nearly all harmful interactions. Therefore it usually undoes the transference repetition. Furthermore it does so by *continuing* the client's impetus at the point where past interactions typically became blocked. If a really present person listens and reflects, the positive impetus which is implicit in all repetitive patterns can reemerge and flow into an interactive completion.

Carl Rogers was quite right to posit "genuineness" as one of his three conditions of therapy (along with "empathy" and "unconditional positive regard").

He was not quite right when he added that the client must "perceive" these three attitudes in the therapist. What I think he should have said is that these attitudes ought not to remain private; they need to be manifested so that they can have an impact, a concrete effect. Human bodies experience their situations *immediately* and *directly*, and not only through the interpretive screen of what they *perceive* or *think* is happening. Many clients begin quite far from being able to *perceive* that anyone understands or cares about them. They cannot even form the thought that someone possibly could. In spite of this lack of perception the concrete interaction will have its effects. The organismic process will move forward and change the person. After enough concrete change, the perceptions of those attitudes can form.

Rogers' method led many therapists to reflect feelings in such a way that they did not actually take them in, or sense them. When Rogers found that his method was being used only verbally, he reacted by going to the opposite extreme: he said (1961) that *only* the therapist's actual attitudes mattered. He said that one need not reflect back what the client says. Reflecting was only one of many ways to manifest the attitude of "empathy."

I feature reflective listening much more centrally than Rogers did. Other ways of expressing empathy might fail to engender the inwardly arising therapeutic process. Without reflecting, bit by bit, neither therapist nor client can easily discover what really is meant and felt, let alone what might come further at the inner edge that opens once a message has been fully received. But Rogers was completely right that the relational conditions are primary in therapy. Listening, focusing, and all other procedures are effective only within a safe, genuine, and trustworthy interpersonal relationship. Everything else is something being tried out by two people who are always more important and more real than any procedure.

In therapy the relationship (the person in there) is of first importance, listening is second, and focusing instructions come only third. If something is wrong in the relationship, it must be dealt with as soon as possible, and all else must wait. And without listening one is not really in continuing touch with a person.

Focusing is not an "intrapsychic process" to be contrasted with interpersonal relating. Such a distinction misses the fact that we are alive in our situations and relationships with others, and that we live bodily in our relations. What do we find when we focus? Isn't it how we are living in the world right then? One can focus alone, but if one does it with another person present, it is deeper and better, *if* that relationship makes for a deeper and better bodily ongoing process. If not, then focusing is limited by the context of that relationship. Whatever is going wrong in the relationship will affect the whole inner quality of the focusing.

Long ago I wrote that focusing is "the motor of therapy." Have I revised that and am I now saying that it comes only third? No, what I mean is that focusing *instructions* come third. All therapy requires making inward touch with the edge of what is concretely there, and focusing makes that specific and deliberate, so that therapy is much more effective.

Focusing does involve certain attitudes toward whatever comes up from inside. These are relational attitudes toward oneself. Focusing employs those attitudes, and also helps one to discover them, if one did not already have them.

In the second half of this book, I have tried to show how all other avenues of psychotherapy become experiential when they are integrated in relation to focusing rather than remaining separate contents.

In conclusion I need to say that this has been only one therapist's ways of modifying the many methods to fit them with focusing and the inwardly arising process. Others are arriving at more ways to do this. As the years go by, we are acquiring richer and better ways.

CHAPTER 24

Should We Call It "Therapy"?

THE WORD "THERAPY" is often applied to anything that is done by a trained therapist. I disagree. We must distinguish *therapy* from what I call a therapist's "administrative role." Let me give an example of what I mean by administrative role: When a court renders a judgment, it stands not because it was a good judgment, but because a properly appointed judge rendered it. Even if the judge is known to have questionable ability, even if the decision appears unjust on the face of it, it stands because of the judge's proper administrative role. And this has to be so, because society needs a defined way to dispose of such problems. But justice does not depend on a role, and neither does therapy. The definition is always controversial, but it is not based on the judge's or the therapist's administrative role.

The role of "therapist" involves official credentials, knowing how society handles the problems that come up, knowing how to use the right words, the right to diagnose people, sign insurance forms, hospitalize someone, and operate the whole administrative machine. This is a legitimate reality which should have a name. I call it the "administrative role" of the therapist.

Therapy is something else. Even if there was a therapist involved, we must still ask: *Did a therapeutic process happen for the client?* We can differ on what this means and how we determine it, but it is clearly a different question from whether the therapist had proper credentials.

Unfortunately people tend to think that if someone goes regularly to a therapist, whatever happens is therapy. They may never have been in a relationship in which they experienced the little inwardly arising steps of getting better. Therapists differ about therapy, but I can say another thing it is not:

Freud established the principle that an analyst should abandon an interpretation when nothing from the patient's unconscious arises to corroborate it. For instance, in *The Wolf Man* (1915/1971) he reports giving up his interpretation, but it was after having insisted on it for nine months! Of course we forgive pioneers. But one hears countless cases of all sorts of dire, stupid, or hurtful statements that therapists did not have the good sense to retract, and of clients being coerced into life steps against their better judgment. It makes many people think of therapy as something no sensible person would want. But there is a huge difference between a respectful process designed and intended to let content arise from inside, and one in which the "therapy" *regularly consists of* trying to impose ideas and actions from the outside *as a matter of method*. Let us not call something like that therapy.

Let us work to change the public conception of "going into therapy," which still often means putting oneself into the hands of someone who takes charge and thinks that taking charge is possible. It means giving that person's comments and advice greater status than one gives one's own or other peoples' comments and advice. It means that one is "in treatment," which means that the mere doctor–patient structure *is* something.

Here is a story about this: A well-trained and intuitively gifted therapist I know very well sent her young daughter into therapy. The mother tells me some ugly things the therapist said, and of intrusive treatments he proposed, which she only barely managed to stop. Meanwhile she tells me nothing of what her little daughter says about her trouble. "What does *Janie* feel about it, don't *you* listen to her?" I ask. "Well, you're not supposed to treat your own child," she says—quite rightly, of course. But should she not listen? When she is so talented? I cannot ask her about it. I am silenced by too much that would take hours to explain. Certainly one's therapist cannot be one's mother. I agree she must find a therapist who can help. But she isn't looking for one; she is putting up with this one! What is she doing letting such a person get at her child? The answer is that he is a therapist, and she believes in *therapy*! She answers, "Well, Janie has to have *some* therapy."

I see that she thinks that some therapy is better than none, that there is such a thing as therapy that consists of going to see someone who is called a therapist. I found myself telling her, "Look. There is no such thing as therapy! Except when it doesn't work, then it's therapy" (Rohlfs, 1990).

Of course I have long written the opposite, that we ought *not* to call it therapy just because two people meet in a room and one of them is a therapist. But when I saw that even this good therapist used the word "therapy" for the external doctor–patient trappings, I felt I had to abandon the word. The helpful process is so different, and has so little to do with this empty doctor–patient structure that it moved me to think that if *this empty thing* is therapy, therapy means that the helpful process is not happening. If this is how the word "therapy" is commonly used, we ought not to use it. If we use it, let us correct its public meaning.

We must spell out what therapy means, both in public and in training, so as not to produce a self-satisfied role that is empty at its center. If the distinction were plainly made, I think most therapists would agree that we are not only administrators; we attempt to help, and that therapy has not actually happened when we have not succeeded in helping.

The second issue I raise about the meaning of therapy may be more controversial. I think that we need to emphasize the inherent equality in any relationship between persons as persons. There can be inequality in roles. If one has the role of therapist, teacher, parent, and so on, one must accept inequalities of roles (and how it might be necessary), but in terms of relating one must know that the inequality is unreal.

For example, as a "professor" I cannot relate to students in a real way. How can we have a real interaction when I hold the power over whether the student graduates? I have to use the power responsibly, since a Ph.D. gives someone power over others. The society gives me the role of insuring that academic credentials are not given just to anyone. It is a socially necessary role that someone has to perform. But I need students to perceive that I despise the false respect I am supposed to be accorded. For example, I may know more about many things, but we do not need to pretend that I know more about a topic to which the student has just devoted two years of study.

I want students to understand that I don't need them to make it seem that I did not lose an argument. Unreal role relating is such a waste of time and life. What it is about does not really exist! Why work hard for something unreal? Better to lie on a beach! Real relating is inherently equal. You have to know that there is someone in that body over there, a different creature living a life in a way you can never encompass. So you must wait; you cannot control or displace what comes from there. If you skip that, you are alone and the connection is only pretended.

Among therapists I often get very warm responses to statements such as these. They feel helped by my saying these things out loud. It shows the terrible fact that the false notion of "therapy" can oppress even therapists who understand what I have said here very well. They have been made to feel that they must attempt to wear a false front in order to practice.

The deeper issues involved are difficult to make explicit. Focusing-oriented therapy is Client-Centered therapy. It is difficult to communicate across the immense gulf that separates the client-centered conception of therapy from others. Rogers eliminated the therapist's sitting unseen behind the patient, the medical model, the "patient" as a different kind of being from the "doctor"; he eliminated diagnosis, "treatment," history taking—the entire structure. But the point is not simply for there to be a change in these therapist behaviors; how can we convey what these changes mean?

Even in Client-Centered therapy, so vastly more healing, more livable and real, many of our colleagues practice a kind of formal dance: They say only certain kinds of things and keep themselves competently hidden, not behind a couch but still behind a well-working routine. In this way they bring back the old difference between doctor and patient after all.

There are now also Focusing Teachers (capital letters intended) who bask protectedly in their certified knowledge of focusing instructions, perpetuating the same old doctor–patient structure.

Some beginning clients just assume that focusing therapy consists of an hour of silent focusing. They say, "Excuse me but I just have to talk this out for a while." This worries me not only because therapy involves much more than focusing, but also because clients who ask a question like this don't feel that *of course* they own the hour.

How should our training communicate this? At the start of classes I introduce this basic understanding with the words "of course." I say specific things such as, "Of course you would stop if the client wants to stop," or "Of course you would not argue with the client about the client's own experience," and then I add: "This is not just about what to do and not to do; it is about the *'of course.'* Today you might not know why I say 'of course,' but if you do not feel this 'of course' pretty soon, then I will have failed."

I find that I am unable to spell out what I mean, even in my own classes. I depend on the students to grasp it indirectly. The point is not the things I say but what makes them "of course."

Finding the "of course" may not be possible in general statements. It requires a lot of examples, instances, situations. Perhaps our training needs to include a specially instituted activity to find this "of course." Training programs might include as a major dimension "real-making" (or some such phrase), and specific aspects of it could be collected, discussed, and consulted about. The specifics of real-making need to become a substantial and explicit part of our practice.

We cannot solve the problem with general principles. It is not a matter of some sort of "faith" or "belief," but of very specific inwardly differentiated experiences and observations, for example, those I offered in the preceding chapter. General attitudes will not fill a course's worth of work. The current training of therapists includes many courses on less vital topics, but there is not even one full course on therapists' attitudes. Instead, the different therapies are defined by different kinds of "interventions." The literature *can* present and compare them, but it is difficult to generate course material on basic attitudes. Carl Rogers defined therapy *totally* in terms of therapist attitudes. Yet even in Client-Centered training most of the time is taken up with the precision of listening, and now also with focusing instructions. About the all-important attitudes there is not enough detail to fill a course. We need the type of specificity that I generated for focusing. I took something that was known to many people, but vague, and I differentiated many strands of it: the bodily attention, the attitudes, the steps, and many distinctions and details at each step. It will take time and more than one person to do that for the topic of therapists' attitudes.

We also need specific details to make recognizable the false aspects of the therapist role, for example, always having to be right. Trainees could quickly perceive that they are unreal.

Trainers and students could collaborate in a project of articulating detailed experiences of real-making by communicating inward differentiations; they do this now, but I would ask them to collect them, sort, organize, and keep them, thus extending the material we now have.

Such collaboration would incorporate another dimension that Carl Rogers always provided in the training he offered: Rather than ready, cut-and-dried content, he always presented the method as still in the process of being developed. It provided the excitement of collaborating, contributing, and thinking on the edge of what is known. He began each course by handing out a long list of available "resource materials" (tapes, books, etc.,) and invited students to decide how to begin, what to use, and how to proceed. It enabled us to experience and instance exactly the kind of process with people that he wanted to teach.

Realness does not equate therapy with friendship, or deprive it of its distinctive structure and limits. I have said that the structure and limits crucially protect the client. The therapist carries certain responsibilities, whereas the client is left more free than in other settings. All feelings are welcomed, but possible actions are highly restricted. That keeps therapy from becoming like other relationships. The limits on action make depth possible. Limiting the relationship in breadth, fencing it off on the left and right, defines a central channel between client and therapist in which they can relate more deeply and in a more real way than we usually do in our needful and twisted personal relationships where we hear each other so poorly, and so much of what we say and feel is projection.

The narrow but more real channel has been widely misunderstood and not sufficiently articulated. Therapy is a real life-relationship between two people; it is not a substitute or "symbolic" representation of a relationship. It is true that childhood lacks fill themselves in, but this is possible only as part of real contact. I hope this book has shown some of this, but we need a whole branch of our field to concern itself directly with how one person approaches another if it is to be therapy.

Focusing involves certain attitudes toward the felt sense and whatever comes up from inside. Such attitudes are *relational*, like those of a client-centered therapist toward a client. Focusing requires self-responses that create a climate of safety and receptivity to anything that arises from inside (along with making room separately for other reactions that also must be acknowledged).

We should not make focusing seem mysterious. By "focusing" we mean spending time with the at first unclear body sense of a problem, so that new steps come. Focusing is a little door. Some people want to give the name "focusing" to everything they find through this door. No, focusing is just attending to the bodily uneasiness of a problem. We need to keep this simple, so people can find it. But we need to articulate something large and deep here, the basic set of what we call "therapy," understood more deeply from focusing. "Focusing-oriented therapy" is not therapy that includes brief bits of focusing instruction. Rather, it means letting that which arises from the focusing depths within a person define the therapist's activity, the relationship, and the process in the client.

But there are difficult philosophical problems with this conception of therapy. The person with inner continuity at the focusing level seems unknown to the culture. The culture assumes that human beings are nothing but what it inculcates in them. The dominant view has long been that nothing *can* arise from inside. If something seems to do so it is said to be only the result of society, social class, history, and language. If something has gone wrong with our "socialization," it is believed that only some other form of socialization can repair it. But although each of us is socialized, what arises bodily from behind and beneath and beyond the socialization is more intricate, and can make more sense and be more ethical than our cultural training.

According to old assumptions, the body is merely a machine. Currently there is a great deal of concern with the body, but most people have not yet discovered that special kind of bodily sense that is the sense *of* a situation.

Why does focusing work? How does "the process" come to be so wise? It is the body that is so "wise," but of course it is not the body reduced to physiology, not the body-as-machine, but rather the body from out of which you are living. This body is not one thing while you are another, a second thing. Your body enacts your situations and constitutes them largely before you can think how. When your attention joins this living, you can pursue many more possibilities and choices than when you merely drive the body as if it were a machine like the car. It lives inherently with others. It is born into interaction and physically implies moves toward and with people. When it first arrives, it implies nursing and being held, and after it absorbs all the complex human circumstances, it can imply an intricate new move in an unheard-of predicament.

The interactional nature of the body-in-situations is contrary to most theories. But even if we reject the theories, the old assumptions remain; they are built into common words and phrases. In my philosophy I find a way to devise phrases and sentences in which words come to be used in new ways, so that we can go on from here, to think further. I have built a theory with concepts of a new kind that have both logical and experiential connections. With those concepts I am able to build a new understanding of the physical body as continuous with, and capable of, animal behavior, then of language, and at last of focusing.

Bibliography
and Resources

Allen, F. H. (1942). *Psychotherapy with Children*. New York: Norton.

Alperson, E. (1980). Contacting Bodily-Felt Experiencing. In J. E. Shorr, G. E. Sobel, P. Robin, and J. A. Connella (Eds.), *Imagery: Its Many Dimensions and Applications*. New York: Plenum Press.

Amodeo, J., and Wentworth, K. (1986). *Being Intimate: A Guide to Successful Relationships*. London: Penguin.

Beebe, J. (1992). *Integrity in Depth*. College Station: Texas A & M University Press.

Boukydis, C. F. Z. (1990). Client-Centered/Experiential Practice with Parents and Infants. In G. Lietar, J. Rombauts, and R. VanBalen (Eds.), *Client-Centered and Experiential Psychotherapy in the Nineties*. Leuven, Belgium: Leuven University Press.

Campbell P. A., and McMahon, E. M. (1985). *Biospirituality*. Chicago: Loyola University Press.

Depestelle, F. (1996). A Primary Bibliography of Eugene Gendlin. *Tijdschrift voor Psychotherapie, 1*.

Egendrof, A. (1981). Consciousness and Mastery. *The CEA Critic, 44*(1).

Ellis, A. (1962). *Reason and Emotion in Psychotherapy*. New York: Lyle Stuart.

Fenichel, O. (1945). *The Psychoanalytic Theory of Neurosis*. New York: Norton.

Finlay de Monchy, M. (1995). The Horrified Position: An Ethics Grounded in the Affective Interest in the Unitary Body as Psyche/Soma. *Body & Society, 1*(2).

Focusing Biblothek, DAF, D-97082 Würzburg, Frankfurter Strasse 10.

Focusing Connection, Bulletin. Focusing Resources, 2625 Alcatraz Ave. #202, Berkeley, CA 94705-2702.

Focusing Folio. Journal of the Focusing Institute, 800-799-7418.

Focusing Institute. Training centers in various cities, tapes, and other resources, 800-799-7418.

Freud, S. (1926/1936). *The Problem of Anxiety*. New York: Norton.

Freud, S. (1911/1957). Formulations Regarding the Two Principles in Mental Functioning. In *Collected Papers*, Vol. 4 (pp. 13–21). London: Hogarth Press.

Freud, S. (1923/1960). *The Ego and the Id*. New York: Norton.

Freud, S. (1928/1959). *Beyond the Pleasure Principle*. New York: Bantam.

Freud, S. (1940/1949). *Outline of Psychoanalysis*. New York: Norton.

Freud, S. (1915/1971). *The Wolf Man*. New York: Basic Books.

Friedman, N. (1995). *On Focusing*. 259 Massachussetts Avenue, Arlington, MA 02174, 1995.

Gendlin, E. T. (1962). *Experiencing and the Creation of Meaning*. New York: Free Press. (Reprinted by Macmillan, 1970; Japanese translation, 1994; paperback, Northwestern University Press, 1996).

Gendlin, E. T. (1964). A Theory of Personality Change. In Worchel and Byrne (Eds.), *Personality Change*. New York: Wiley. (Reprinted in J. Hart and T. Tomlinson (Eds.), *New Directions in Client-Centered Therapy*. Boston: Houghton-Mifflin, 1970. Also reprinted in A. Mahrer and L. Pearson (Eds.), *Creative Developments in Psychotherapy*. New York: Aronson, 1974.)

Gendlin, E. T. (1965). Expressive Meanings. In J. Edie (Ed.), *Invitation to Phenomenology*. Chicago: Quadrangle Books.

Gendlin, E. T. (1965/1966). Experiential Explication and Truth. *Journal of Existentialism*, 6, 131–146. (Reprinted in F. R. Molina (Ed.), *The Sources of Existentialism as Philosophy*. Englewood Cliffs, NJ: Prentice Hall, 1969.)

Gendlin, E. T. (1967). Values and the Process of Experiencing. In A. Mahrer (Ed.), *The Goals of Psychotherapy*. New York: Appleton-Century-Crofts.

Gendlin, E. T. (1968a). Experiential Groups. In G. M. Gazda (Ed.), *Innovations to Group Psychotherapy*. Springfield, IL: Charles Thomas. (Also in *Journal of Research and Development in Education, 1*(2).)

Gendlin, E. T. (1968b). The Experiential Response. In Hammer (Ed.), *Interpretation in Therapy: Its Role, Scope, Depth, Timing and Art*. New York: Grune and Stratton.

Gendlin, E. T. (with Beebe, Cassens, Klein, and Oberlander). (1968c). Focusing Ability in Psychotherapy, Personality, and Creativity. In J. M. Shlien (Ed.), *Research in Psychotherapy*, Vol. 3. Washington, DC: American Psychological Association.

Gendlin, E. T. (1971). A Phenomenology of Emotions: Anger. In D. Carr and E. Casey (Eds.), *Explorations in Phenomenology*. The Hague, The Netherlands: Martinus Nijhoff.

Gendlin, E. T. (1972). Therapeutic Procedures with Schizophrenic Patients. In M. Hammer (Ed)., *The Theory and Practice of Psychotherapy with Specific Disorders*. Springfield, IL: Charles Thomas.

Gendlin, E. T. (1973). Experiential Phenomenology. In M. Natanson (Ed.), *Phenomenology and the Social Sciences*. Evanston, IL: Northwestern University Press.

Gendlin, E. T. (1975). The Newer Therapies. In S. Arieti (Ed.), *American Handbook of Psychiatry*, Vol. 5 (chap. 14). New York: Basic Books.

Gendlin, E. T. (1978/1979). Befindlichkeit. *Review of Existential Psychology and Psychiatry*, 16(1–3): 43–71.

Gendlin, E. T. (1981). *Focusing*, Second Edition. New York: Bantam Books. (Translations: Danish, Dutch, French, German, Hungarian, Japanese, Spanish, Swedish.)

Gendlin, E. T. (1982). Two Phenomenologists Do Not Disagree. In Bruzina and Wilshire (Eds.), *Phenomenology: Dialogues and Bridges*. Albany: State University of New York Press.

Gendlin, E. T. (1983). Dwelling. In R. C. Scharff (Ed.), *Proceedings of the Heidegger Conference*. University of New Hampshire. (Reprinted in H. Silverman, A. Mickunas, T. Kissel, and A. Lingis (Eds.), *The Horizons of Continental Philosophy: Essays on Husserl, Heidegger and Merleau-Ponty*. Dordrecht, The Netherlands: Kluwer, 1988.)

Gendlin E. T. (1984). The Politics of Giving Therapy Away. In D. Larson (Ed.), *Teaching Psychological Skills: Models for Giving Therapy Away*. Monterey, CA: Brooks/Cole.

Gendlin, E. T. (1984). The Client's Client. In J. M. Shlien and R. Levant (Eds.), *Client-Centered Therapy and the Person-Centered Approach*. New York: Praeger.

Gendlin, E. T. (with Grindler, D., and McGuire, M.). (1984). Imagery, Body, and Space. In A. A. Sheikh (Ed.), *Imagination and Healing*. New York, Baywood.

Gendlin, E. T. (1986a). *Let Your Body Interpret Your Dreams*. Wilmette, IL.: Chiron.

Gendlin E. T. (1986b). Process Ethics and the Political Question. In A-T. Tymieniecka (Ed.), *Analecta Husserliana*, Vol. 20 (pp. 265–275). Boston: Reidel. (Reprinted in *Focusing Folio*, 5(2): 68–87.)

Gendlin, E. T. (1986c). What Comes after Traditional Psychotherapy Research? *American Psychologist*, 41(2): 131–136.

Gendlin, E. T. (1987). A Philosophical Critique of the Concept of Narcissism. In D. Levin (Ed.), *Pathologies of the Modern Self* (pp. 251–304). New York: New York University Press.

Gendlin, E. T. (1988). Obituary for Carl Rogers. *American Psychologist*, 43(2).

Gendlin, E. T. (1989). Toward a Bodily Human Nature. *Discours Social/Social Discourse*, 2(1–2).

Gendlin, E. T. (1990). The Small Steps of the Therapy Process: How They Come and How to Help Them Come. In G. Lietar, J. Rombauts, and R. VanBalen (Eds.), *Client-Centered and Experiential Psychotherapy in the Nineties*. Leuven, Belgium: Leuven University Press.

Gendlin, E. T. (1991a). Crossing and Dipping: Some Terms for Approaching the Interface between Natural Understanding and Logical Formation. In M. Galbraith and W. J. Rapaport (Eds.), *Subjectivity and the Debate over Computational Cognitive Science* (pp. 37–59). Buffalo State University of New York, Center for Cognitive Science. (Also in *Minds and Machines*, 5: 547–560, 1995.)

Gendlin, E. T. (1991b). On Emotion in Therapy. In J. D. Safran and L. S. Greenberg (Eds.), *Emotion, Psychotherapy, and Change* (pp. 255–279). New York: Guilford. (Reprinted in *The Focusing Folio*, 2(1): 1–49. Also in *Hakomi Forum*, Winter 1992, Hakomi Institute, P.O. Box 625, Branchville, NJ 07826.)

Gendlin, E. T. (1992a). The Primacy of the Body, Not the Primacy of Perception. *Man and World*, 25(3–4): 341–353.

Gendlin, E. T. (1992b). Thinking beyond Patterns: Body, Language and Situations. In B. den Ouden and M. Moen (Eds.), *The Presence of Feeling in Thought* (pp. 25–151). New York: Peter Lang.

Gendlin, E. T. (1992c). The Wider Role of Bodily Sense in Thought and Language. In M. Sheets-Johnstone (Ed.), *Giving the Body Its Due* (pp. 192–207). Albany: State

University of New York Press. (German translations in *Deutsche Zeitschrift für Philosophie, 41*(4), 1993, and *Brennpunkt, 17*, no. 63, 1995.)

Gendlin, E. T. (1996a). *A Process Model*. Unpublished manuscript. (In eight parts, 422 pages.)

Gendlin, E. T. (1996b). The Use of Focusing in Therapy. In J. K. Zeig (Ed.), *The Evolution of Psychotherapy*. New York: Brunner/Mazel

Gendlin, E. T. (in press). *Language Beyond PostModernism: Fourteen Commentaries on the Philosophy of Eugene Gendlin, and Gendlin's Replies*. (D. Levin, Ed.). Evanston, IL: Northwestern University Press.

Gordon, T. (1970). *Parent-Effectiveness Training*. New York: P. H. Wyden.

Grindler, D. (1984). Focusing with a Cancer Patient. In A. A. Sheikh (Ed.), *Imagination and Healing*. Amityville, NY: Baywood.

Grindler, D. (1995). *Exploring Focusing and Bodily Meanings*. Care Cassette, Vol. 22, 106. The College of Chaplains, 1701 E. Woodfield Rd., Schaumburg, IL 60173.

Grove, D. (1995). *In the Presence of the Past*. David Grove Seminars, RR5, Box 215 AA, Eldon, MO 65026.

Hart, J. T., and Tomlinson, T. M. (Eds.). (1970). *New Directions in Client-Centered Therapy*. Boston: Houghton Mifflin.

Hendricks M. N., and Cartwright, R. (1978). Experiencing in Dreams. *Psychotherapy, Theory, Research, and Practice, 15*(3): 292–298.

Hendricks, M. N. (1984). A Focusing Group: Model for a New Kind of Group Process. *Small Group Behavior, 15*: 155–171.

Hendricks, M. N. (1986). Experiencing Level as a Therapeutic Variable. *Person-Centered Review, 1*: 141–162.

Hendrix, H. (1988). *Getting the Love You Want*. New York: Holt.

Hinterkopf, E., and Brunswick, L. (1981). Teaching Mental Patients to Use Client-Centered and Experiential Therapeutic Skills with Each Other. *Psychotherapy: Theory, Research, and Practice, 18*: 394–402.

Iberg, J. R. (1981). Focusing. In R. J. Corsini (Ed.), *Handbook of Innovative Psychotherapies*. New York: Wiley.

Jaekins, H. (1962). *Fundamentals of Co-Counseling*. Seattle: Rational Island Press.

Jüchli, E. (1995). *GFK Texte*, Vols. 1 & 2, Weierhofgasse 9, CH-9500 Wil, Switzerland.

Johanson, G., and Taylor, C. (1988). Hakomi Therapy with Emotionally Disturbed Adolescents. In C. Schaefer (Ed.), *Innovative Interventions in Child and Adolescent Psychotherapy*. New York: Wiley.

Jung, C. G. (1930/1976). *Vision Seminars*. Zurich: Spring Publications.

Jung, C. G. (1956). *Two Essays on Analytical Psychology*. New York: Meridian.

Katz, R. (1981). Focusing with the Critic. *Focusing Folio, 1*(3).

Klein, M. H., Mathieu, P. L., Kiesler, D. J., and Gendlin, E. T. (1969). *The Experiencing Scale: A Research and Training Manual*. Bureau of Audio-Visual Instruction, the University of Wisconsin, Madison.

Kohut, H. (1977). *The Restoration of the Self*. New York: International Universities Press.

Lazarus, A. A. (1971). *Behavior Therapy and Beyond*. New York: McGraw-Hill.

Levin, D. M. (1985). *The Body's Recollection of Being*. London: Routledge.

Liejssen, M. (1990). On Focusing and the Necessary Conditions of Therapeutic Personality Change. In G. Lietar, J. Rombauts, and R. VanBalen (Eds.), *Client-Centered and Experiential Psychotherapy in the Nineties*. Leuven, Belgium: Leuven University Press.

Lietar, G. (1988). Bibliographical Survey, 1950–1987. Katholieke Universiteit, Leuven, Belgium.

Lietar, G., Rombauts, J., and VanBalen, R. (Eds.). (1990). *Client-Centered and Experiential Psychotherapy in the Nineties*. Leuven, Belgium: Leuven University Press.

McGuire, K. (1981). *Building Supportive Community: Mutual Self-Help Through Peer Counseling, Training Manual*. Focusing Northwest, 3440 Onyx Street, Eugene, OR 97405.

McGuire, K. (1991). Affect in Focusing and Experiential Psychotherapy. In J. D. Safran and L. S. Greenberg (Eds.), *Emotion, Psychotherapy, and Change* (pp. 255–279). New York: Guilford.

McGuire M. (1984). Making a Space. In A. A. Sheikh (Ed.), *Imagination and Healing*. Amityville, New York: Baywood.

McGuire, M. (1990). *Caring Touch Training Manual*. Focusing Institute Publications, 800-799-7418.

McMahon, E. M. (1993). *Beyond the Myth of Dominance*. Kansas City: Sheed & Ward.

Müller, D. (1995). Dealing with Self-Criticism: The Critic Within Us and the Criticized One. *Focusing Folio, 14*(1).

Moustakas, C. (1996). Being-In, Being-For, Being-With. *Psychotherapy Book News, 30*.

Neagu, G. (1988). The Focusing Technique with Children and Adolescents. In C. Schaefer (Ed.), *Innovative Interventions in Child and Adolescent Psychotherapy*. New York: Wiley.

Olsen, L., and Gendlin, E. T. (1970). The Use of Imagery in Experiential Focusing. *Psychotherapy: Theory, Research and Practice, 7*(4).

Perl, S. (1994). A Writer's Way of Knowing: Guidelines for Composing. In A. Brand and R. Graves (Eds.), *A Writer's Way of Knowing: Writing and the Domain Beyond the Cognitive*. Portsmouth, NH: Boynton Cook.

Perls, F. (1969). *Gestalt Therapy Verbatim*. Lafayette, CA: Real People Publishing.

Prouty, G. (1976). Pre-Therapy, A Method of Treating Psychotic and Retarded Patients. *Psychotherapy: Theory, Research, and Practice, 13*(3).

Prouty, G. (1994). *Theoretical Evolutions in Person-Centered/Experiential Therapy: Applications to Schizophrenic and Retarded Psychoses*. Westport, CT: Praeger.

Rank, O. (1929/1945). *Will Therapy and Truth and Reality*. New York: Knopf.

Rogers, C. R. (1961). *On Becoming A Person*. Boston: Houghton Mifflin.

Rohlfs, A. (1990). Fraudulent Degrees or Fraudulent Assertions? *Journal of Mental Health Counseling, 12*(1).

Safran, J. (1990). *Interpersonal Process in Cognitive Therapy*. New York: Basic Books.

Seeman, J. (1954). Counselor Judgments of Therapy Process and Outcome. In C. R. Rogers and R. Dymond (Eds.), *Psychotherapy and Personality Change*. Chicago: University of Chicago Press.

Seeman, J. (1983). *Personality Integration*. New York: Human Sciences Press.

Sherman, E. (1984). *Working with Older Persons*. Boston: Kluwer-Nijhoff.

Sherman, E. (1986). A Phenomenological Approach to Reminiscene and Life Review. *Clinical Gerontologist, 3*: 3–16.

Shlien, J. M., and Levant. R. (Eds.). (1984). *Client-Centered Therapy and the Person-Centered Approach*. New York: Praeger.

Skinner, B. F. (1953). *Science and Human Behavior*. New York: Macmillan.

Stern, Daniel N. (1985). *The Interpersonal World of the Infant*. New York: Basic Books.

Stern, Donnel. (1983). Unformulated Experience. *Contemporary Psychoanalysis, 19*(1).

Stern, Donnel. (in press). *Unformulated Experience*. Hillside, NJ: The Analytical Press.

Sullivan, H. S. (1940). *The Interpersonal Theory of Psychiatry*. New York: Norton.

Ullman, M., and Zimmerman, A. (1979). *Working with Dreams*. New York: Delacorte.

Weiser, A. (1994). *The Focusing Student's Manual* and *The Focusing Guide's Manual*. Focusing Resources, 2625 Alcatraz Ave. #202, Berkeley, CA 94705-2702.

Weiser, A. (in press). *The Power of Focusing: A Practical Guide to Emotional Self-Healing*. Oakland, CA: New Harbinger.

Welwood, J. (1996). *Love and Awakening: The Sacred Path of Intimate Relationships*. New York: Harper Collins.

Wexler, D. A., and Rice, L. N. (Eds.). (1974). *Innovations Client-Centered Therapy*. New York: Wiley.

Wiltschko, J. Focusing Biblothek, DAF, D-97082 Würzburg, Frankfurter Strasse 10.

Wolfus, B., and Bierman, R. (1996). *An Evaluation of a Group Psychotherapy Program for Incarcerated Male Batterers*. Ontario Correctional Institute, 109 McLaughlin Rd. South, Brampton, Ontario L6V 2P1, Canada.

Zimring, F. M., and Balcombe, J. K. (1974). Cognitive Operations in Two Measures of Handling Emotionally Relevant Material. *Psychotherapy: Theory, Research, and Practice, 11*(3).

Index

on dreams, 281–282
functions hypothesized by, 66–67, 215
on superego, 256
Jungian psychoanalysis
active daydreams, 19, 170, 173, 214–215
avenues used in, 170
dreams and, 200, 202, 203, 204–205, 208
procedures, 169–170

K

Katz, R., 255
Kohut, H., 9
Kohutian therapy, 169

L

Laughter, 96, 137
Lazarus, A. A., 214
Life-forward direction
biological basis for, 280–281
negatives as movement in, 56, 293–294
therapist response to, 137, 259–263
values and, 264–275
Listening; see Reflective listening
Logic, experience and, 14

M

"making space", 90–91, 93, 115, 117–118,
121, 143
Massage therapy, focusing and, 182
Meditation, 65–66, 225, 273
Morality, superego and, 251–252
Moreno, J. L.,192
Mother-child preparedness, 280–281
Movement; see Therapeutic movement

N

Negative thoughts, 56, 238–239; see also
Superego
Nodding, involuntary, 84

O

Openings, in felt sense, 26, 34–35, 59, 63
Operant behavior therapy
action steps, 173–174, 227–237
experiential use of, 230–232
reinforcement, 233
Organisms, filling in capacity of, 276–282
Orientations; see Therapeutic
orientations

P

Pain, putting down, 143
Parent-child preparedness, 280–281
Pathology
as lack of experiencing, 38
life-forward movement and, 262
Patients; see Clients
Perception, vs. bodily sensing, 297
Playfulness, 137, 147
Pointing responses
examples of, 47–48, 150
vs. focusing instructions, 50
Positive life energy, negatives as, 56
Posture changes, energy flow and, 185–191,
225–226
Preconscious, 18–19
Preparedness, organismic, 280–281
Present experiencing, 14–15, 67, 223–
224
Primal therapy
catharsis in, 222, 223
felt sense and, 67
Problems
alternate views of, 239, 240
content mutation of, 27, 36, 88, 95, 115,
123
spiritual values and, 273–275
unclear edges in, 17–18, 72–73
Process steps; see Experiential process
steps
Projection, 296
Psychoanalysis; see also Freudian
psychoanalysis; Jungian psychoanalysis;
Psychotherapy
dead ends in, 9
transference in, 294
Psychodrama, 192
Psychosexual concepts, 256
Psychosomatic illness, 64
Psychotherapy; see also specific type of
therapy; Therapeutic movement
authoritarianism in, 273, 285, 300–302
balance in, 109–110
behavior therapy and, 237

Psychotherapy (*continued*)
compared to fresh thinking, 245
dead ends in, 7–15
disjunctions during, 51–52, 106, 110–111, 291–294
focusing as motor of, 297–298
frame for, 109–110, 286–291
meaning of therapy in, 299–304
necessary conditions for, 287–289, 296–297
overuse of focusing in, 108
priorities in, 172, 177–178, 297–298
theoretical orientations in, 169–174, 179–180, 240
therapeutic avenues in, 170–180

R

Rational-emotive therapy, 241
Reason, compared to felt sense, 58
Reevaluation counseling, 223
Reflective listening
analogy with driving, 28, 106
author's emphasis on, 297
client's inward response to, 11–12
described, 45–46
as foundation for focusing, 111
implicit interaction during, 284
importance of, 297
transference and, 296
use by orientation, 9, 169
Reframing, 9, 242–244
Regression, 223
Reinforcement, 233
Relaxation level, 65–66, 214, 224, 225
Religion, values and, 273–275
Repetition compulsion, 47
Resistance, 52
Rest periods, 112–113
Right and wrong, sensing of, 265–275
Rogers, C.
client-centered therapy and, 301–302, 303
on conditions for therapy, 287–289, 296–297
reflection of feeling method, 9
Role play
body energy in, 192–194, 197–198, 255
dreams and, 195–197, 206, 208, 209
essential contribution of, 193
experiential version of, 195–198
focusing and, 194
superego and, 254–255

Roles
of clients, 104–106, 110, 132–140
inequality in, 301
of therapists, 45–56, 104–106, 109–110, 299

S

Safety, for clients, 123–124, 289–290
Self; *see also* Growth and development
development of, 21–23, 37, 56, 80
finding parts of, 119–120, 288–289
inner child in, 217–220
Sensation function, Jung's, 66
Sensing; *see* Bodily sensing
Sighing, 89
Silence, 46, 290–291
Simonton's imagery sequence, 173, 213–214
Skinner, B.F., 227
"spacing out", felt sense and, 65
Spirituality, values and, 273–275
Spontaneity, in role play, 194
Stanislavsky, K., role play and, 194, 195
Strain
during focusing, 116
holistic quality of, 84
Stuckness; *see* Dead-end discussions; Dead-end feelings
Superego
combatting, 238–239, 247–248, 253–258, 272
described, 248–249
Freud on, 247, 249, 251, 256
signs of attacks by, 249–253
Systematic Desensitization, 170, 173, 214

T

Tantrums, 222
Therapeutic avenues
defined, 170
focusing and, 171, 174–180
gaining familiarity with, 172–174
link between, 174–176
procedures grouped by, 170–171
Therapeutic movement
analogy with driving, 28, 106
bodily sensing and, 1–2, 9, 20
border zone and, 69